AGING
IN GOOD HEALTH

EDITED BY
SUE E. LEVKOFF, YEON KYUNG CHEE,
AND SHOHEI NOGUCHI

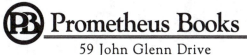

Prometheus Books

59 John Glenn Drive
Amherst, New York 14228-2197

Published 2003 by Prometheus Books

Inquiries should be addressed to
Prometheus Books
59 John Glenn Drive
Amherst, New York 14228–2197
VOICE: 716–691–0133, ext. 207; FAX: 716–564–2711
WWW.PROMETHEUSBOOKS.COM

07 06 05 04 03   5 4 3 2 1

Library of Congress Cataloging-in-Publication Data

Aging in good health / Sue E. Levkoff, Yeon Kyung Chee, and Shohei Noguchi, editors.
    p. cm.
    Originally published: Aging in good health : multidisciplinary perspectives. New York :
Springer Pub., 2001.
    Includes bibliographical references and index.
    ISBN 1–59102–026–3 (alk. paper)
    1. Aged—Health and hygiene. 2. Aged—Mental health. 3. Aged—Psychology.
I. Levkoff, Sue. II. Chee, Yeon Kyung. III. Noguchi, Shohei.

RA777.6 .A35 2002
613'.0438—dc21

2002036617

Printed in the United States of America on acid-free paper

Contents

Contributors

Alan L. Balsam, Ph.D., M.P.H.
Director, Public Health and
  Human Services
Massachusetts Department of
  Public Health, Brookline
Assistant Adjunct Professor
Boston University School of
  Public Health, Harvard Medi-
  cal School, Tufts School of
  Nutrition
Boston, MA

**Margaret Bergmann, M.S.,
G.N.P.**
Gerontological Nurse
  Practitioner
Hebrew Rehabilitation Center
  for Aged
Boston, MA

Raymond Bossé, Ph.D.
Lecturer
Harvard School of Dental
  Medicine
Boston, MA

Carolyn L. Bottum, M.P.H.
Director, Bedford Council on
  Aging
Bedford, MA

Francis G. Caro, Ph.D.
Professor and Director of the
  Gerontology Institute
University of Massachusetts at
  Boston
Boston, MA

Yeon Kyung Chee, Ph.D.
Instructor in Social Medicine
Department of Social Medicine
Division on Aging
Harvard Medical School
Boston, MA

Xing-jia Cui, M.D.
Research Fellow in Psychiatry
Harvard Medical School
Beth Israel Deaconess Medical
  Center
Boston, MA

Naomi K. Fukagawa, M.D.
Associate Professor of Medicine
Associate Program Director of
the General Clinical Re-
search Center
College of Medicine
University of Vermont
Burlington, VT

Muriel R. Gillick, M.D.
Associate Professor in Medicine
Harvard Medical School
Hebrew Rehabilitation Center
for Aged
Boston, MA

Jerry H. Gurwitz, M.D.
Executive Director, Meyers Pri-
mary Care Institute
Associate Professor of Medicine
University of Massachusetts
Medical School
Worcester, MA

Suzanne B. Hanser, Ed.D.
Chair, Music Therapy
Department
Berklee College of Music
Boston, MA

**Jonathan Howland, Ph.D.,
M.P.H.**
Professor of Social Behavioral
Sciences
School of Public Health
Boston University
Boston, MA

Ruth Kandel, M.D.
Instructor in Medicine
Harvard Medical School
Hebrew Rehabilitation Center
for Aged
Boston, MA

Margie E. Lachman, Ph.D.
Professor of Psychology
Director, Life-Span Develop-
mental Psychology
Laboratory
Department of Psychology
Brandeis University
Waltham, MA

Sue E. Levkoff, Sc.D.
Associate Professor of Psychia-
try, Social Medicine, Health
and Social Behavior
Brigham and Women's
Hospital
Harvard Medical School
Harvard School of Public
Health
Boston, MA

Alan J. Lieberman, Ph.D.
Clinical Psychologist
Instructor in Psychology
Harvard Medical School
Boston, MA

Robert Morris, D.S.W.
Kirstein Professor Emeritus
Brandeis University
Senior Fellow at the Gerontology Institute
University of Massachusetts at Boston
Boston, MA

Shohei Noguchi
President
Mejiro Human Science College
Mejiro Life Science College
Chuo College of Law
Tokyo, Japan

Elizabeth Walker Peterson, M.P.H., O.T.R./L
Clinical Assistant Professor
Department of Occupational Therapy
University of Illinois at Chicago
Chicago, IL

Amy E. H. Prue
Research Assistant
College of Medicine
University of Vermont
Burlington, VT

Paula A. Rochon, M.D., M.P.H., F.R.C.P.C.
Scientist, Kunin-Lunenfeld Applied Research Unit
Baycrest Centre for Geriatric Care
Departments of Medicine and Public Health Sciences
University of Toronto
Toronto, Canada

Myles Sheehan, S.J., M.D.
Associate Dean
Stritch School of Medicine
Loyola University Medical Center
Maywood, IL

Diana Laskin Siegal, M.P.A.
(Retired)
Director, Elder Health Program
Massachusetts Department of Public Health
Boston, MA

Margery Hutton Silver, Ed.D.
Clinical Instructor in Psychology
Associate Director of the New England Centenarian Study
Department of Psychiatry
Division on Aging
Harvard Medical School
Boston, MA

Maria A. Fiatarone Singh, M.D.
Associate Professor
School of Nutrition Science and Policy
Jean Mayer USDA Human Nutrition Research Center on Aging
Tufts University
Boston, MA

Lauren E. Storck, Ph.D., C.G.P.
Clinical Psychologist
Clinical Instructor
Department of Psychiatry
Harvard Medical School
Boston, MA

**Linda Thalheimer, O.T.R./L,
  M.H.A.**
Long-Term Care Specialist
Private Practice
Natick, MA

George E. Vaillant, M.D.
Professor of Psychiatry
Harvard Medical School
Brigham and Women's
  Hospital
Boston, MA

Patricia Flynn Weitzman, Ph.D.
Instructor in Social Medicine
Department of Social Medicine
Division on Aging
Harvard Medical School
Boston, MA

Rosalie S. Wolf, Ph.D.
Executive Director, Institute on
  Aging
Assistant Professor
Departments of Medicine, Com-
  munity Medicine, and Family
  Practice
University of Massachusetts Me-
  morial Health Care System
Worcester, MA

Foreword

As I speculate on why I was asked to write the foreword for *Aging In Good Health, Multi-Disciplinary Perspectives*, I might assume that it is because I am a subject for study. In this role, I can't help but sound an optimistic note about the process of aging. I recently was privileged to become an octogenarian. Some years ago—long before I thought I might attain such exalted status—while writing a chapter on human development, I came upon an observation by the British writer Frank Swinnerton:

For me, it is great privilege to be an octogenarian. The high fevers of life are over, and unless his facilities are badly rusted (which is not the experience of my octogenarian friends) the man of eighty-odd begins every day free from the anxieties, angers and frustrations which beset his juniors. He is no longer love-sick; he has not to jostle with the crowds on the train or street car; he had time to "stand and stare." Further satisfactions follow. He is still richly alive; and having experienced nearly a hundred years of rich and turbulent history; sees the present in perspective as more than a detail in the tremendous stream of time.

Today, I probably would have a bit of a disagreement about "standing and staring." For example, by university statutes I became emeritus, but I didn't retire. More and more, my colleagues remain energized in most of their customary activities as they become emeritus. We are engaged in a national dialogue about raising the age level for social security and retirement eligibility.

It is not fortuitous that concerns over aging in our society are so prominent, for we are growing older faster than we are growing younger (and the baby boomers haven't yet arrived). A few demographic trends should be noted: life expectancy has increased from

48 years at the turn of the century to 75.8 years in 1995. We must continue to strive to reduce the 5-year lag for men as well as the relative lag among minorities of diverse ethnic backgrounds. These demographic changes weren't entirely anticipated. I can recall reading articles by respected demographers in the 1970s suggesting that the great gains in life expectancy were over because of the striking reductions in mortality—especially from the infections diseases—in the early decades of the century. They were predicting that there would be little increase in the period beyond age 65. The data, of course, have proven them wrong. The period beyond 85 years constitutes the single most rapidly growing group in our population. We haven't yet fully made an accommodation to these changes.

We are interested in the long-term goal of not only extending the length of life, but also promoting health and the quality of life during these additional years. This book should prove useful to health professionals from various disciplines as they help both younger and older persons alike to learn to take control of health and life styles which enable them to maintain independence for as long as possible. Certainly health habits related to stress; alcohol and medication use; exercise and nutrition; have much to do with function as we grow older. This book is a wonderful guide to better health by bringing together knowledge based on the latest research in all of these areas.

Being free of illness does not necessarily ensure quality of life, though. Mobility, independence, cognitive function, psychological state, social and family relations or networks, assume great importance. Significantly, the elderly often do not associate absence of illness with health. In fact, good health has been defined in functional, nonmedical terms.

This book, with its optimistic tone toward problem solving, moves us on the road to a redefinition of issues facing older people. Professional workers should find it very helpful and refreshing.

Recently research studies show that it is possible to improve and to maintain physiological performance, sense of well-being and quality of life, and we are understanding more about how to enhance function. The goal of vital aging is now very much within our reach. This is an interesting and exciting time indeed.

Julius B. Richmond, M.D.
Professor of Health Policy, Emeritus
Harvard Medical School
Former U.S. Surgeon General and
Former Assistant Secretary of Health,
U.S. Department of Health and
Human Services

Introduction

Sue E. Levkoff, Yeon Kyung Chee, and Shohei Noguchi

Survival to advanced age is one of the great accomplishments of the modern era. The increased longevity of Americans means that demands for elder care benefits will soon surpass the demand for childcare benefits. Minority groups, in particular, will see growth in their aged populations. Non-Hispanic Whites, who currently make up three-quarters of the population, will constitute only 60% of the population in 2030, and 53% in 2050 (Day, 1993). The African American population will double in size by 2050. Demographic changes will be even more dramatic for Latinos. Latinos represent the fastest growing segment of the elderly population, with the Latino population as a whole predicted as emerging by 2010 as the second largest ethnic group in the United States (Day, 1993). The increase in the population aged 85+ has also been striking. At the turn of the 20th century, the average life expectancy for an American man was 46.3 years; and for an American woman, 48.3 years (National Institutes of Health, 1992). The life expectancy of men and women living now has practically doubled (Day, 1993), with gains for women even greater than those for men. In fact, by the middle of this century, it is estimated that women will outnumber men by 3 to 1 in age groups over 85 (Day, 1993).

These demographic shifts will have a number of significant consequences for the shaping of social and public policy in the United States. For example, the increase in groups aged 85 and older will necessitate significant expansions in services to address health issues seen in the very old, including frailty, dependency, and institutional-ization (U.S. Department of Health & Human Services, 1997). Since most of the oldest old will be women (Day, 1993), increased products and services to address health conditions found more frequently in women, e.g., breast cancer, thyroid disorders, incontinence, kidney disease, and osteoporosis, will also be needed (U.S. Department of Health & Human Services, 1997). More attention will also need to be paid to issues relevant to all segments of the aging population, including increased health care costs, disability, later retirement, and caregiving for the impaired.

The exact nature of the health needs of the expanding elderly population will relate, in part, to the general state of psychological wellness in this group. We know that depression, for example, is typically underreported and undertreated in older individuals. About 3% of Americans over the age of 65 have a formal diagnosis of depression. Yet it is estimated that as much as 15% of the elderly population suffers from persistent depressive symptoms (Lebowitz, 1995). The most likely causes of depression in older adults are chronic illness, medication side effects, genetic predisposition, low self-esteem, and loss of a spouse or close confidant (Haber, 1999; Oxman, Berkman, Kasl, Freeman, & Barrett, 1992). Depression not only interferes with one's engagement in and enjoyment of daily activities, but may increase susceptibility to other illnesses (Haber, 1999). Thus, older adults are at risk for getting trapped in a vicious cycle of mental and physical illness, such that chronic illness can lead to depression, and depression can lead to an exacerbation of chronic illness, which can lead to deeper depression, and so on. Additionally, chronic illness and depression can increase the likeli-hood that an older adult, particularly older women, will begin to abuse alcohol (Gomberg, 1995; Schonfeld & Dupree, 1991). Good mental health is clearly a necessary prerequisite for successful aging.

Another prerequisite for successful aging is a strong social support system. Community dwelling older adults with stronger social net-works express greater life satisfaction, less depression, and less loneli-ness than those with fewer contacts (Antonucci, Fuhrer, & Dartigues, 1997; Oxman et al., 1992). Research has shown, however, that it is not the presence of a social network per se that protects health and well-being, but rather the older adult's subjective perception of how well cared for he/she is by members of the network (George, Blazer,

Hughes, & Fowler, 1989; Oxman et al., 1992). It is the quality of the relationships within an older adult's social support network rather than the sheer quantity of members that counts. As women age, they are more at risk than men to become widowed, live alone, live in poverty, or have a chronic disability (U.S. Department of Health & Human Services, 1997). Thus, the strength of older women's social networks may be of particular importance to their continued well-being. This may be especially true for elderly African American women, who are more prone to chronic disability, and to aging without a spouse or available adult children than older White women (Ford, 1999). Elderly African American women with no spouse or with family members less available for help are the most likely to experience a scenario in which, newly faced with a disabling illness, they have to seek out new ways of socializing, of getting from one place to another, and of staying active within their churches and communities. These changes can be hard to manage, as can decisions about seeking practical assistance and social support. Thus, once a disabling illness strikes an older African American woman, the impact it can have on her social support system can place her at great risk for a rapid and irreversible decline.

The complicated picture of the interaction between social, psychological, and physical aspects of aging may lead policymakers and providers to view the impending graying of our society with trepidation. Certainly the health statistics cited here can lead to rather bleak conclusions about the prospects of aging in the United States. But those conclusions would be erroneous. It is important to keep in mind that despite the increased risk of illness that aging brings, research shows that most older adults lead productive, happy lives, without significant levels of disability or illness (Rowe & Kahn, 1998). Disability in older Americans is declining as a whole (National Institutes on Aging, 1999). Continuing advances in medical technology and pharmaceutical product development are likely to maintain that trend. More and more, chronological age is a less powerful predictor of health care use and service needs than progressively disabling disease (Rowe & Kahn, 1998), which research suggests will occur at increasingly later points in the life span of Americans. Indeed, most elderly people live active lives. For example, almost one in five Americans over the age of 65 engages in unpaid volunteer activities, which is a higher percentage than in most other industrialized nations

(Wei & Levkoff, 2000). Obviously society can reap significant economic benefits from adding as many vital years as possible to the lives of its citizens. Public policy should focus not only on prolonging life, but also on maintaining and extending health, resilience, and vigor.

In order to develop services and policy that help individuals maintain health, resilience, and vigor into old age, one must first ask the question: What is successful and productive aging? Although there are numerous possible answers to this question depending on one's vantage point, perhaps the best way to think of successful aging is conceptually, i.e., as arriving at a level of physical, social, and psychological well-being in old age. Productive aging perhaps can be thought of practically, as engagement over a lifetime in paid or unpaid activities that produce goods or services valued by the self and by society. Activities deemed personally and socially productive in old age do not necessarily fall into the same categories as for younger adults, and can include leisure activities and grandparenting. Both the notions of successful and productive aging assume an underlying foundation of good mental health and social support. Each of the chapters in this book deals explicitly or implicitly with the ways in which good mental health and strong social support connect to aspects of functioning, such as retirement, caregiving, engagement in art and music, or the practice of good nutritional habits. Rather than endorsing a particular definition of aging in good health, however, the intent of this volume is to stimulate thought about what constitutes aging in good health, so that the reader can create his/her own definition and apply it to his/her own efforts to promote the well-being of older individuals in our society.

More specifically, this book seeks to integrate aging issues from salient disciplinary perspectives to project how America is likely to age in the 21st century, and provide a forum to systematically consider how population aging will impact upon our future society, in both global and local terms. Topics for the forum are selected based on their importance to the practice of gerontology and geriatrics, and their applicability to a broad range of settings. This book is a product of linkages formed between researchers and practitioners in aging. The twenty chapters are organized into the following four basic content areas that address the integration of research and practice to appeal to researchers, practitioners, and students who are interested in well-being and independence of people as they grow older:

1. Psychological understandings of aging: The six chapters in this section examine the role of negative life events in late life adaptation; the complex process of life review among older adults; the totality of spirituality in old age; emotional health and maturity; music therapy with a geriatric population; and family relational ethics and caregiving.
2. Sociological understandings of aging: The four chapters in this section provide an overview with a sociological look at older women's aging; planning and consequences of retirement; aging in the rural context; and elder abuse in domestic settings.
3. Biomedical understandings of aging: The six chapters in this section focus on polypharmacy; nutritional assessment and recommendations; physical activities in old age; fear and prevention of falls; maximizing functional capacities by rehabilitation; and reconceptualization of alcohol abuse and intervention.
4. Service provision for the elderly: The four chapters in this concluding section encompass information on improving physician-patient communication; ethical issues in geriatric care; exemplary services in the community; and volunteerism.

The book offers reflections on aging in good health from experts in a wide range of disciplines, including theology, journalism, psychology, psychiatry, sociology, social work, public health, geriatrics, and gerontology. The multidisciplinary cadre of authors parallels the close linkages between social science, demography, and public health that have characterized research on aging in the last several years. Together with the authors, we hope that this book will help readers identify potential connections among different content areas and theoretical perspectives on aging, and in so doing leave them with a broader understanding of vital aging for use in clinical practice and policy planning.

REFERENCES

Antonucci, T., Fuhrer, R., & Dartigues, J. (1997). Social relations and depressive symptomatology in a sample of community-dwelling French older adults. *Psychology and Aging, 12,* 189–195.

Day, J. C. (1993). *Population projections in the United Sates by age, sex, race, and Hispanic origin: 1993–2050. Bureau of the Census, Current Population Reports, P25-1004.* Washington, DC: Government Printing Office.

Ford, A. (1999). Older Black women, health and the Black helping experience. *African American Research Perspectives, 5,* 1–9.

George, L. K., Blazer, D. G., Hughes, D., & Fowler, N. (1989). Social support and the outcome of major depression. *British Journal of Psychiatry, 154,* 478–485.

Gomberg, E. S. L. (1995). Older women and alcohol use and abuse. In M. Galanter (Ed.), *Recent developments in alcoholism: Alcoholism and women* (pp. 61–79). New York: Plenum.

Haber, D. (1999). *Health promotion and aging: Implications for the health professions* (2nd ed.). New York: Springer.

Lebowitz, B. (1995, Spring). Depression in older adults. *Aging and Vision News, 7,* 2.

National Institutes of Health (1992). *Report of the National Institutes of Health: Opportunities for research on women's health, NIH Pub. No. 92-3457.* Washington, DC: Government Printing Office.

National Institute on Aging (1999). *Research highlights in the demography and economics of aging, Issue No. 5.* Washington, DC: Government Printing Office.

Oxman, T., Berkman, L., Kasl, S., Freeman, D., & Barrett, J. (1992). Social support and depressive symptoms in the elderly. *American Journal of Epidemiology, 135,* 356–368.

Rowe, J. W., & Kahn, R. L. (1991). *Successful aging.* New York: Pantheon Books.

Schonfeld, L., & Dupree, L. W. (1991). Antecedents of drinking for early and late onset elderly alcohol abusers. *Journal of Studies on Alcohol, 52,* 587–592.

U.S. Department of Health and Human Services (1997). *Women's health: Report of a survey and recommendations.* Washington, DC: Government Printing Office.

Wei, J., & Levkoff, S. E. (2000). *Aging well: The complete guide to physical and emotional health.* New York: Wiley.

PART I

Psychological Understandings of Aging

CHAPTER 1

Stressful Life Events and Late Adulthood Adaptation

Xing-jia Cui and George E. Vaillant

E xperiencing life-changing events is part of human existence. As Hinkle (1973) pointed out: "to be alive is to be under stress." It is well recognized that stressful life events are closely associated with an individual's physical and psychological health. Therefore, understanding successful and productive aging requires appreciation of successful adaptation to stressful life events at advanced age.

For many years, the studies of stressful life events focused primarily on extraordinary taxing or catastrophic events such as incarceration in concentration camp, war, famine, or hurricane. Since the 1960s, the studies have been extended to include single, well-defined, and usually occurring events such as death of a beloved one, unemployment, financial strain, or marital failure. It has been widely reported that a stressful life event has a strong association with various physical illnesses, for example, diabetes mellitus (Stenstrom, Wikby, Hornquist, & Anderson, 1993), headache (De Benedittis & Lorenzetti, 1992; Passchier, Schouten, Van Der Donk, & Van Romounder, 1991), Graves' disease (Harris, Creed, & Brugha, 1992; Winsa et al., 1991), low birth weight (Mutale, Greed, Maresh, & Hunt, 1991; Wadhwa, Sandman, Porto, Dunkel-Schetter, & Gartie, 1993), herpes zoster (Schmader, Studenski, MacMillan, Grufferman, & Cohen, 1990), duodenal ulcer (Ellard, Beaurepaire, Jones, Piper, & Tennant, 1990; Hui, Shiu, Lok, & Lam, 1992), and seizure (Webster & Mawer, 1989). Similarly, many other studies have revealed a link between stressful life events and many psychiatric disorders, for example, schizophrenia (Bebbington et al., 1993; Day et al., 1987), neurotic impairment (Blazer, Hughes, & George, 1987), addiction (Gorman & Brown, 1992), postpartum psychosis (Marks, Wieck, Checkley, & Kumar, 1991), and depression (Brown & Harris, 1989; Paykel, 1994; Tennant, Bebbington, & Hurry, 1981).

In recent decades, investigators have begun to realize that the relationship between stressful life events and their health consequences is more complicated and elusive than it appears. Meanwhile, conceptualization of stressful life events has been widened to include not only a single traumatic event but also daily hassles or moderate chronic stress as well as no event at all, as in the case of loneliness (Wong, 1990). Moreover, some of the stressful life events are noted to be beneficial to physical or psychological health of human beings (Leenstra, Ormel, & Giel, 1995), and Han Selye coined a term "eustress" to distinguish it from "understress," which has the connotation of a negative effect (Kasl, 1992). In addition, more and more studies have demonstrated that the relationship between stressful life events and their consequences in mental and physical health is mediated or confounded by various psychosocial factors, for example, social support and network (Levkoff & Wetle, 1984; Paykel, 1994), personality traits (Wilkie, Eisdorfer, & Staub, 1982), and alcohol drinking (Krause, 1995).

Comparatively, elderly persons usually experience less stressful life events than the young as a result of diminishing social involvement at advanced age. Moreover, elderly persons could be more experienced and resourceful in handling some stressful changes because they are more likely to have experienced them previously. However, some older age relevant and inevitable stressful life events, for example, retirement, spouse death, relocation, and physical illness, can pose grave challenges to older people. These events, compounded by social network and financial resources shrinking at older age, if not adequately addressed, could impair the physical and psychological health of elderly persons, and the resultant impairment of health could, in return, engender more stressful events. Consequently, the vicious circle could lead to deterioration of individual's health or even death.

In this section, we are going to review literature about the stressful life events that often happen to older people and their potential deleterious consequences, and then we will elaborate on some of the important psychosocial factors that may affect successful adaptation.

STRESSFUL LIFE EVENTS AND THEIR HEALTH CONSEQUENCES FOR OLDER AGE

The studies of stressful life events among elderly persons are often conducted with focus on either cumulative stressful life events or on a single landmark event. The former approach pays attention primarily to a grand total of stressful life events, including major and minor events or chronic stress, which occur in a specific period, whereas the latter approach is usually implemented by following up the elderly person prospectively after a single salient event like retirement, widowhood, relocation, and so forth.

Cumulative Stressful Life Events

Late adult depression is often noted to be closely associated with cumulative stressful life events (Emmerson, Burvill, Finlay-Jones, & Hall, 1989; Krause, 1985; Wilkie, Eisdorfer, & Staub, 1982). In a longitudinal community study of noninstitutionalized people 65 years of age or older, Glass and colleagues (Glass, Kasl, & Berkman, 1997) reported that after adjusting for baseline depressive symptoms; relevant social demographic variables; and chronic medical conditions such as myocardial infarction, high blood pressure, stroke, cancer, diabetes, and hip fracture the total number of stressful life events occurring during the follow-up period was noted to have a significant association with depressive symptoms. There was a dose-effect relationship between the number of cumulative life events and change of depressive symptoms. Similarly, some studies revealed that a predominate portion (approximately 80%) of the elderly depressive patients associated the onset of their depression with specific life change events (Post, 1972). Heikkinen and his colleagues (1995) reported that most common stressful life events preceding suicide among elderly persons are retirement and somatic disease. More specifically, other studies of elderly persons have detected the association of depressive symptoms with financial strain (Krause, Jay, & Liang, 1991; Krause & Liang, 1993), chronic stress (Billings, Cronkite, & Moos, 1983), daily hassles (Russell & Cutrona, 1991), being a crime victim (Kasl, 1992), and acute stressful events (Colenda & Smith, 1993; Husaini et al., 1991; Murphy, 1982).

In a prospective study, we have observed that cumulative negative life events together with family history of depression are both independent predictor for depression (Cui & Vaillant, 1996). Meanwhile, we observed that depression increase the likelihood of future negative life events (Cui & Vaillant, 1997). The difficulty with the study in this area is that it is hard to control for confounding variables, such as, over-reporting bias due to depression and poor physical health, organic brain syndrome, and alcohol abuse, which may increase both depression and stressful life events. Many elder drug and alcohol addicts acquired their addictive behavior at young age. However, addicts with late onset have more possibility of organic brain syndrome and health problems in general (Rosin & Glatt, 1971; Wilkie, Eisdorfer, & Staub, 1982).

By using the Social Readjustment Rating Questionnaire (SRRQ) in late 1960s, Holms and Rahe observed the relationship between the magnitude of the life events and the risk of physical health outcomes (Rahe et al., 1974; Rahe & Arthur, 1978). Their studies indicated that if the total life event experienced fall between 150 to 199 Life Change Units (LCU), 37% of people would have health problems, and this percentage rose to 51 if the total event score ranges from 200 to 299 and to 79% if the score increases to 300 or more (Holmes & Masuda, 1974). In addition, an association between seriousness of illness and magnitude of life change was also noted (Holmes & Masuda, 1974). However, precaution has been taken before taking conclusion regarding such relations because of the methodologic limitations of those studies, which included information bias, poorly defined life events, moderate or low correlation coefficient, and possible alternative explanations (Rabkin & Struening, 1976) and failure to control for alcohol abuse as a potent cause of both stressful events and impaired immune function (Cui & Vailliant, 1996). Furthermore, Mechanic pointed out that the stressful life events could trigger an individual's help-seeking behavior, and therefore seeing doctor at a difficult time as a way of coping rather than for truly physical impairment (Mechanic, 1974). Empirically, in a longitudinal study, we failed to observe the association between cumulative life events and subsequent decline in physical health (Cui & Vaillant, 1996).

SPECIFIC LIFE EVENTS IN THE ELDERLY

Retirement

Traditionally, retirement is considered as a stressful life event. Indeed, retiring from active professional work is an important transition in the life process that requires certain physical and psychological adjustment. As Carp (1977, p. 141) suggested: "The sheer scope and pervasiveness of changes must forecast physical illness, according to the Holmes and Rahe paradigm." There are studies providing some indirect evidence that support this belief. It is reported that retirement is associated with the higher suicide rate among the white men at age 65 or older (Miller, 1979) and high mortality at old age (Adams & Lefebvre, 1981). In addition, some studies indicated that retirement can affect family incomes (Parnes, 1981), marital relationships (Hill & Dorfman, 1982) and the sense of well being (Thompson, 1973). However, since most of preceding studies were cross-sectional in design, no casual inference can be reliably deduced. For instance, one's retirement and suicide may be both precipitated by major depressive disorder. Similarly, one may take retirement due to physical health problems, which can likely lead to death.

The vast majority of studies of retirement, however, have failed to demonstrate that retirement has any remarkable adverse impact on poor physical and/or mental health. In a longitudinal study of 58 married couples, Crawford (1972) demonstrated that retirement caused no significant changes in subjective feeling in health, in physician visits, or in appetite and body weight. Likewise, retirement produced no changes in subjective feelings in health or in physician visits among wives of the study subjects (Crawford, 1972). After comprehensive literature review, Kasl (1980, p. 152) concluded " . . . only a minimal general impact of retirement on mental health and wellbeing." In a study of the stressfulness of retirement, Matthews and colleagues asked retirees to rate the stressfulness of 34 important life events that they had experienced. Retirement ranked 28th among the 34 events on the list (Matthews & Brown, 1987). In a similar study, which examined 1516 male participants, Bossé and colleagues found that among those retiring in the past year, respondents' and spouses' retirement were rated the least stressful from a list of 31 possible events. Only 30% of the participants thought retirement was stressful at all (Bossé, Aldwin, Levenson, & Workman-Daniels, 1991).

For some people, retirement is freely chosen. Others experience retirement as compulsory. Some people willingly and happily give up their working role and pursue interests or hobbies that they could not pursue during their working years. For others, working is a major life pursuit. For them, retirement leaves time that they do not know how to fill. Financially, some people are well prepared for retirement. For others, retirement results in a major decrease in income. Some people must retire due to incompetence, economic downturn, or poor physical health. Others retire through free choice. Thus, it is not surprising that as they pass from working to nonworking status retirees undergo vastly different experiences.

Nevertheless, for some people, retirement is stressful. In a study comparing dissatisfied with satisfied retirees, Blau and his colleagues (1982) reported that the former had less education, less adequate income, saw friends less often, and reported poorer premorbid physical and mental health. In a similar study of retirees, Matthew and Brown (1987) found that retirement is stressful for men whose retirement is involuntary or are of low socioeconomic status or had experienced more premorbid stressful life events. Other factors identified as stressful include: where the predictability and control over the retirement is lost; when it occurs too early or "off time"; when retirement disrupts social support, financial stability or residential pattern; finally, the person's preretirement feelings and attitudes toward the loss of the work role (Levkoff & Wetle, 1984).

Death of a Spouse

Like retirement, for many older people, death of a spouse, or widowhood, is an inevitable event. It has been considered as one of the most stressful life events at advanced age. Conceivably, losing a lifetime partner is a traumatic life change, which entails immense lifestyle, mental, and physical adjustment. For some people, death of a spouse represents the loss of dependable financial resource and a concomitant decline in the economic status, while for others, it may represent a decline in social interaction and a concurrent decline in social involvement.

Various studies demonstrated that health problems, especially depression, happen to the elderly widow or widower following the death of spouse (Gallagher, Thompson, & Peterson, 1981–1982). The most common reaction to death of a spouse at any age is bereavement, which manifests primarily the constellation of grief or depressive symptoms, which sometimes meet criteria for major depression. The difference between bereavement and depression is primarily based on the duration of symptoms. By following up a group of widows, Clayton (1972) reported that 35% of widows manifested full depression within 1 month and that 17% were still depressed 1 year later. In a similar prospective study of 350 widows or widowers, Zisook and Shuchter (1991) found that 24% of study subjects met criteria for depressive episode at 2 months, 23% did so at 7 months, and 16% did so at 13 months.

Even though death of a spouse at advanced age is a traumatic event, its causal relationship with adverse health consequences is, however, illusory or mediated by other factors. For example, Atchley (1975) reported that income loss was a major mediating variable. Morgan (1976) also found poor adaptation to widowhood to be associated with low income. The additional contributing factors that have been identified to be relevant to the adaptation of widowhood include age of widowed person, availability of alternative role, characteristics of coping styles, adequacy of the social network, and religious commitment (Gallagher et al., 1981–1982; Levkoff & Wetle, 1984).

Relocation

Relocation at older age involves various types of moves: from one home to another home, from one community to another community, from home to institution, from one institution to another institution. No matter what the reason for the move, it is understandable that relocation requires elderly persons to adjust to the new physical and social environment, which could be challenging and stressful. The moves involving healthy people in the community clearly have different meaning in comparison with the moves that involve frail individuals in institutions.

In a prospective study, Lander and colleagues (1997) followed up 78 residents with and without cognitive, mood, or other psychotic disorders who were involved within institutional relocation due to the renovation of a health facility. The study demonstrated that after relocation a significant increase was observed in the number of medical visits, weight loss, and fall rate. For the residents with cognitive impairment, a significant difference before and after relocation was seen in self-care and withdrawn behavior. In a similar study, Friedman et al. (1995) followed up 210 nursing home residents who moved from a 125-year-old facility to a newly constructed facility. They found that the fall rate per resident increased from 0.34 in the 3 months before the move to 0.70 falls in the 3 months after the move. In addition, fall-related injuries were significantly increased from 0.06 per resident per quarter to 0.15.

Forced relocation due to an event like the closing of nursing care facility is relatively stressful because social relocation is involuntary, unexpected, and out of control of the elderly persons. In a follow-up study that tracked 69 older people who were forced to relocate, Beirne et al. (1995) found that the 65% of the relocated residents who were unable to return after the recertification of the facility suffered health deterioration or death. Similarly, after the closing of three public chronic disease hospitals in Massachusetts, it was found that relocation increased both the rate of incontinence and mortality (Caro et al., 1997). However, the association between relocation and its health consequence is not linear in character. Various factors, including psychosocial, environmental and physical factors, were identified to confound this association (Armer, 1996; Mirotznik, 1995; Reinardy, 1995).

FACTORS MEDIATING THE STRESSFUL LIFE EVENTS AND THEIR CONSEQUENCES

Three salient intervening factors mediating the successful adaptation to stressful life events among elderly persons are control over events, defense styles, and social support.

Control Over Events

Events, which happen suddenly and unexpectedly, have much more profound morbid impact than anticipated and well-prepared-for events. Therefore, the timing of a life event is a crucial determinant for its stressfulness. Usually death of a spouse is more devastating to mood at 40 than at 80. Without preparation, people experiencing stressful events are more overwhelmed by the experience. In contrast, people can minimize the effect of a stressful event if it can be anticipated, and they can rehearse and seek social support or professional counsel. For example, the death of the husband who has been suffering from a chronic fatal disease for many years might have far less effect on an elderly woman than unexpected death of a child or grandchild. For that reason, Neugarten argued that it is the unanticipated life events, the "off-time" event, that should be classified as the stressor (Wilkie, Eisdorfer, & Staub, 1982).

The controllability of life events is another factor that may mitigate their impact on health. Several investigators argued that when people feel in control of life change they are less likely to be negatively affected by them. Reinardy (1995) examined 502 elderly residents after their admission to a nursing home. They found that the people who decide to move and want to move were more satisfied with service and more actively participating in nursing home activities. In a similar study, Iwasiw et al. (1996) observed that adjusting to a long-term care facility was easier if the elderly residents had actively participated in the decision to be admitted. But, of course, the effect of such controllability is to a certain extent determined by premorbid mental and physical health. The premorbid nondepressed or intellectually intact persons are less likely to be placed in a nursing home against their will.

Several investigators suggested that it is the perception of understanding or mastery rather than the actual ability to control that determine the health consequence of the event (Wilkie et al., 1982). However, Rodin and Langer (1980), in an experimental study that controlled for premorbid status, demonstrated that the critical factor affecting the health of nursing home residents was the involvement of the decision making and taking responsibility.

Defense or Coping Styles

Defense refers to a variety of self-protective coping reactions to external stresses. The aims of defense are to enable people to retain mental and physical equilibrium, that is, homeostasis, at the time of experiencing stressful life events. These strategies and mental mechanisms play a vital role in mediating the relationship between stressful life events and adverse health outcomes. People may use different defense strategies to cope with different stress situations, and these strategies (e.g., projection or altruism) may not be under conscious control (Vaillant, 1992).

Specifically, the defense responses and coping strategies employed by elderly persons for the stressful life change can be classified into three categories: (a) eliciting help from appropriate others by mobilizing social support; (b) voluntary cognitive efforts such as information gathering, anticipating danger, and rehearsing response to danger; and (c) involuntary ego mechanism of defense (Vaillant, 1994). Generally, the former two strategies of defenses are reality oriented and active problem solving so that in most cases they are effective and adaptive. The consequences of involuntary ego defenses, however, are variable depending on the level of maturity of the adopted mechanisms. Empirical studies suggest that defenses like projection, neurotic denial, and acting out led to sacrifices in adjustment in every aspect of living, and on the other hand, the mature defenses such as suppression, sublimation, and altruism led to sacrifice in none (Vaillant, 1976). For example, a woman who lost her husband recently could mitigate her grief by helping other women who have same experience (altruism) or organizing a nice memorial service for her deceased husband (suppression and sublimation). On the contrary, a bereaved woman could make her situation deteriorate by seeking attention through various somatized complains (hypochondriasis) or excessive spending, drinking, or gambling (dissociation).

Defense styles over the life span are not static. Maturation and experience lead to using more mature defenses. Impaired central nervous system (CNS) integration due to Alzheimer's disease, bipolar illness, and alcohol abuse is associated with less mature defenses. For some individuals, reaction formation and displacement replace the adolescent hypochondriasis, and, in turn, might be replaced by altruism by age 60. Similarly, for an alcoholic, the process might be reversed. An altruistic urge might become phobic (displacement) and then hypochondrical in response to change (Vaillant, 1976). In general, elderly persons tend to become less egocentric, more concerned with other people's difficulties, and mature in the defense selection.

Physical impairment at advanced age may limit use of some strategies that entail physical vigor or intellectual competence. For example, the people who like to use physical exercise to alleviate stress might have difficulty because of physical illness. A life-long bookworm would have less difficulty from arthritis but more from cataracts.

Social Support

It has been long speculated that social supports can be instrumental for the adaptation of stressful life events among aging individuals. More and more empirical evidence for this hypothesis has been accumulated in recent years, albeit research scientists do not have consensus in the definition of social support. Various studies among the aging population have noted beneficial effects of social support on morbidity and mortality (Berkman & Syme, 1979), morale, cognitive functioning, hospital, long-term care, cardiovascular disease, and physical health (Jackson & Antonucci, 1992; Stansfeld, Rael, Head, Shipley, & Marmot, 1997). Similarly, it has been reported that lack of a confiding relationship is a vulnerability factor that is associated with risk of depression in response to life events (Emmerson et al., 1989; Lowenthal & Haven, 1968; Murphy, 1982). A difficulty with most such studies is that they fail to control for objective physical health, alcohol abuse, and major depression—all of which increase the likelihood of poor morale, lack of confidence, and poor subsequent physical health. Such confounders need to be controlled before final conclusions about the relationship between social support and physical/mental consequence can be drawn. For example, in a 50-year prospective study of 223 men, Vaillant and colleagues have observed that the strong association between social support and physical health was very much attenuated after controlling prior smoking, depression, preexisting health problems, and alcohol abuse (Vaillant, Meyer, Mukamal, & Soldz, 1998).

Another difficulty is related to the measurement of social support. Jackson and Antonucci (1992) have argued that to grasp the complexity of social support, appropriate attention should be paid to following factors: (a) the nature of support (e.g., aid, affect, or affirmation); (b) the source of supports (e.g., spouse, close friends, or neighbor community); and (c) the perception of supports by recipient (e.g., does the recipient feel aided or smothered?). It was noted that it is the quality rather than quantity and it is the subjective perception rather than objective magnitude of social support that plays the more important role in health consequences (Duff & Hong, 1982; Field & Minkler, 1988). Additionally, different sources of support could exert different effects on health outcomes. For example, in certain circumstances, friends may be more instrumental in maintaining physical health than family members (Vaillant et al., 1998).

Finally, assuming social support does affect health, what is the mechanism of its effectiveness? Two explanations have been proposed, one in psychological and the other in biological. Many researches have speculated that social support can cause changes in coping resources (Pearlin, 1989) and in self-esteem and personal efficacy (Krause, 1990). Others have suggested that social support can induce feeling of autonomy and control in older persons (Schaie, Rodin, & Schooler, 1990; Schulz, 1976). Jackson and Antonucci (1992) have hypothesized that effective social support provides social interaction, and a confiding relationship between the support recipient and the provider, induces positive change on the personal efficacy of the recipient.

Physiologically, even though there is no direct supporting evidence, several hypotheses linking psychoimmunology (Ader, Cohen, & Felton, 1991) and the pituitary-hypothalamic axis (Cassel, 1976; Cobb, 1976; Post, 1974) have been posited. For example, House (1988) suggested that "social relationships" and contacts, mediated through the amygdala, activate the anterior hypothalamic zone; stimulate the release of growth hormone; inhibit the posterior hypothalamic zone; and depress the secretion of adrenocorticotropic hormone (ACTH), cortisol, and catacolamines. At present, the evidence for such postulation depends more on an animal experiment than on the demonstration of these effects in humans.

CONCLUSION

In summary, stressful life events are very influential variables for physical and mental health of older people. However, the association of stress with health is not linear. Many other biological, psychological, and social factors could either mediate or confound such relationships. In addition, the outcomes of stress can also be potential causes of stressful life events. Therefore, these complicated associations pose daunting challenges for researchers who try to disentangle the relationships between various stress relevant variables. To address this question, we expect that more refined measurement of life events and other psychosocial variables, longitudinal in study design, and multidimensional statistical modeling techniques will be needed in future studies.

REFERENCES

Ader, R., Cohen, N., & Felton, D. (1991). *Psychoneuroimmunology*. San Diego, CA: Academic Press.

Adams, O., & Lefebvre, L. (1981). Retirement and mortality. *Aging and Work, 4*, 115–120.

Armer, J. M. (1996). An exploration of factors influencing adjustment among relocation rural elders. *Image: The Journal of Nursing Scholarship, 28*, 35–39.

Atchley, A. C. (1975). Dimensions of widowhood in later life. *The Gerontologist, 15*, 176–178.

Bebbington, P., Wilkins, S., Jones, P., Foerster, A., Murray, R., Toone, B., & Lewis, S. (1993). Life events and psychosis: Initial results form Camberwell Collaborative Psychosis Study. *British Journal of Psychiatry, 162*, 72–79.

Beirne, N. F., Patterson, M. N., Galie, M., & Goodman, P. (1995). Effect of a fast-track closing on a nursing facility population. *Health and Social Work, 20*, 116–123.

Berkman, L. F., & Syme, S. L. (1979). Social networks, host resistance, and mortality: A nine-year follow-up study of Alameda County residents. *American Journal of Epidemiology, 109*, 186–204.

Billings, A. G., Cronkite, R. C., & Moos, E. H. (1983). Social-environmental factors in unipolar depression: Comparison of depressed patients and non-depressed controls. *Journal of Abnormal Psychology, 92*, 119–133.

Blau, Z. S., Oser, S. T., & Stephens, R. C. (1982). Patterns of adaptation in retirement: A comparative analysis. In A. Kolker & P. E. Ahmed (Eds.), *Coping with medical issues: Aging* (pp. 119–138). New York: Elsevier.

Blazer, D., Hughes, D., & George, L. K. (1987). Stressful life events and the onset of a generalized anxiety syndrome. *American Journal of Psychiatry, 144*, 1178–1183.

Bossé, R., Aldwin, C. M., Levenson, M. R., & Workman-Daniels, K. (1991). How stressful is retirement: Findings from the Normative Aging Study. *Journal of Gerontology, 46*, 9–14.

Brown, G. W., & Harris, T. O. (1989). *Life events and illness.* New York: Guilford.

Caro, F. G., Glickman, L. L., Ingegneri, D., Porell, F., Stern, A. L., & Verma, K. (1997). The impact of the closing of three Massachusetts public chronic disease hospitals: A multidimensional perspective. *Journal of Community Health, 22*, 155–174.

Carp, E. M. (1977). Retirement and physical health. In S. Kasl & V. Reichsman (Eds.), *Advances in psychosomatic medicine: Epidemiological studies in psychosomatic medicine* (pp. 140–159). Basel: S. Karger.

Cassel, B. (1976). The contribution of the social environment to host resistance. *American Journal of Epidemiology, 104*, 107–123.

Clayton, P. J. (1972). The depression of widowhood. *British Journal of Psychiatry, 120*, 71–78.

Cobb, S. (1976). Social support as a moderator for life stress. *Psychosomatic Medicine, 38*, 300–314.

Colenda, C. C., & Smith, S. L. (1993). Multivariate modeling of anxiety and depression in community-dwelling elderly persons. *American Journal of Geriatric Psychiatry, 1*, 327–338.

Crawford, M. P. (1972). Retirement as a psychosocial crisis. *Journal of Psychosomatic Research, 16*, 375–380.

Cui, X-. J., & Vaillant, G. E. (1996). Antecedents and consequence of negative life events in adulthood: A longitudinal study. *American Journal of Psychiatry, 152*, 21–26.

De Benedittis, G., & Lorenzetti, A. (1992). The role of stressful life events in the persistence of primary headache: Major events vs. daily hassles. *Pain, 51*, 35–42.

Duff, R. W., & Hong, L. K. (1982). Quality and quantity of social interactions in the life satisfaction of older Americans. *Sociology and Social Research, 66*, 418–434.

Ellard, K., Beaurepaire, J., Jones, M., Piper, D., & Tennant, C. (1990). Acute and chronic stress in dodenal ulcer disease. *Gastroenterology, 99,* 1628–1632.

Emmerson, J. P., Burvill, P. W., Finlay-Jones, R., & Hall, W. (1989). Life events, life difficulties, and confiding relationships in the depressed elderly. *British Journal of Psychiatry, 155,* 787–792.

Field, D., & Minkler, M. (1988). Continuity and change in social support between young old and old-old or very-old age. *Journal of Gerontology, 43,* 100–106.

Friedman, S. M., Williamson, J. D., Lee, B. H., Ankrom, M. A., Ryan, S. D., & Denman, S. J. (1995). Increase fall rates in nursing home residents after relocation to a new facility. *Journal of the American Geriatrics Society, 43,* 1237–1242.

Gallagher, D. E., Thompson, L. W., & Peterson, J. A. (1981–1982). Psychosocial factors affecting adaptation to bereavement in the elderly. *International Journal of Aging and Human Development, 14,* 79–94.

Glass, T. A., Kasl, S. V., & Berkman, L. F. (1997). Stressful life events and depressive symptoms among the elderly. *Journal of Aging and Health, 9,* 70–89.

Gorman, D. M., & Brown, G. W. (1992). Recent developments in life-event research and their relevance for the study of addiction. *British Journal of Addiction, 87,* 837–849.

Harris, T., Creed, F., & Brugha, T. S. (1992). Stressful life events and Graves' disease. *British Journal of Psychiatry, 161,* 535–541.

Heikkinen, M. E., Isometsa, E. T., Aro, H. M., Sarna, S. J., & Lonnqvist, J. K. (1995). Age-related variation in recent life events preceding suicide. *Journal of Nervous and Mental Disorder, 183,* 325–331.

Hill, E. A., & Dorfman, L. T. (1982). Reaction to housewives to their retirement of their husband. *Family Relation, 31,* 195–200.

Hinkle, L. E. (1973). The concept of "stress" in the biological and social science. *Science, Medicine, and Man, 1,* 31–48.

Holmes, T. H., & Masuda, M. (1974). Life change and illness susceptibility. In B. S. Dohrenwend, & B. P. Dohrenwen (Eds.), *Stressful life events: Their nature and effects* (pp. 45–71). New York: Wiley.

House, J. S., Landis, K. R., & Umberson, D. (1988). Social relationship and health. *Science, 241,* 540–545.

Hui, W. M., Shiu, L. P., Lok, A. S., & Lam, S. K. (1992). Life events and daily stress in duodenal ulcer disease: A prospective study of patients with active disease and in remission. *Digestion, 52,* 165–172.

Husaini, B. A., Moore, S. T., Castor, R. S., Neser, W., Witten-Stoval, R., Linn, J. G., & Griffin, D. (1991). Social density, stressors, and depression: Gender differences among the black elderly. *Journal of Gerontology,* *46,* 236–242.

Iwasiw, C., Goldenberg, D., MacMaster, E., McCutcheon, S., & Bol, N. (1996). Residents' perspectives of their first 2 weeks in a long-term care facility. *Journal of Clinical Nursing, 5,* 381–388.

Jackson, J. S., & Antonucci, T. C. (1992). Social support process in health and effective functioning of the elderly. In M. L. Wykle, E. Kahana, & J. Kowal (Eds.), *Stress and health among the elderly* (pp. 73–95). New York: Springer.

Kasl, S. V. (1980). The impact of retirement. In C. L. Cooper, & R. Payne (Eds.), *Current concerns in occupational stress* (pp. 137–186). New York: Wiley.

Kasl, S. V. (1992). Stress and health among the elderly: overview of issues. In M. L. Wykle, E. Kahana, & J. Kowal (Eds.), *Stress and health among the elderly* (pp. 5–31). New York: Springer.

Krause, N. (1990). Stress, support, and well being in later life: Focusing on salient social roles. In M. A. P. Stephens, J. H. Crowther, S. E. Hobfoll, & D. L. Tennenbaum (Eds.), *Stress and coping in later-life families* (pp. 71–97). New York: Hemisphere.

Krause, N. (1995). Stress, alcohol use, and depressive symptoms in later life. *Journal of Gerontology, 35,* 296–307.

Krause, N., Jay, G., & Liang, J. (1991). Financial strain and psychological well-being among the American and Japanese elderly. *Psychology & Aging, 6,* 170–181.

Krause, N., & Liang, J. (1993). Stress, social support, and psychological distress among the Chinese elderly. *Journal of Gerontology, 48,* 282–291.

Lander, S. M., Brazill, A. L., & Ladrigan, P. M. (1997). Intrainstitutional relocation: Effects on resident's behavior and psychosocial functioning. *Journal of Gerontological Nursing, 23,* 35–41.

Leenstra, A. S., Ormel, J., & Giel, R. (1995). Positive life intrainstitutional relocation: Effects on resident's behavior and change and recovery from depression and anxiety: A three stage longitudinal study of primary care attenders. *British Journal of Psychiatry, 166,* 333–343.

Levkoff, S., & Wetle, T. (1984). Adaptation to transition in late adulthood: Implication for health education. *International Quarterly of Community Health Education, 4,* 191–200.

Lowenthal, M. F., & Haven, C. (1968). Interaction and adaptation: Intimacy as a critical variable. *American Sociological Review, 33,* 20–30.

Matthews, A. M., & Brown, K. H. (1987). Retirement as a critical life event. *Research on Aging, 9,* 548–571.

Mechanic, D. (1974). Discussion of research programs on relations between stressful life events and episode of physical illness. In B. S. Dohrenwend, & B. P. Dohrenwend (Eds.), *Stressful life events: Their nature and effects* (pp. 87–97). New York: Wiley.

Miller, M. (1979). *Suicide after sixty: The final alternative.* New York: Springer.

Mirotznik, J. (1995). Response of noninterviewable long-term care patients before and after interinstitutional relocation. *Psychological Reports, 76,* 1267–1280.

Morgan, A. (1976). Reexamination of widowhood and morale. *Journal of Gerontology, 31,* 687–695.

Murphy, E. (1982). Social origins of depression in old age. *British Journal of Psychiatry, 141,* 135.

Mutale, T., Greed, F., Maresh, M., & Hunt, L. (1991). Life events and low birth weight-analysis by infants preterm and small for gestational age. *British Journal of Obstetrics & Gynecology, 98,* 166–172.

Paykel, E. S. (1994). Life events, social support and depression. *Acta Psychiatrica Scandinavia, 377*(Suppl), 50–58.

Parnes, H. (1981). *Work and retirement.* Cambridge, MA: MIT Press.

Passchier, J., Schouten, J., Van Der Donk, J., & Van Romunder, L. K. (1991). The association of frequency of primary headache with personality and life events. *Headache, 31,* 116–121.

Pearlin, L. L. (1989). The sociological study of stress. *Journal of Health and Social Behavior, 30,* 241–256.

Post, F. (1972). The management and nature of depressive illness in late life. A follow-through study. *British Journal of Psychiatry, 121,* 389–395.

Post, R. M. (1974). Molecular biology of behavior. *Archives of General Psychiatry, 54,* 607–608.

Rabkin, J. G., & Struening, E. L. (1976). Life events, stress and illness. *Science, 194,* 1013–1020.

Rahe, R. H., & Arthur R. J. (1978). Life change and illness studies: Past history and future directions. *Journal of Human Stress, 3,* 3–15.

Rahe, H. R., Floistad, I., Bergan, T., Ringdal, R., Gerhardt, R., Gunderson, E. K. E., & Arthur, R. J. (1974). A model for life changes and illness research. *Archive of General Psychiatry, 31,* 172–177.

Reinardy, J. R. (1995). Relocation to a new environment: Decisional control and the move to a nursing home. *Health and Social Work, 20,* 31–38.

Rodin, J., & Langer, E. (1980). Aging labels: The decline of control and the fall of self-esteem. *Journal of Social Issues, 36,* 12–29.

Rosin, A. J., & Glatt, M. M. (1971). Alcohol excess in the elderly. *Quarterly Journal of Study of Alcohol, 32,* 52–59.

Russell, D. W., & Cutrona, C. E. (1991). Social support, stress, and depressive symptoms among elderly: Test of a process model. *Psychology and Aging, 6,* 190–201.

Schaie, K. W., Rodin, J., & Schooler, C. (1990). *Self-directedness: Cause and effects throughout the life course.* Hillsdale, NJ: Erlbaum.

Schmader, K., Studenski, S., MacMillan, J., Grufferman, S., & Cohen, H. J. (1990). Are stressful life events risk factors for herpes zoster? *Journal of American Geriatrics Society, 38,* 1188–1194.

Schulz, R. (1976). Effects of control and predictability on the physical and psychological well-being of the institutionalized age. *Journal of Personality and Social Psychology, 33,* 563–573.

Stansfeld, S. A., Rael, E. G. S., Head, J., Shipley M., & Marmot, M. (1997). Social support and psychiatric sickness absence: A prospective study of British civil servants. *Psychological Medicine, 27,* 35–48.

Stenstrom, U., Wikby, A., Hornquist, J. O., & Andersson, P. O. (1993). Recent life events, gender, and the control of diabetes mellitus. *General Hospital Psychiatry, 15,* 82–88.

Tennant, C., Bebbington, P., & Hurry, J. (1981). The role of life events in depressive illness: Is there a substantial causal relation? *Psychological Medicine, 11,* 379–389.

Thompson, G. B. (1973). Work versus leisure roles: An investigation of morale among employed and retired men. *Journal of Gerontology, 28,* 339–344.

Vaillant, G. E. (1976). Natural history of male psychological health. *Archive of General Psychiatry, 33,* 535–545.

Vaillant, G. E. (1977). *Adaptation to life.* Boston: Little, Brown.

Vaillant, G. E. (1992). *Ego mechanisms of defense.* Washington, DC: American Psychiatric Press.

Vaillant, G. E. (1994). Ego mechanisms of defense and personality psychopathology. *Journal of Abnormal Psychology, 103,* 44–50.

Vaillant, G. E., Meyer, S. E., Mukamal, K., & Soldz, S. (1998). Are social support in late midlife a cause or a result of successful physical aging? *Psychological Medicine, 25,* 1159–1168.

Wadhwa, P. D., Sandman, C. A., Porto, M., Dunkel-Schetter, C., & Garite, T. J. (1993). The association between prenatal stress and infant birth weight and gestational age at birth: A prospective investigation. *American Journal of Obstetrics and Gynecology, 169,* 858–865.

Webster, A., & Mawer, G. E. (1989). Seizure frequency and major life events in epilepsy. *Epilepsia, 30,* 162–167.

Wilkie, F. L., Eisdorfer, C., & Staub, J. (1982). Stress and psychopathology in the aged. *Psychiatric Clinics of North America, 5,* 131–143.

Winsa, B., Adami, H. O., Bergstrom, R., Gamstedt, A., Dahlber, P. A., Adamson, U., Jansson, R., & Karlsson, A. (1991). Stressful life events and Graves' disease. *Lancet, 338,* 1475–1479.

Wong, P. T. P. (1990). Measuring life stress. *Stress Medicine, 6,* 69–70.

Zisook, S., & Shuchter, S. R. (1991). Depression through the first year after the death of a spouse. *American Journal of Psychiatry, 148,* 1346–1352.

CHAPTER 2

The Significance of Life Review in Old Age

Margery Hutter Silver

I n many cultures, older people enjoy telling their life stories. However, there is more to this storytelling than just sharing memories. It may be the expression of a complex psychological process—*life review*—that is related to the last stage of life and is activated by the physical, social, and other changes that take place in old age.

In life review, memories of the past seem to increase and become more intense. As elderly persons sift through these memories and come to understand them in new ways, they can make meaning of their lives. This can be done alone, but for many individuals, life review is more helpful when another person is present to hear their memories. In this way, they can resolve old conflicts and accept losses, as well as celebrate their accomplishments. This can lead to acceptance of one's self and one's entire life cycle. In this way, coming to terms with what their life has been can give people greater capacity to accept their present lives, cope with their challenges, and find satisfaction and meaning.

LIFE REVIEW OR REMINISCENCE?

To discuss life review, it is important to distinguish between life review and reminiscence. Reminiscence is simply recounting memories, such as a grandmother's recollection of the first trolley cars as she boards the MTA with her granddaughter or the memories evoked by hearing a particular song. In life review, in contrast, there is a psychological process, conscious or unconscious, that may result in a person seeing his or her life in a somewhat different way. People reminisce during life review, but in life review, something internal is also happening. This is an important distinction that makes it imperative for clinicians who are working with older patients to understand the theory underlying life review and the research on the effects of life review.

This chapter will discuss the major theorists who have written about life review. It will then present major findings emerging from research studies of the life review. The use of life review therapy in clinical practice will be described, including practical suggestions for approaching patients and initiating the life review process. A case study will be included to illustrate the process and outcome of a course of life review therapy.

LIFE REVIEW THEORIES

A number of theorists have expounded on the positive effects of the life review. The concept of life review as a developmental process that is universal and normative is most fully articulated in the writings of psychiatrist Robert Butler, former Director of the National Institute of Aging (1963). Reintegration of past experience through spontaneous or purposive memories leads to making sense of one's life as a whole. Its successful outcome results in resolution and in serenity and wisdom (Butler, 1963). Butler emphasizes the adaptive and therapeutic aspects of life review, and he believes that it is more effective "in the presence of acceptance and support from others" (Lewis & Butler, 1974, p. 166). A therapist can tap into an ongoing process and participate in it with the older person to "enhance it, to make it more conscious, deliberate, and efficient."

The developmental stage theory of Erik Erikson has also been associated with life review. In each of Erikson's eight psychosocial stages, there is a struggle between two opposite characteristics; for example, in the first stage, the infant stage, it is trust vs. mistrust (1950). In the final stage, old age, the struggle is between integrity and despair. Integrity is achieved by "acceptance of one's one and only life cycle and of the people who have become significant to it," as well as accepting one's death.

Acceptance of one's one and only life cycle implies a review of one's past, although Erikson does not specifically label it life review. Life review is further implied in his powerful essay "Reflections on Dr. Borg's Life Cycle" (1976), which he calls "a memoir that begins with the end." In it, he interprets Ingmar Bergman's film *Wild Strawberries* as a life review precipitated by the integrity vs. despair conflict of the last stage of life. Dr. Borg's journey back in time is discussed as a symbolic movement backward through earlier life stages. In the end, Dr. Borg even sees his parents differently, accepting his past and achieving resolution of the final stage of life.

Other theorists have conceptualized processes that might be called life review. For example, Bertrand Cohler of the University of Chicago (1980), describes "the personal narrative," the reconstruction of one's life story at developmentally significant points in one's life. The individual's interpretation of events changes over time. Revisions must be made in terms of life events and social and biological changes to "make sense of the life history as a whole" (p. 8). Similarly, Roger Gould (1978) speaks of "assumptions" that we recast at particular phases of life.

George Pollock's work on the mourning-liberation process in old age further illuminates the concept of life review (1978). Pollock, a well-known geropsychiatrist, suggests that this process may be closely related to life review. As people grow older, there are more crises, more losses, but they do not have to lead to psychological incapacity if they initiate a successful mourning process. As people review their lives, they must mourn for parts of the self that are lost or changed, for lost others, for unfulfilled hopes and aspirations. The ability to work through grief and loss can be liberating and can result in "creative freedom, further development, joy, and the ability to embrace life (1978, p. 42). If a person can do that, there is a "liberation" from the past, "that enhances life, allows the person to change and develop, and releases creativity."

RESEARCH STUDIES

There are a number of research studies that relate life review to the successful outcome of the integrity vs. despair stage of Erikson's theory, including a study that shows that high reminiscers have higher integrity scores (Boylin, Gordon, & Nehrke, 1976). A strong association between reminiscence and mourning has been found, which supports Pollock's theory that mourning is related to life review (McMahon & Rhudick, 1964). This study also found that high reminiscing was associated with low depression.

The adaptive effects of life review have been considered in a number of studies. A review of 97 studies of the effects of reminiscence found positive outcomes in 70 of the 97 and negative outcomes in only seven (Haight, 1991). High amounts of reminiscence were associated with low incidence of depression in several research studies (Fallot, 1979–80; McMahon & Rhudick, 1964). High reminiscence has also been associated with good cognitive functioning and with a high survival rate (McMahon & Rhudick, 1964). Furthermore, high reminiscence has been correlated with good adjustment and high morale (Havighurst & Glasser, 1972) and positive mood (1979–80).

Two other important findings have emerged from life review and reminiscence research. The first is support of Butler's contention that life review is more successful when done in the presence of others. A study of styles of reminiscence (Marshall, 1974) revealed that subjects who were most often alone (low social resources) were less likely than those who talked frequently to others to have a successful outcome, which was defined as "a view of the past which could be fairly called 'integrity' in Erikson's definition of that term" (1975, p. 126). The second is that people who show sadness during the life review are more likely to have a successful outcome. Ego integrity was highly correlated with dysphoric affect in a study by Boylin and colleagues (1976). This may mean that those who can tolerate remembering bad times and bad feelings are more likely to go through the healthy mourning that is part of life review.

THEMES OF THE LIFE REVIEW

Discovery of the themes of the life review was the goal of a previous study I conducted (Silver, 1982). Little had been written about what people actually talked about or what were the usual themes or preoccupations of individuals as they reviewed their lives. Twenty elderly women aged 65 to 85 who were participants in an adult day health center were seen for 12 sessions of life review. Tape recordings of the life review sessions were analyzed to find the most frequently occurring themes. The three themes that occurred most frequently—mourning, integrity, and caring and being cared for—will be discussed here.

Mourning and loss, which, as mentioned above, had been associated with the life review in the writings of Pollock (1978), was the most frequent theme. The women in the study not only mourned the loss of loved ones, but the loss of physical capacity, competence, independence, physical appearance, the way things used to be. Many mourned their past selves—who they used to be.

The second prominent theme was the integrity vs. despair struggle of Erikson's life-stage model. The women in the study, through life review, struggled to come to terms with their life as it had been. This included accepting themselves, both their present selves and their past selves, as well as accepting transience and the nearness of death.

The third theme that emerged from the life reviews of these elderly women was a new finding: the struggle to balance giving and accepting care. As these older women became less able to care for themselves, they needed to accept care without giving up and becoming completely helpless and demanding. At the same time, they needed to be able to maintain a sense of dignity and self-worth and to continue to care for others.

Adult children have a similar task. They must learn to care for parents without infantilizing them. Many of the conflicts in families come from the struggles of both older parent and adult child to successfully adapt to these care-related developmental tasks. Similarly, conflicts with other care givers, such as nursing home staff or home health aides, are often related to the difficulties an elderly person may experience in learning to accept care.

This issue of how to balance giving and accepting care is a very common and extremely important one in clinical work with elderly patients. Sometimes it is effective to help clients to identify ways they are still providing care. For example, a retired man who can no longer "care" for his family by supporting them financially may not recognize that he still is providing care—by giving his daughter emotional support when she has problems or by giving his grandson advice on what profession to choose. Helping him to reconceptualize what he is doing as an important way of caring can help him feel productive and needed, leading to increased self-esteem and in some cases helping to decrease depression.

HELPING ELDERLY INDIVIDUALS
THROUGH LIFE REVIEW

Life review can be a helpful approach to increasing the well being and life satisfaction of elders in the community who may tell their stories to families, friends, in group settings, or to a professional. It can help them to negotiate major transitions that individuals must often go through in old age; for example, the transition from living independently at home to being cared for in a nursing home or from married life to a being single when a spouse dies.

In nursing home settings, life review can be very useful in a number of ways, such as:

1. Establishing rapport and relationships between residents and staff. The resident benefits by having the support of a listener, and staff benefits as well by an opportunity to know the resident as a complex, whole person, not just a catalogue of illnesses.
2. Building self-esteem. During life review, the resident can review accomplishments, getting back in touch with his or her sense of competence.
3. Cognitive stimulation and reinforcement. Research has shown that the act of reminiscing can improve memory. As a supportive listener reflects back memories and asks questions, memories are reinforced.
4. Life review groups. Groups can become more than just reminiscence groups. With a skilled facilitator who can foster trust and

encourage group process, a group can develop that attempts to understand the significance of their memories and make meaning of their lives.

FACILITATING LIFE REVIEW

As stated earlier, life review is a natural process. It is not a "technique," but a developmentally important activity of the later years that can be facilitated by a psychotherapist or counselor. It is more important to understand its theoretic basis and therapeutic potential than to use a particular approach. Different styles may be effective for different clinicians. In the research project mentioned previously (Silver, 1982), the subjects were simply told that the listener wanted to hear their life stories. They could begin where they wanted to and should talk about what was important to them. This method does not always work, but there are other ways to encourage people to start talking about their memories.

Daniel Asnes, a geriatric psychiatrist, uses *Life Validation Techniques.* He learns about the period of history when the elderly patient lived and focuses on his or her place in the larger historic context. This approach helps elderly patients to increase their self-esteem and to make meaning of their lives, a part of the Eriksonian task of old age, achieving integrity as opposed to despair.

A variation of this approach, which is easily implemented with geriatric patients, is to show them headlines from old newspapers or books that illustrate historic events. A headline from their adolescence or early twenties is most effective. Then the psychotherapist, counselor, or other listener asks, "Do you remember this? You must have been about 16. What were you doing then?" Usually individuals will start talking about the event and how it impacted their lives or about other aspects of their life at that time. This helps stimulate their memories so that they start to review their lives.

Tape recording a person's memoirs is another approach to life review. For example, Hannah, an 81-year-old widow with severe memory impairment and little insight, was referred because of her disruptive behavior in a nursing home. The staff reported that she would wheel herself in her wheelchair to a spot near the entrance and stop visitors, then tell them what a terrible place the nursing home was.

Needless to say, this was upsetting to the staff and administration. An interview revealed that the disruptive behavior might be related to depression. (Anger and acting out toward caregivers is often a facet of depression in elderly persons.)

To begin treatment, Hannah was given an appointment book to keep track of her nursing home schedule. Since she had been a busy career woman, the appointment book helped her feel more in control and helped revive her image of herself as a successful career woman. Each week her appointment to tape her memoirs was written in the book. During her weekly life review appointment she talked about her memories, which were tape-recorded. Many of them focused on her career in real estate, and as she came to be more in touch with that successful past self, her self-esteem seemed to increase. After 5 or 6 weeks, there was a reduction in her disruptive behavior, and she appeared less depressed. She asked that the tapes be given to her daughter, and she was thrilled by the legacy that she could leave her family. The taping also provided her with cognitive stimulation, structure, and memory reinforcement, since in each session we reviewed the tape from the previous session.

Music can also be very helpful in getting people started. As the music plays, the counselor can ask questions like: How old were you when you listened to this song? Where were you? Who was important to you? Ethnic music can draw out people who originally came from other countries or other cultures. For example, Mrs. X, a 79-year-old woman who was born in Greece, would not talk to the counselor treating her depression for several weeks. It was not until the counselor played a tape of Greek music that she began to talk about her life. Similarly, books and magazines that remind people of their homelands or the places they lived when they were young can also stimulate memories.

Family photographs are an invaluable catalyst for life review. Psychotherapists or counselors can ask family members to bring in pictures, then look at them with the patient and ask questions to reminiscence. For example, Betty, a 67-year-old divorced participant in an adult day health program, was referred for psychotherapy for depression and somaticization. For the past four years, Betty had spent Christmas and her own birthday in the hospital with a variety of illnesses, including hypertensive episodes and pneumonia. She also suffered from severe psoriasis, a skin condition thought to be related to stress. Betty was delighted to share her memories with an empathetic listener, but after 4 or 5 weeks, she did not seem to be gaining any insight from her memories. Then one day she was asked to bring in family photographs. As she looked through the box, she suddenly held up a picture of a man and said, "There's the handsome so and so." It was her ex-husband, whom she had never mentioned. She began to talk about him, her anger at him, the pain of her divorce. From that time, she began to make real progress in therapy.

Genograms are another excellent tool for initiating life review. They can put people in touch with their generativity by documenting the descendants who give meaning to their lives. They also provide cognitive stimulation. Often individuals like to hang these on their wall, and they serve as a concrete reminder of the therapy and what the patient has gained.

Individuals who are more cognitively intact can be stimulated by talking about major life events or by reviewing turning points, transitions, or crossroads. What metaphor is used depends on what has meaning for that particular person. Creating a metaphoric framework for one's life story not only helps give it meaning, but the act of organizing and recalling provides cognitive stimulation.

CASE STUDY: LIFE REVIEW WITH A 77-YEAR-OLD MAN WITH COGNITIVE DEFICITS

Joe Green was a 77-year-old White male nursing home resident with a history of chronic alcoholism. He was referred for psychotherapy at the request of the charge nurse because of social isolation, demandingness, uncooperativeness, and possible depression.

The major problem that precipitated the referral was Joe's refusal to take medication from the charge nurse on his unit. This situation usually developed into a shouting match with the nurse and ended in a stand-off.

On neuropsychological examination, Joe demonstrated moderate short-term memory problems. His medical history was significant for congestive heart problems, peripheral neuropathy, arthritis, and hearing impairment. He was married with four children; his wife lived in a nursing home in a distant state, and they had no contact with each other. He had worked as an upholsterer and had owned his own business.

Treatment was approached from several different perspectives, including addressing the conflict with the nurse by applying family systems theory and focusing on the relationship between the nurse and Joe. The psychotherapist taught her some cognitive behavioral techniques and convinced her that she was reinforcing Joe's behavior by shouting at him when he was noncompliant. The attention, even though it was negative, served to increase Joe's uncooperative and confrontational behavior.

Joe's depression was approached in a different way. He was scheduled for weekly psychotherapy using a life review approach. The primary focus of Joe's life review was his accomplishment in starting his own successful small business. Out of this came not only an increase in his self-esteem but an opportunity to review with him the social skills he had used in business relationships and to discuss how to apply them to his relationships with the staff and other residents. He also talked about his alcoholism and his other faults with great regret. In telling about his pride in his children's accomplishments, however, he came to terms with some of his guilt and regret, deciding that he must have been in some ways a good father because his children had turned out so well.

Joe also reminisced about his relationships with women and how he had always been a ladies' man. Initially, he was very flirtatious with the psychotherapist. As she worked on setting limits and repeatedly defining the relationship of counselor and client to him, he acted more appropriately in the sessions. Joe at this time began to develop a good relationship with his daughter for the first time and said with great pride and some surprise that this was the first time that he was able to have a relationship with a woman that was not sexual. At this time he also began to get along better with female residents in the nursing home.

During Joe's 4 months of life review therapy, his self-esteem increased, and his depression decreased. With the decrease in depression, he became less irritable and therefore less demanding. Because of this and because he was able to draw on his formerly successful social skills, his relationships with his family and with nursing home staff and residents improved. This decreased his isolation, which further decreased his depression.

CONCLUSION

As the case of Joe illustrates, life review can be a very effective approach to therapy with elderly persons. Because it is a natural process that a psychotherapist or counselor can tap into, it is easier to overcome the resistance of an elderly person to whom the idea of psychotherapy may be quite foreign. When life review is allowed to unfold as a natural process in which elderly persons express what they wish at their own pace, it may be less threatening than more probing therapies. It may also allow the elderly persons' own psychological defenses to protect them from being overwhelmed by painful memories that exacerbate depression.

Finally, an individual does not have to be without cognitive impairment or capable of great insight to benefit from life review. Hannah and Joe, both of whom had some cognitive impairment, recalled past strengths and accomplishments on which they could draw to improve the quality of their lives and that made their lives seem meaningful and significant.

REFERENCES

Boylin, W., Gordon, S. K., & Nehrke, M. F. (1976). Reminiscing and ego integrity in institutionalized elderly males. *The Gerontologist, 16*, 118–124.

Butler, R. N. (1963). The life review: An interpretation of reminiscence in the aged. *Psychiatry, 26*, 65–76.

Erikson, E. H. (1950). *Childhood and society*. New York: Norton.

Erikson, E. H. (1976). Reflections on Dr. Borg's life cycle. *Daedulus, 105*, 1–27.

Fallot, R. D. (1979–1980). The impact of mood on of verbal reminiscing in later adulthood. *International Journal of Aging and Human Development, 10*, 385–400.

Gould, R. (1978). *Transformations*. New York: Simon & Schuster.

Haight, B. K. (1991). Reminiscing: The state of the art as a basis for practice. *International Journal of Aging and Human Development, 33*, 1–32.

Havighurst, R. J., & Glasser, R. (1972). An exploratory study of reminiscence. *Journal of Gerontology, 27*, 245–253.

Lewis, M. I., & Butler, R. N. (1974). Life review therapy: Putting memories to work in individual and group psychotherapy. *Geriatrics, 29*, 165–173.

Marshall, V. W. (1975). Age and awareness of finitude in developmental gerontology. *Omega, 6,* 113–129.

McMahon, A. W., & Rhudick, P. J. (1964). Reminiscing: Adaptional significance in the aged. *Archives of General Psychiatry, 10,* 294.

Pollock, G. H. (1978). Process and affect: Mourning and grief. *International Journal of Psychoanalysis, 59,* 255–276.

Silver, M. H. (1982). *Life review as a developmental process: Themes of caring, mourning, and integrity in life review therapy with low-income elderly women.* Ann Arbor, MI: University of Michigan Microfilms.

CHAPTER 3

Spirituality in Later Life

Myles N. Sheehan

This chapter raises many questions on spirituality in later life. What is spirituality? What is special about spirituality in later life? How does one define successful and productive aging in a spiritual context? It also raises questions of perspective. Who is defining spirituality for whom and who is defining aging in good health.

My perspective is that of a physician who specializes in geriatric medicine and who is also a Roman Catholic priest. Thus, spirituality and successful aging, as well as some of the challenges aging poses to a spiritual life will be interpreted within a Christian and Catholic viewpoint from someone whose experience of aging comes from contact with many older people who are facing enormous challenges to their lives as they age. The Catholic viewpoint of the chapter is not meant to devalue, denigrate, or exclude the myriad of other religious traditions or spiritualities: Far from it. Spirituality is not synonymous with religion, and there are many individuals without formal belief systems or participation in an organized religion who lead lives that are deeply spiritual. At the same time, approaching spirituality from an overly broad perspective can devalue the spiritual experience by ignoring the particular facets of a tradition that give meaning, depth, and richness. A spirituality within the Roman Catholic tradition can be a rich source to understand how spirituality provides a way to consider spirituality and aging.

Spirituality is a human experience in which we all face life in a way that is more than the sum of our physical reactions. It has a number of dimensions. For some, spirituality is a way in which a person feels part of something larger than her or his individuality. This something can be, depending on the individual, called God, or nature, or a sense of purpose. Spirituality also provides a way in which the individual can interpret the meaning and significance of life. When a person grapples with questions of understanding life choices or circumstances, wonders about what will happen with death and if there is anything beyond the grave, or attempts to integrate the good and bad experiences of a life to answer questions about the personal significance of one's own journey, then the individual is facing personal spiritual issues. Spirituality also is reflected in habits, rituals, gestures, and symbols that can help a person interpret and manage existence. Buckley, in considering different types of Christian spirituality, analyzes the components that make up Christian spirituality:

> Every Christian spirituality is a statement about (1) God, about (2) what it means to be a human being, and about (3) the way or the means or the journey by which the human is united with the divine . . . each of these three topics or variables will be given their value or assume their meaning by a complex of four interplaying influences. What is the *experience* out of which these values originate, the experiences critical to this spirituality? What is the *expression* through which these experiences are both shaped and articulated, the fundamental experiences reaching their own completion in their cognate expression? What is the *hermeneutics* or the *theology* through which this experience and its correlative expressions are explored and explained, the reflection which brings experience under concept? And finally, what are the ways, the *instrumentalities*, and the counsels by which this experience—expression—explanation are placed in communication, are made available to others? Without inquiry into these three variables and the four questions that disclose the process by which they are given their values, every spirituality can be reduced to cliches about the divine and the human and every unitive journey into a pastiche of acceptable aphorisms. Neither the *topics* of God, the hu-

man person, and the means toward unity nor the *questions* which deal with experience, expression, explanation, and communication form anything but a set that permits the discipline of spirituality to achieve some accuracy and depth of understanding. (Buckley, 1989)

In considering a spirituality of aging, Buckley's model focuses attention on the experience of aging, the expression of the aging experience, and a theology that would bring understanding to this experience and expression. Successful aging implies that the experience of aging can be good, it is an expression of aging as a positive experience, and it raises the question of what is the meaning of that *success* and its experience. In what follows, I will look carefully, from a Christian perspective, at what successful aging might mean and how that influences a spirituality of aging. The focus is on the underlying theology that brings understanding and expression to the experience.

"O God, you have taught me from my youth and till the present I proclaim your wondrous deeds; and now that I am old and gray, O God, forsake me not till I proclaim your strength to every generation that is to come" (Ps 71, 17–18). The author of Psalm 71 proclaims an optimistic view of aging. Old age is another thread in the fabric of the psalmist's life, a life that has been lived in faithfulness to God. Old age is a time to look to the future and to bring the past in contact with the future, proclaiming the experience of God's fidelity and wondrous deeds of liberation. Yet that is not the only voice in the Psalter that speaks of aging. Psalm 90 describes old age as the final chapter of a meaningless saga: "Seventy is the sum of our years, or eighty if we are strong, and most of them are fruitless toil for they pass quickly and we drift away" (Ps 90, 10). For the author of this psalm, old age is a time to drift away. There is no prayer for an ongoing relationship with God. There is no hope of transcendent experience to connect the past with the future. Is old age a time when God's presence can be experienced or is it a time of fading and doom? The clashing voices of these two psalms are heard in our current experience of aging.

This clash must be at the center of any reflection on the aging process. Gerontology, the study of aging in its biological, social, and psychological elements, has produced an abundance of data on the processes involved in aging, the experiences of older persons, and what it feels like to grow old. There is a striking resonance between the data of gerontology and the differing points of view of the two psalmists. Aging is a mix of good news and bad news, fulfillment and loss, hardship and satisfaction.

Although frequently neglected, reflection on human relationship with God is part of any adequate consideration of the experience of humanity. Gerontology, the scientific study of human aging can be broadened by considering theological questions of meaning and method. Discerning God's activity in aging and reflecting on how God is and is not present at the end of the life span is part of the work of theology. How does Christian faith influence our understanding of growing older? The fundamental aspects of Christian faith both question and are questioned by what we know about growing old. Our understanding of God, the meaning of salvation, the significance of Christ, and the mystery of the Cross are all elements that must be in dialogue with our knowledge of the aging process from biology, medicine, psychology, and the social sciences. Without this dialogue, theology becomes out of touch with experience and a field like gerontology withdraws from humanity. In learning about aging, traditional Christian symbols are seen as having meaning and response in the light of questions about aging. The symbols of faith objectify our understanding and provide a structure for interpreting the aging process. In even considering a topic like successful aging, we are engaged in asking new questions about aging. Our faith provides us with insights in how we can approach these questions and provide tentative answers. Christian faith provides the symbols to interpret human experience. That has been a continuous experience since the death and resurrection of Jesus were proclaimed by Peter on Pentecost (Acts 2:14–41). If the faith cannot provide the substance for interpreting the human experience of aging at the threshold of the twenty-first century then the interpreters are faithless or the faith is false.

Geriatric medicine considers illnesses and syndromes. It deals with decline, struggles for independence, and death. Although the variability of aging and the potential for reversible illness has been emphasized, morbidity and death come for all. Behind the demographics about independence, age span, and an expanding elderly population there remain ghosts of dependence, death, and old persons leading lives, in the words of Psalm 90, filled with "fruitless toil" before they "drift away." Focusing on the problems of older people, however, may make aging appear bereft of opportunities for new life after youth and middle age are done. Betty Friedan describes what possibilities and hope can be discovered in age:

> I think it is time we start searching for the fountain of age, time that we stop denying our growing older and look at the actuality of our own experience, and that of other women and men who have gone beyond denial to a new place in their sixties, seventies, eighties. It is time to look at age on its own terms, and put names on its values and strengths as they are actually experienced, breaking through the definition of age solely as deterioration or decline from youth. Only then will we see that the problem is not age itself, to be denied or warded off as long as possible, that the problem is not those increasing numbers of people living beyond 65, to be segregated from the useful, valuable, pleasurable activities of society so that the rest of us can keep our illusion of staying forever young. Nor is the basic political problem the burden on society of those forced into deterioration, second childhood, even senility. The problem is not how we can stay young forever, personally, or avoid facing society's problems politically by shifting them onto age. The problem is, first of all, how to break through the cocoon of our illusory youth and risk a new stage in life, where there are no prescribed role models to follow, no guideposts, no rigid rules or visible rewards, to step out into the true existential unknown of these new years of life now open to us, and to find our own terms for living it. (Friedan, 1993)

Friedan is eloquent in voicing the need to move to new models of aging. She looks to understand aging not on the basis of old paradigms but as experienced by those who find new life as they age. They live not by the standards of youth or middle age but in a way unique to older age: rich, gratifying, and filled with personal growth. The problem is that the "true existential unknown of these new years of life" may frustrate dreams and bring times of pain. Friedan acknowledges the problem of trying to find, as we age, "our own terms for living it." Aging on one's own terms can be lifegiving if one rejects the terms imposed by a society obsessed by youth. The great difficulty is determining what it means to age on one's own terms in the face of decline, illness, and death.

Friedan is critical of gerontology's preoccupation with disease and disability. She rightly notes that such a fixation creates an expectation that growing old means growing sick. The kind of information usually considered worthy of study by geriatrics and gerontology are topics like dementia, nursing home care, medication use, and syndromes like incontinence and falls. Friedan emphasizes opportunities for new careers, interests, and relationships. One wonders, however, what happens to those who are old, sick, and suffering when aging is looked at as a time for new life and new opportunity?

Any discussion of aging that evades the negativity of the aging process is illusory and misleading. Nicholas Lash, a contemporary English theologian, describes the responsibility of the theologian, a responsibility shared by all Christians "for continually attempting to grasp the 'heart of the matter,' to concentrate attention on the single mystery of God and his grace. And the heart of the matter is that all theological construction, all positive expression of faith in God, which cannot stand the strain of exposure to negativity, is suspect of illusion" (Lash, 1986). Considering the topic of gerontology from the perspective of theology requires both a firm look at the negative aspect of aging as well as a willingness to grasp what Lash calls the " 'heart of the matter,' the single mystery of God and his grace."

Aging is not all negativity. As Friedan points out, it is a time for new possibilities and untapped potential. Old age can be a time of peace, comfort, growth, and satisfaction. Ignoring this reality risks accepting ageist assumptions that elderly persons are all ill, demented, feeble, and a drain on society. But aging marks a limit in the experience of being human. Death comes for all and this limit to our life span serves as a marker that makes aging different than the other periods of human life. Aging may well be a time of extreme negativity. Lash describes this negativity as "experience of mortality, of loneliness and the loss of meaning; of all forms of physical and mental suffering and of the recognition of the sheer finitude, impermanence and ambiguity of all particular human achievement" (Lash, 1986). But both the Christian believer and the gerontologist would object to characterizing aging solely as negativity, letting death be the final word on this stage of the human journey. Death, however, from both the theological and gerontological perspective, remains a frightening end to life. Yet, in faith, those who call themselves Christian must agree with Lash that aging and its terminus remains a place to grasp the heart of the matter, the mystery of God's grace. As Lash says, "This is, I think, a terrifying suggestion. But it does at least seem consonant with the claim that the transformative power of the creator spiritus is at work—not 'even' here, but above all here, in particularity and tragedy. I do not see what belief in the incarnation of the Word, in the divinity of the crucified, can mean if it does not mean this" (Lash, 1986).

Neglecting the negativity leaves us out of the experience of those who do not age successfully. It also can leave us blind to the possibility of God's involvement in the particular tragedies that are part of the aging of many individuals. Tracy Kidder, in a book on life in a nursing home, comments: "Ideal aging—these days known as 'successful aging,' often depicted in photographs of old folks wearing tennis clothes—leaves out a lot of people. It is estimated that nearly half of all the Americans who make it past 65 will spend more time in a nursing home. The celebration of successful aging leaves out all of them. Ultimately, of course it leaves out everyone" (Kidder, 1993). Thus aging in good health and spirituality in a Christian context includes all older people, regardless of whether they are vigorous and active or depressed and frightened. The story of how an older person tries to relate to God in the events of life is a spiritual one; its success is not measured by external markers but by the ability of the relationship to sustain the individual as they age and face death.

A major theme in the history of the Church has been who is left out and who is let in. The early Church struggled with what to do with gentiles. The Church of the first centuries argued about what to do with those who sinned and those who had lapsed in time of persecution. The Church during the Reformation split over who could belong to the Church and who constituted the Church. Leaving people out of the experience of the Church has always been a serious matter. In recent years, attention has focused on the lack of serious consideration of the experience of women. As Schussler-Fiorenza points out in her book, *In Memory of Her*, the story of the woman who anointed Jesus before his death had long been ignored (Schussler-Fiorenza, 1983). Women's experiences do not count in a paradigm where women are ignored. The experience of suffering elderly persons does not count in a paradigm that emphasizes success, achievement, and youth. Forgetting the voices of women has lessened the experience of the Church. Likewise, leaving out the stories of negativity that are also part of aging leaves out three crucial items: the experience of those older persons who suffer, Christian responsibility to suffering elderly persons, and the presence of God in these elderly persons.

A church that worships one who was crucified cannot avoid the experience of suffering that is often the lot of elderly persons. Tragedy is a dimension of aging. Christian faith recognizes the dimension of tragedy within the paschal mystery. Orthodox Christian faith condemned the docetist heresy: Christ only appeared to die a human death on the cross. Just as the docetists were scandalized by human suffering, the trend in our culture is to pretend that tragedy does not exist:

> The reason why . . . [we] should think about tragic pain is because, as a culture, we are rapidly losing an understanding of tragedy—which means that we are losing one important way of thinking about human life. It is easy today to regard tragedy as merely a vanished literary form: an oversized fossil, like epic. It is quite possible . . . that the ruling systems of thought in our time are inherently antitragic, in the sense that, like medicine, they draw strength from the vision of continuing progress toward a utopian future. As a culture we do not take kindly to the tragic vision. We tacitly reject it, even as medicine almost blindly resists the biological fact of death, strapping terribly damaged, infirm, or unconscious bodies onto machines that pump the blood and keep the cells alive until it takes a court order to allow death to reenter the world. Yet tragedy, as Emerson wrote, is all around us. The problem is not that tragedy has vanished or become impossible. It is worse than that. We no longer recognize tragedy when we encounter it. Richard Selzer wrote that to perceive events as tragic is to wring from them beauty and truth. The corollary is also true: not to perceive tragedy . . . is to wring from it next to nothing. We simply gaze with a numbed fascination at a meaningless set of actions we cannot comprehend, then shift our attention elsewhere. (Morris, 1991)

As Christians, the cross is a transcendent symbol of suffering that cuts across generations. It also provides a remarkable commentary on what success means in the context of Christian spirituality. Jesus died a young man, but his death provides a focus for the experience of elderly persons. Dorothy Soelle writes: "To meditate on the cross means to say good-bye to the narcissistic hope of being free of sickness, deformity, and death. Then all the energies wasted on such hopes could become free to answer the call for the battle against suffering" (Soelle, 1975). Taking seriously the experiences of pain and suffering that affect people as they age does not mean, from either a gerontological or a theological perspective, a lugubrious fascination with pain and tragedy that borders on sadomasochism. It does mean that the experience of illness, loneliness, dementia, and impending death is seen as part of the human story that all people of all ages should attend to. Soelle questions contemporary society's inability to pay attention to suffering:

> One wonders what will become of a society in which certain forms of suffering are avoided gratuitously, in keeping with middle-class ideals. I have in mind a society . . . in which . . . relationships between generations are dissolved as quickly as possible, without a struggle, without a trace. Such blindness is possible in a society in which banal optimism prevails, in which it is self-evident that suffering doesn't occur. (Soelle, 1975)

Paying attention to the totality of the experience of aging avoids a fixation on physical ability, independence, economic comfort and security and, in its place, emphasizes the reality of human experience. Such attention to elderly persons carries with it the germs of revolution. Simone de Beauvoir comments about aging:

> Old age exposes the failure of our entire civilization. It is the whole man that must be remade. It is the whole relationship between man and man that must be recast if we wish the old person's state to be acceptable. A man should not start his last years alone and empty-handed. Society cares about the individual only in so far as he is profitable. Once we have understood what the state of the aged really is, we cannot satisfy ourselves with calling for a more generous 'old-age policy', higher pensions, decent housing and organized leisure. It is the whole system that is at issue and our claim cannot be otherwise than radical change in life itself. (De Beauvoir, 1973)

Changing life is a daunting goal. Yet one of the claims of Christianity is that the power of God can change societies and structures. A spirituality of aging must encompass a theology of suffering and a true theology of liberation:

A true acceptance of suffering is never a self-sufficiency which would be at peace and satisfied already now in the devil's inn. The acceptance of suffering by giving oneself over to it rather than facing it with tranquillity arises out of a different relationship to the future. The God who says, "Behold, I make all things new" (Rev 21:5), cannot himself exist now without suffering over what is old. What is promised is not only a restoration of elemental goodness after the storm of power, but the abolition of all power by which some men dominate others, all anguish. This is why, in the Christian understanding of suffering, mysticism and revolution move so close to one another. (Soelle, 1975)

The transformative power of God present in negativity and tragedy is not reserved solely for those who are the subject of pain and suffering. Looking at the struggles of aging as only the problems of those who age evades the potential for all people to be transformed. Loneliness, poverty, poor medical care, and unnoticed suffering need not be the fate of many individuals at the end of their lives.

Karl Rahner, in describing Christian hope regarding the future, comments that "What we know about Christian eschatology is what we know about man's present situation in the history of salvation. We do not project something from the future into the present, but rather in man's experience of himself and of God in grace and in Christ we project our Christian present into its future" (Rahner, 1978). Aging is the future of all persons. It is rapidly becoming a future for American society. Are there human experiences of aging that we can identify at this time that recognize "God in grace and in Christ?"

Contemplating aging in the light of faith provides a richness of images. These images need to be supplemented not with the comments of academic gerontologists and theologians, but by the experience of people who are old and who live their lives in faith. With this caution as a background, three types of experience can be considered.

First, there are some of the experiences emphasized by Betty Friedan. An older woman discovers new resources and finds aging a new time in her life. She is able, in the words of Friedan, "to risk a new stage in life, where there are no prescribed role models to follow, no guideposts, no rigid rules or visible rewards, to step out into the true existential unknown of these new years of life" (Friedan, 1993). One need not look for an explicitly Christian experience to see in the kind of adventurous living that Friedan describes a willingness to accept life as good and the world as a place where life triumphs over death.

Second, reflect on the examples of excellent care given to older persons who have not aged successfully from a physical or cognitive perspective. I was struck one day, while working at a nursing home, to find an elderly Jewish woman with advanced Alzheimer's disease whose hair had been neatly braided into cornrows. The silver blue of her wispy hair usually was in some sort of cloud-like style, floating about her head. The aides who cared for this woman were mainly young women from the Caribbean. The love shown in the gesture of styling this woman's hair sounded clear and sweet, even above the dissonance of an old Jewish lady with a hairdo more commonly seen in women of African heritage. Love and care are possible between generations, races, and cultures. The power of God can be seen in a relationship where a young Black woman cares for an old Jewish woman with love and affection, especially when the older woman is totally helpless and unable to respond with more than a smile.

Third, contemplate the death of an older person. Is this a time when God is not present? Does Christian revelation no longer have anything to say about death? Or does death reveal an encounter with mystery? Individuals who worship a human crucified on a cross as a central theme in the story of God's relationship with humanity must recognize the presence of God in Christ, even, or, perhaps, especially in a death where the person is alone and has received inadequate care.

These three experiences are not meant as constituting the whole of experience. There is no omniscient, universal view of aging. Gerontology emphasizes diversity. Aging is a time for new life when younger persons may see only decline. Decline and death remain realities for all. Too much of aging is filled with suffering brought about by social structures and paradigms that care little about human persons. But the God found in Christ can be found in all of these snapshots of aging, not in a glorification of suffering, but in a human experience of life, reflection, and compassion. The challenges for older persons are numerous. The hope is that they experience conditions where they can echo the voice of the psalmist of Psalm 71 who continues to "proclaim God's wondrous deeds." In the context of Psalm 71, the wondrous deeds of God refer to Israel's liberation from slavery and the creation of a new people in a new land. For younger persons, the challenge of aging is to participate in the experience of liberation. First, by treating older persons as persons and not as relics either destined for the scrap heap or venerated as antiques. Second, and for the purposes of this essay, is to cooperate with God's creative Spirit. Aging and the suffering that is often a part of it is not a time to retreat into what Soelle calls "theological sadomasochism." The death of an older person who has received inadequate care and whose passing seems unnoticed requires a reaction not of simpering piety about God's presence. Rather, in recognizing God's solidarity with the elderly person's suffering, a Christian will accept that God's choice to be human, suffering, and frail requires a response that is no less magnanimous. The old, the poor, the sick, the unwanted are all places of encounter with God. Our task is to respond in ways that alleviate suffering, loneliness, and discrimination. A spirituality of aging that is successful looks not only to those who play tennis when they are old, but to those who can find in their experience of aging, positive and negative, meaning and a relationship with God. Successful aging and spirituality is not simply a private affair for the aging individual. It requires, from a Christian perspective, the engagement of others to care for those who are failing so that they may experience the nearness of God as their life ends.

REFERENCES

Buckley, M. J. (1989). Seventeenth-century French spirituality: Three figures. In L. Dupre & D. E. Saliers (Eds.), *Christian spirituality: Post-reformation and modern* (pp. 28–68). New York: Crossroad.

De Beauvoir, S. (1973). *The coming of age*. New York: Warner Paperback Library.

Friedan B. (1993). *The fountain of age*. New York: Simon and Schuster.

Kidder, T. (1993). *Old friends*. Boston: Houghton Mifflin.

Lash, N. (1986). *Theology on the way to emmaus*. London: SCM Press.

Morris, D. B. (1991). *The culture of pain.* Berkeley, CA: University of California Press.

Rahner, K. (1978). *Foundations of Christian faith.* New York: Seabury.

Schussler-Fiorenza, E. (1983). *In memory of her.* New York: Crossroad.

Soelle, D. (1975). *Suffering.* Philadelphia: Fortress Press.

CHAPTER 4

Emotional Health and Socioeconomic Stress

Lauren E. Storck

> Blow, winds, and crack your cheeks! Rage! Blow!
>
> Depression is so mysteriously painful and elusive as to verge close to being beyond description.
>
> It is like a squeezing powerful pain in my chest that never goes away and I can't stand the pain. Don't waste your time on me. I try to hurt myself with other pain, just to get some relief from the first pain.

D epression is a depressing topic whether it be found in medicine, psychology, great literature, or everyday life, and it can be devastatingly more oppressive for older people. The selection of quotations above from (1) King Lear (Shakespeare, 1608, Act III, Scene II), (2) a poetically written personal account of depression by a well-known writer (Styron, 1990), or (3) a simpler and brutally honest patient journal (2000), will teach anyone who is interested in depression and aging that depression takes many forms and can range, in its most difficult stages, from raging self-hatred to excruciating emotional pain.

Depression, in spite of being the second most prevalent illness of all physical and emotional disorders in the general population, second only to cardiovascular disease, is still significantly confusing and difficult to believe in, for a good number of people from all walks of life. Although it accounts for death, loss of work, ruined relationships, violence, and less obvious suffering in many forms, the illness of depression is underdiagnosed and undertreated, especially for elderly people (Alexopoulos, 1997; Gallo & Lebowitz, 1999; Gurland, Cross, & Katz, 1996; U.S. Department of Health and Human Services, 1999).

For the elderly person and the family, onset of depression in late life is doubly difficult to fathom, sometimes buried within multiple physical signs and complaints of aging. However, using a psychological perspective, it is useful to remember that new psychological challenges during aging can be stressful and confusing in the best of circumstances and for healthy individuals too.

A psychological perspective includes dividing aging challenges into their behavioral, cognitive, and emotional components. For example, some new behaviors will help one to adjust to alterations in sensory and motor systems, such as learning to use different reading or walking aides. Other behaviors such as shopping and cooking may require some adjustments and energy saving steps. Cognitively, planning for the future and thinking about how to make it satisfying and comfortable is a major psychological challenge. New learning and patience are required to deal with new medical insurance and other technologies. Emotionally, one can reasonably expect, for example, some physical disease in oneself or one's spouse that will temporarily interfere with everyday routines and be stressful, for a while, or periodically. There will be sorrow and grief when there are losses of friends and relations due to disabilities, relocations, or deaths. In addition, it is likely that some family entanglements and misunderstandings from the past will resurface, adding confusion, and emotional strain. Finally, the awareness that life will be limited and the acceptance of the fact that some form of help will be required, in the form of either physical, financial, social, or emotional assistance, can be emotionally frustrating and upsetting, unless balanced by the knowledge that people want to help and one will be remembered. These profound psychological events affect all aging people and are not, in themselves, the illness called depression.

DEPRESSION DEFINED

For the elderly person, however, these many adjustments can mask or be confused with depression, and more worrying, for the elderly person who suffers from undiagnosed and untreated depression, these normal psychological challenges can exacerbate depressive illness, be it major clinical depression, minor depression with a range of depressive symptoms, or a third type of depression, sometimes called double depression. Double depression is the unfortunate combination of a major depressive episode, or repeated episodes, on top of underlying depressive symptoms (Wells, Sturm, Sherbourne, & Meredith, 1996). Furthermore, since underlying and undiagnosed depressive illness may have gone undetected for many adult years, the elder person who experiences depression requires careful and thorough evaluation of all emotional and physical symptoms and complaints.

For older people, there is often little experience with any psychological science, and it is also understandable that any possibility of "mental" problems after a long and productive life would feel insulting or be embarrassing. Yet depressive illness exists, and it needs better detection and treatment, especially for growing numbers of aging people. If depression, often accompanied by an anxiety problem, is not treated promptly and appropriately, the health and life of the elder person is at serious risk (U.S. Department of Health and Human Services, 1999).

Although the prevalence of major depression is reported to be lower in late life than it is in midlife, the prevalence of depressive symptoms in elderly persons remains worrisome and high (Hagnell, Lanke, Rorseman, & Ojesjo, 1982), especially for women who suffer at twice the rate of men (Eaton et al., 1989; Weissman et al., 1988). For example, among several separate community-based studies of older adults, one study found that 15% of older adults report "significant dysphoria" (Blazer & Williams, 1980). Another report stated that 27% of their large sample of older adults reported depressive symptoms, with 8% suffering from clinically significant depressive symptoms that were associated predominantly with physical problems (Blazer, Hughes, & George, 1987). Another study found that up to 35% of older primary care patients reported depressive symptoms (Gurland et al., 1996).

These percentages represent very large absolute numbers of people suffering from depression that interferes with a satisfying daily life. Furthermore, depression may also alter the body's physical or biological pathways in some manner that leads to greater likelihood of somatic illness (U.S. Department of Health and Human Services, 1999). There is little doubt that depressive illness, by itself or combined with other behavioral or physical illness, is an important and growing health concern as our elderly populations increase in numbers.

Other prevalence studies demonstrate that depression affects about 25% of all elderly people with chronic illness, especially patients with heart disease, stroke, cancer, lung disease, arthritis, Alzheimer's disease, and Parkinson's disease (Borson, 1995). These often chronic and disabling illnesses are common enough in late life without the added burden of depression.

Interestingly, suicide rates are positively correlated with age in spite of the fact that the incidence of major depression decreases with age. This correlation is largely due to higher suicide rates among White men over age 60 in most Western cultures (Blazer, 1999). This highlights at least two important issues for further investigation: (a) suicide may be underreported in many groups of elders for many different reasons (e.g., religious customs, accident reports rather than suicide attributions, and so on); and (b) minor depression or a combination of depressive symptoms and certain other life events may contribute in significant ways to suicide or shortened life in many groups of elderly people, not only in adult White males.

Depression (a major or clinical depression) is defined in the American Psychiatric Association's *Diagnostic and Statistical Manual of Mental Disorders,* 4th Edition (*DSM-IV*), as a depressed mood with or without loss of interest or pleasure (in one's usual activities, relationships, pursuits), plus four of the following (three if *both* depressed mood and loss of interest or pleasure are present):

Weight loss or weight gain
Insomnia or hypersomnia
Psychomotor agitation or retardation
Fatigue or loss of energy
Feelings of worthlessness or guilt

Difficulty concentrating
Recurrent thoughts of death or suicidal ideation*

TREATMENT

Major depression in any person, and when it is recognized in an elderly patient, requires appropriate treatment as soon as possible. This is usually medication or a combination of medications to prevent further deterioration of mood. Although most medical textbooks concentrate on these important physiological interventions (and sometimes recommend further somatic treatments such as electroconvulsive therapy if medications do not alleviate the suffering), it is often wise to include some counseling along with biological treatments. At a minimum, supportive, educational, and sympathetic instructions, on a regular basis, for medication compliance should be included in treatment planning. If possible, the family who is available and interested in helping should be included as well, on a regular basis (Blazer, 1999). Depression is a confusing and difficult illness for a family to understand, and family support is one of the priceless and most effective treatments available for sufferers of depression (Styron, 1990). Hospitalization is sometimes required as well, and it is often more comforting than not to the very depressed patient who realizes that hospital safety, structure, and medications may be lifesavers.

Of equal concern are the debilitating and unhealthy consequences of minor depression which encompass a broad range of symptoms and complaints including those listed above, as well as other categories of illness such as adjustment disorders (prolonged bereavement), excessive sadness, agitated behaviors, frequent somatic complaints, and hypomanic-type behaviors, for example, increased spending or unwarranted suspiciousness (Blazer, 1999). These depressive symptoms, a few or many, often subtly accumulate over two

---

*(These lists are modified from Blazer, D.G. (1999). Depression. In W. R. Hazzard, J. P. Blass, W. H. Ettinger, J. B. Halter, & J. G. Ouslander (Eds.), *Principles of Geriatric Medicine and Gerontology* (4th ed.) (pp. 1331–1340). New York: McGraw-Hill, and are adaptations from the American Psychiatric Association (1994), *Diagnostic and Statistical Manual of Mental Disorders* (4th ed.), Washington DC: Author.) Reprinted with permission of McGraw-Hill.

or more years, and are frequently not recognized early enough. Additional symptoms may include irritability, apathy, cognitive difficulties, and other sleep disturbances. Depression is often comorbid with physical disease, each independently making the other worse. To thoroughly assess and select treatments for any depressive illness in late life, the practitioner requires knowledge across the following categories:

Mood disorders (major depression as above, a single episode or recurrent);

Adjustment disorders (adjustment disorder with depressed mood, uncomplicated bereavement);

Organic mood disorders (primary degenerative dementia with associated major depression; organic mood disorder, depressed; secondary to physical illness, e.g., hypothyroidism, stroke, carcinoma of the pancreas; secondary to pharmacologic agents, e.g., methyldopa, propranolol);

Psychoactive substance-use disorders (alcohol abuse and/or dependence; sedative, hypnotic, or anxiolytic abuse and/or dependence);

Somatoform disorders (hypochondriasis, somatization disorder).*

Clearly, the differential diagnosis of depressive symptoms in late life, according to DSM-IV, requires careful and thorough evaluation by a highly trained and experienced practitioner in order to select the proper treatment, or in many cases, the best combination of treatments. Left untreated, depression leads to further illness, disability, and dysfunction, including, at times, expensive institutional care or mortality.

ADAPT—AGING, DEPRESSION, ANXIETY, PRIDE, 'TIL WE MEET AGAIN: A CASE STUDY

Ms. N. H. finally telephoned. Her adult son had spoken with a good friend who was a professional and lived distantly, also far away from my own locale. This professional had called me many months previously, inquiring if I could be available to see his friend's mother.

It required efforts to confer, including voicemail and messages exchanged. When I reached him, he was on a car phone.

I include these details to emphasize that we are all busy people, including the patient, each in our own manner, and it takes vigor, modern communications, a certain amount of financial comfort, as well as experience in social networking to set up a first appointment, especially for the older person. The senior is more reluctant to telephone himself or herself. Oftentimes, it is adult children who want to help. Most of us want to provide the best professional effort we can, although we constantly wish it were easier for patients to find us, and that we were better supported by medical, business, and government understanding of the value and efficacy of mental health services in addition to somatic medicine.

She did not call for several months, but she did call. This too is typical of many elderly people, wanting to take their own time and make their own decisions, even when the depression or anxiety makes that process itself problematic. Depressed mood interferes with recognizing the depression, muddles precise thinking and decision making, and threatens self-esteem when self-critical thoughts are already present, such as "what have I done wrong?"

In addition, many elderly people do not believe in psychological therapy at all. The benefits of talking with a stranger about private suffering or revealing personal and family issues that have become too stressful, is preconceived as similar to talking with friends, or experienced as a potential betrayal to the family. When the distress of depression becomes too painful, however, or with repeated suggestions from family, the elderly adult may be encouraged to "be bold and give it a try."

When we met, she was composed, depressed, well-spoken, and reluctant to share details with a stranger. She was also doubtful that treatment for her discomfort would help, since she had tried counseling previously with little effect, she said, when her husband suddenly died a few years previously. However, as we introduced ourselves to each other and I assessed the state and seriousness of her depression, she relaxed just enough to share her grief, her loneliness, her financial fears, and the despair behind her eyes. She made another appointment.

Many patients appear to be rather "normal" to the inexperienced or impatient gaze. They are composed, do not necessarily look worried, and do not readily share their serious symptoms. Even patients with major or clinical depression, in the aging years, may behave and communicate with practiced aplomb, irrespective of their formal education or internal distress, until sufficient time is spent in building trust and assessing moods, behaviors, and thoughts.

Being widowed, in spite of apparent financial comforts in the past, the patient was left with few assets. A legally complicated situation and other family matters left her struggling to decide where to live and necessitated that she be employed even at her current age of 67. She was betwixt and between many things, we agreed, between jobs, without her best and only husband, far away from her three adult children, each with their own personal or health worries, she said. She was also far removed from her place of birth and from some friends, although she had a few friends close enough. She also had spiritual faith and belonged to a congregation, but found no solace there currently. Her actual landlady, with whom she thought she had developed an authentic new friendship, had just announced that she was selling the apartment and her tenant, the patient, would have to find something else fairly quickly.

This patient was perhaps lucky because she had no serious health problems herself, she said, not being comfortable with the idea that depression or anxiety was a real health problem. With many other older patients who still have spouses or family nearby, even under the same roof, there are frequently obvious and chronic health issues to deal with everyday. Serious physical, behavioral, and emotional concerns include, for example, cardiovascular illness, diabetes, arthritis, cancer, mental illness, caregiving duties for multiple relatives or children and grandchildren in addition to self and spouse, sensory and motor losses such as visual or hearing deficits which make communication very difficult and stressful, increasing minor or major memory lapses or confusions, due to identified or unidentified neurophysiological deficits. For the patient here, none of these issues were apparent, "merely" the depression and anxiety disorders, the real health issues for her, including exaggerated but real loneliness and terror of financial ruin.

I am combining real facts from about four different patients here in order to protect their privacy. If the reader feels that this person is someone he or she knows, I can assure you that this sketch is a composite. I can also be quite sure that most readers will already know someone in similar circumstances.

This patient was "lucky" in another way—she was well educated and had been able to include many enriching lifetime experiences. As part of a couple, she had been able to afford many pleasures, including travel, healthy food, good healthcare, safe neighborhoods, and access to information and good social supports. As a young mother, she had raised her children with the emotional and financial support of her husband, family, and friends. These experiences, bolstered by socioeconomic advantage, helped her build self-esteem and self-confidence.

After three meetings, she felt stronger and more confident. She declined further sessions for now, started a more satisfying job, and said she would telephone in the future if necessary. Not hearing from her for a few months, I followed up with two brief telephone calls, inviting her to let me know how she was feeling, and asking whether she wanted another appointment. No further intervention was needed.

Oftentimes, a few supportive and psychoeducational sessions will be sufficient to allow the older person to find new hope and turn more productively to available inner resources as well as available family and friends.

ANOTHER SCENARIO: SOCIOECONOMIC STRESS SYNDROME AND DEPRESSION

For most elderly people, income and financial security are reduced, sometimes dramatically, especially for widows. This economic reality provokes reasonable anxiety and worry, sometimes escalating to significant nervousness and less than optimal spending and planning. Many elderly people have also managed with less social and economic advantages throughout their lives, and this section describes a different scenario of depression, a situation that, unfortunately, affects more elderly with fewer resources.

Using a second case example, a socioeconomic stress syndrome, or *SESS*, is introduced (Storck, 1998; Storck, 1999) as a way to explore possible links between depression and socioeconomic realities. SESS is a new theoretical approach to understand better the complex interactions between psychological distress, including depression, and medical illness, and also to design new psychomedical interventions to alleviate illness and suffering. Formulations of SESS are based on recent qualitative studies carried out by the author from clinical interviews (Storck, 1999), as well as additional analyses (post-hoc) of in-depth interviews of caregivers of Alzheimer's patients (Hinton, Fox, & Levkoff, 1999) from a large study on aging in several cultural groups.

IS THERE HOPE?—A CASE STUDY OF A WOMAN WHO ENDURES

Esperanza swam for her life. She survived stormy weather to reach safe haven across a shore. The place she left was rife with poverty and abuse, too oppressive for someone of her curiosity and courage. The youngest of nine children, she worked hard to survive, working day and night, without exaggeration, eventually serving a husband who developed serious cancer and cardiovascular complications. Nurturing her own children, she suffered more frequent bouts of depression and migraine, in addition to serious gastrointestinal illness.

This story too is a composite of real case histories, combining facts from several patients seen in psychological and medical treatments over the past few years. Again, if you feel like you know who this person is, be assured she is not the person you know, for she is either from Asia, South America, Africa, the Caribbean, other islands, or from a distant European country. She is from the United States too, from a river or mountain region, or from an urban or suburban neighborhood where working class or disadvantaged families struggle to pay the rent and ignore racial, class, or religious insults and injuries, verbal or physical barriers to growth and health.

Importantly, her family and class values may be very different from commonly accepted values in other families. For example, family loyalty is considered a most precious commodity, of higher value than career mobility or money. Expression of emotions and sharing community dinners are considered to be of higher value than working extra time and passing examinations in school, especially when her people are often silenced in job interviews, passed over for promotions, or unrecognized for efforts in spite of hours, sweat, sacrifice, and determination to get ahead.

Esperanza came into the clinic as a free-care patient. Fortunately, her mental health team spoke her language. She was able to form a trusting bond with her psychologist, although he was a doctoral trainee. This city system still had enough resources to offer intensive supervision to the trainee and extensive services to the patient. These included necessary medical examinations and treatments, knowledgeable social services for employment and housing, as well as regular individual and group supportive psychotherapy that included cognitive and psychodynamic understanding, as well as collaborative dialogue. Esperanza was able to begin to heal the wounds from years of suffering.

At this time in her life, she was no longer being abused by her husband or his family, no longer being called "stupid" by her deceased parents, and no longer feeling required to lie to others or deceive herself about her own skills and competence as a human being, woman, mother, and employable intelligent person.

Esperanza's family and class values differ from many professional expectations and assumptions. For example, her desire for further education was postponed to pay the rent. Her inclination to use half a tablet of medication was sensible in order to save money for food. Her missing a medical appointment was due to lack of carfare plus a family argument at home. Her values and loyalty to family, including elders in her neighborhood, took precedence over her own physical and emotional needs.

Socioeconomic conditions, especially when continual or chronic, interfere with health and life, as most people readily understand. What is further damaging to health, is when traumatic socioeconomic stress and experiences cannot be verbalized or examined with understanding, and then socioeconomic stress itself becomes the illness, probably via some form of psychological dissociation (Storck, 1999).

Class divisions and class experiences are not easily talked about in a culture that is supposed to be class-free. Socioeconomic insults, for example being called "White trash," or daily economic stress such as postponing utility bills to buy food or books, are emotionally painful and injurious, leading to depressive symptoms if not to major clinical depression, especially for many women, including elderly women and their adult children.

Elderly citizens from all socioeconomic strata face longer life and related financial considerations. It is suggested that a socioeconomic stress syndrome inhibits healing from depression and comorbid disease categories, until it is recognized and addressed in a healing dialogue (Storck, 1999).

It is not suggested that the physician can alleviate social and political problems in any direct way. It is argued that the practitioner can take time to validate economic stress where it exists, recognize a socioeconomic stress syndrome, and then make an informed choice about prescribing mental health or psychoeducational services when needed (Storck, 1999). With educated and focused psychological and psychosocial supports, the patient can heal from SESS and more serious depressions may be prevented (Storck, 1999).

This is not to suggest either that all clinical depression or depressive illness is due to SESS alone, or to similar syndromes. But when economic concerns and class divisions within society affect many elderly people in our communities, especially women, we are obligated to seek ways to understand better and discuss socioeconomic stress in medical and psychological interviews. How to do this with professional empathy, without embarrassing patients, and how to provide mental health services that address these specific issues in order to alleviate SESS and depression remain as crucial issues to be investigated further.

CONCLUSION

Clinical depression and depressive symptoms which appear in a variety of emotional, cognitive, and behavioral manifestations are serious and underdiagnosed health concerns for all of us, especially for the elderly population. In addition, it is proposed that a socioeconomic stress syndrome also interacts with health and disease, and that this syndrome includes many forms of depression, and can contribute to prevention, assessment and treatment.

If recognized, thoroughly evaluated, and treated by one or by a judicious combination of pharmacological, psychological, and social supports, many forms of depression can abate and suffering can be reduced substantially. Good treatments are available, and new formulations will make good health more possible than ever.

REFERENCES

Alexopoulos, G. S. (1997). Epidemiology, nosology, and treatment of geriatric depression. Paper presented at Exploring Opportunities to Advance Mental Health Care for an Aging Population. Meeting sponsored by the John A. Hartford Foundation. Rockville, MD.

American Psychiatric Association (1994). *Diagnostic and Statistical Manual of Mental Disorders* (4th ed.). Washington, DC: Author.

Blazer, D. G. (1999). Depression. In W. R. Hazzard, J. P. Blass, W. H. Ettinger, J. B. Halter, & J. G. Ouslander (Eds.), *Principles of geriatric medicine and gerontology* (4th ed.) (pp. 1331–1340). New York: McGraw-Hill.

Blazer, D. G., & Williams, C. D. (1980). Epidemiology of dysphoria and depression in an elderly population. *American Journal of Psychiatry, 137*, 439.

Blazer, D. G., Hughes, D. C., & George, L. K. (1987). The epidemiology of depression in an elderly community population. *The Gerontologist, 27*, 281–287.

Borson, S. (1995). *Comprehensive textbook of psychiatry.* Baltimore, MD: Williams & Wilkins.

Eaton, W. W., Kramer, M., Anthony, J. C., Dryman, A., Shapiro, S., & Locke, B. Z. (1989). The incidence of specific DIS/SM-III mental disorders: Data from the NIMH Epidemiologic Catchment Area Program. *Acta Psychiatrica Scandinavica, 79*, 163–178.

Gallo, J. J., & Lebowitz, B. D. (1999). The epidemiology of common late-life mental disorders in the community: Themes for the new century. *Psychiatric Services, 50*, 1158–1166.

Gurland, B. J., Cross, P. S., & Katz, S. (1996). Epidemiological perspectives on treatment of depression. *American Journal of Geriatric Psychiatry, 4*(Suppl 1), 7–13.

Hagnell, O., Lanke, J., Rorsman, B., & Ojesjo, L. (1982). Are we entering an age of melancholy? Depressive illnesses in a prospective epidemiological study over 25 years: The Lundby Study, Sweden. *Psychological Medicine, 12*, 279–289.

Hinton, W. L., Fox, K., & Levkoff, S. E. (1999). Introduction: Exploring the relationships among aging, ethnicity, and Family dementia caregiving. *Culture, Medicine, and Psychiatry, 23*, 403–413.

Shakespeare, W. (1608). *The Tragedy of King Lear.* Washington Square Press Edition, 1960, New York: Washington Square Press.

Storck, L. E. (1998). Social class divisions in the consulting room: A theory of psychosocial class and depression. *Group Analysis, 31,* 101–115.

Storck, L. E. (1999). Dissociative disruptions: Psychological (psychosocial) pathways uncovered in the healing process. *Annals New York Academy of Science, 896.*

Styron, W. (1990). *Darkness visible.* New York: Vintage Books.

U.S. Department of Health and Human Services (1999). *Mental Health: A Report of the Surgeon General.* Washington, DC: Office of Public Health and Science, Government Printing Office.

Weissman, M. M., Leaf, P. J., Tischler, G. L., Blazer, D. G., Kamo, M., Bruce, M. I., & Florio, L. P. (1988). Affective disorders in five United States communities. *Psychological Medicine, 18,* 141–153.

Wells, K. B., Sturm, R., Sherbourne, C. D., & Meredith, L. S. (1996). *Caring for depression.* Cambridge, MA: Harvard University Press.

CHAPTER 5

The Role of Music Therapy in Successful Aging

Suzanne B. Hanser

What has music to do with successful aging?

> For Elizabeth R., a 92-year-old woman who always wanted to study piano, it is a dream come true.
>
> For Hyram P., whose retirement has brought challenging transitions to his new lifestyle, it is a divergent path that he travels with creativity, imagination and optimism.
>
> For Dennis K., a gentleman in the late stages of Alzheimer's disease, it is a familiar stimulus in a strange and bewildering world.

Throughout our lives, music surrounds us. It often accompanies such memorable moments as the time we fell in love or even a deeply spiritual experience at a religious service. It may draw tears of joy or despair. We may wake up to it in the morning; we hear it on the radio in the car; it is ever present in offices and elevators without our choosing to listen. It motivates us to buy more in grocery stores, to slow our pace in airports, and to interact more comfortably at a party. If we attend concerts or religious services, we may have had a peak aesthetic experience when music moves us significantly. If we are musically trained, we have learned a language that communicates very differently from using standard intellectual channels. Perhaps, we have been fortunate to work with a music therapist, thus experiencing directly how music changes our emotions or finding a nonverbal, expressive way to connect to the world.

In each of these examples, music affects our lives, whether we know it or not. There are even more dramatic examples in the research literature, owing to the work of music therapists whose business it is to find music that will change our lives in some small way. Many older adults who wish to use music to achieve specific nonmusical goals, such as overcoming depression, sleeping better, maintaining cognitive functioning, or improving interpersonal relationships, are beginning to seek the services of a music therapist. In addition, adults with cognitive impairments, physical ailments, or psychological problems are being referred to music therapists whose credentials signify advanced training in dealing with their special needs. This chapter describes some of the processes contributing to the effects of music as therapy and offers examples of applications in late life. It presents a brief overview of the field, a synopsis of research on its efficacy with older adults, three cases, a sampling of four clinical strategies, and a format for organizing music therapy groups.

THE EXPERIENCE OF MUSIC AS THERAPY

According to the American Music Therapy Association, music therapy is "an allied health profession in which music is used within a therapeutic relationship to address physical, psychological, cognitive, and social needs of individuals. After assessing the strengths and needs of each client, the qualified music therapist provides the indicated treatment including creating, singing, moving to, and listening to music. Through musical involvement in the therapeutic context, clients' abilities are strengthened and transferred to other areas of their lives" (1997). In their work with older adults, music therapists work in nursing homes, adult day health programs, respite care, senior centers, hospice, geriatric clinics, and community agencies. They serve people at different levels of functioning and with diverse needs.

Cognitively impaired individuals frequently have preserved musical abilities that allow them to recall familiar songs and respond in rhythm well into the latest stages of a disease such as Alzheimer's. People recovering from strokes have had successful gait rehabilitation accompanied by music, which cues tempo, rhythm, and fluidity of movement. Healthy older adults enjoy music as recreation or entertainment, and if they wish to be actively involved in music making, it provides a new arena for exploring their creative energy and talent. Others are distracted from pain by focusing on music that has meaningful associations and elicits positive images. When older adults become frail or develop physical limitations, some still engage in creating, performing, or listening to music, possibly compensating for loss through using specially adapted musical instruments while exercising weak areas of motor control.

THE EFFICACY OF MUSIC THERAPY

Research has documented many specific outcomes of music therapy. Perhaps the greatest body of literature regarding late life is devoted to research supporting its efficacy for individuals with dementia. In addition to a multitude of descriptive studies (Gibbons, 1988; Smith, 1990), a recent review (Brotons, Koger, & Pickett-Cooper, 1997) cites 69 references between 1986 and 1996, of which 42 were empirical studies of the effects of music with people who have dementia. Positive results have been achieved when music therapists targeted objectives such as face-name recognition (Carruth, 1997), cognition (Smith, 1986), socialization (Pollack & Namazi, 1992), reality orientation (Riegler, 1980), and active participation (Christie, 1992; Clair & Bernstein, 1990; Kovach & Henschel, 1996; Smith-Marchese, 1994). Other effects included enhanced quality of life (Lipe, 1991; Silber & Hes, 1986), alertness in patients with advanced dementia (Clair, 1996a), improved social interaction (Newman & Ward, 1993; Olderog-Millard & Smith, 1989; Ward, Los Kamp, & Newman, 1996), greater recall of words when sung as opposed to spoken (Prickett & Moore, 1991), more positive affect (Gaebler & Hemsley, 1991), and better responsiveness (Norberg, Melin, & Asplund, 1986; Sambandham & Schirm, 1995). In a comparison of different therapies for Alzheimer's disease, Rabins (1996) reports modest gains for music therapy, tacrine, and other treatment approaches.

It has been observed that music is a remarkably preserved ability in many people suffering from dementia. There is considerable anecdotal and scientific evidence of individuals in the late stages of Alzheimer's disease experiencing, enjoying, and responding to music even when they are no longer capable of recognizing loved ones or speaking coherently (Beatty et al., 1988; Clair, Bernstein, & Johnson, 1995; Crystal, Grober, & Masur, 1989; Swartz, Hantz, Crummer, Walton, & Frisina, 1989; Swartz, Walton, Crummer, Hantz, & Frisina, 1992). There are cases of active singing after intelligible speech has ceased, classical piano performance accompanied by extreme disorientation in other spheres of life, and rhythmic improvisation by individuals who are incapable of mobility or speech. It seems that music is capable of heightening emotions in cognitively impaired older adults who cry, laugh, and emote as music evokes memories, images, associations, and even spiritual connections (Sacks & Tomaino, 1991). Clearly, music gives a person a unique opportunity to feel and experience a range of emotions in a protected and healthy manner regardless of functional capacity.

Behavioral music therapy interventions have been found to decrease troublesome behaviors such as agitation (Brotons & Pickett-Cooper, 1996; Clair & Bernstein, 1994; Gerdner & Swanson, 1993; Goddaer & Abraham, 1994; Tabloski, McKinnon-Howe, & Remington, 1995; Ward, LosKamp, & Newman, 1996), inappropriate verbalizations (Casby & Holm, 1994), aggressiveness during bathing (Thomas, Heitman, & Alexander, 1997), sleeping problems (Lindenmuth, Patel, & Chang, 1992), and wandering (Fitzgerald-Cloutier, 1992; Groene, 1993). Gero-psychiatric patients also benefit from music therapy, which is frequently the treatment of choice when other methods fail. The literature reports several efficacious techniques in psychiatric settings, including guided imagery and music (GIM) (Blake & Bishop, 1994; Bonny, 1994; Clarkson & Geller, 1996), songwriting (Cordobes, 1997; Ficken, 1976), musical improvisation (Bruscia, 1987; Nolan, 1994; Pavlicevic, Trevarthen, & Duncan, 1994), and music listening with singing (Tang, Yao, & Zheng, 1994).

Rehabilitation programs have benefitted from music therapy strategies. Thaut, McIntosh, Prassas, and Rice (1992) describe how rhythmically cued ambulation with preferred music facilitates efficiency of walking. These techniques have been effective with stroke patients and individuals with Parkinson's disease (McIntosh et al., 1995; Thaut, McIntosh, Prassas, & Rice, 1993).

I have reported positive outcomes related to music therapy for depression (Hanser & Thompson, 1994). Symptoms of depression, distress, and anxiety were reduced significantly in older adults suffering from major or minor depression as compared with no-contact control subjects. These individuals engaged in a protocol described briefly later in this chapter. In another study, Shealy, Cady, and Cox (1995) reported that as many as 85% of their 351 depressed clients were responsive to music, photostimulation, insight meditation, education, and other treatments within 2 weeks, while avoiding drug therapy.

There are also many cases where music therapy has evoked a peak experience in individuals who produce insights about the meaning of their lives at the end of their lives (Lane, 1994; Martin, 1991; Munro, 1984). Because music can be enjoyed both passively through listening and actively through performance, singing, or composition, it allows for many meaningful shared experiences with family, friends, and loved ones. On the subject of music and healthy older adults, Shaw's book, *The Joy of Music in Maturity* (1993) addresses how creative music therapy techniques may be applied. Another book presents intergenerational programs, offering opportunities for young and old to learn about one another and share positive experiences (Shaw & Manthey, 1996). The value of music as therapy in late life is supported by this literature. The following section tells the story of three individuals who have transformed their lives through music.

LATE LIFE CHALLENGES: THREE CASES

Ninety-two-year-old Elizabeth R. was in relatively good health, but lacking motivation to get out of bed in the morning. She was eating less and less and becoming quite weak. Her family, fearing that she was deteriorating physically, referred her to a geriatric mental health team. In the course of their interviews, the team learned that Ms. R. enjoyed listening to music at home, the only pleasurable activity that she could identify. She was diagnosed with major depression and referred to a music therapist. When the therapist learned that Ms. R. had always wanted to take piano lessons, the plan seemed clear. Ms. R. looked forward to weekly piano lessons and enjoyed practicing piano every day, frequently singing along. Pentatonic scale improvisation on the black keys allowed her to experience instant success and an endless number of opportunities for creative expression. Soon, she was inviting friends to come and hear her latest tunes. An early morning practice schedule got her out of bed, and evening improvisation made her loneliest hours pass more quickly and enjoyably. The result was a happier Elizabeth R., who was now socializing frequently, eating regularly, and learning something new each time she sat at the piano.

Hyram P. was a successful executive until his company policy forced him into retirement. Mr. P. had always enjoyed attending concerts with his wife, but never understood very much about music. He decided to enroll in a music appreciation class at the local community college. During class, Mr. P. would invariably hum or sing along with musical excerpts, always right on pitch and with a deep baritone vibrato. The music instructor urged Mr. P. to develop his vocal abilities by joining a choral group. Three months later, Hyram P. had learned to read music and was soloist with his church choir. He commented that his once-feared retirement gave him a brand new vocation and a new life. He had never known such happiness.

Dennis K. has Alzheimer's disease. He has been in a nursing home for 2 years. His wife's regular visits become more and more difficult for her as he becomes more agitated and disoriented. No longer recognized by her husband, Mrs. K. has been experiencing hypertension, stomach ulcers, and other stress-related illnesses. The music therapist working with the couple assists Mrs. K. to compose a song about their relationship. It is cathartic. She cries as she sings it, accompanied by the therapist. She says that she has not had an opportunity to talk about how tormented she feels when she sees her husband deteriorating. She finds the writing and singing liberating. When they sing the song a second time, Mr. K. hums along and looks at his wife in an affectionate way. She is moved by feeling a connection between them that has long been lost.

When music triggers good feelings, as evidenced by these vignettes, it does so without the necessity of following the neural pathways that are involved in more complex intellectual functioning. Indeed, music evokes a multiplicity of behaviors, from such simple maneuvers as toe tapping, humming, arm waving, and drumming with the fingers to more complex conducting, dancing, singing, harmonizing, accompanying, and performing on any number of musical instruments. When the stimulus of music is introduced, these responses often seem to occur "without thought." The heart starts to race, the memories flood, the emotions flow without a conscious attempt to change our bodies or minds. It may be theorized that the emotional response to music is triggered in the amygdala and the hippocampus, short circuiting the prefrontal lobes and eliciting a more natural and automatic response. The way that music is processed in the brain is too complex to be fully understood given the current state of knowledge and technology. However, the pervasiveness of its impact on such systems as hearing, memory, cognition, emotion, and sometimes, language, may begin to account for its ability to touch so many human beings.

A SAMPLING OF MUSIC THERAPY STRATEGIES

Having introduced some basic theory and research in music therapy, this section presents a few specific protocols that have been shown to be efficacious with older adults. The techniques include musical improvisation, music-facilitated stress reduction, music performance, and music at the end of life.

Working From Spontaneity: Musical Improvisation

The interactive musical dialogue that comes alive in clinical improvisation is a significant feature of music therapy (Aldridge, 1989). In a moving account of a musician dying from AIDS, Lee (1996) details the impact of collaborative piano improvisation in creating a nonverbal experience. The impulsiveness that is characteristic of individuals with neurological impairment, and of many who are not, can be transformed into spontaneous performance when improvisation techniques are introduced. There are basic rhythmic improvisations that can be mastered by almost anyone. Claire (1996b) recounts how severely regressed dementia patients engage in *vibrotactile* drumming, a technique designed to stimulate the rhythmic response as well as the sense of touch through vibrating drum heads.

Instrumental improvisation on percussion allows for a failure-free experience for participants. In one method, group members drum against a steady beat, creating a rhythmic composition that allows each person to contribute a new or unique rhythm while building a new rhythmic composition. Against a structured ostinato (an ongoing musical pattern), participants can be creative and original within a structure. Gifted improvisational music therapists contain feelingful expression by imitating and accompanying patterns used by the performer (Bruscia, 1987).

Working From Calm: Mood Music

Music quickly sets a mood when people take time to select a piece that is meaningful and listen to it while observing its effect on their thinking, feeling, and behaving. A cognitive behavioral approach was applied by this author to cue elevated mood, muscle relaxation, and pleasant imagery in a variety of settings with older adults (Hanser, 1987, 1988, 1996; Hanser & Clair, 1995; Hanser & Thompson, 1994). In this protocol, individuals identify recorded music that is relaxing and evokes positive associations, memories, and visual images. They listen to different types of music while attending to differential effects on their bodies and minds. They learn and practice the following eight techniques in music-facilitated stress reduction:

(1) A musical workout—gentle exercise to preferred music;
(2) Music massage—facial massage to calming music;
(3) Building a bond with music—progressive muscle relaxation to specific music to accompany waves of tension and relaxation;
(4) Painting peaceful images—guided imagery which lets the music evoke a desirable place;
(5) Creative problem solving—special imagery to provide a relaxing environment for approaching problems or worries;
(6) Lullaby and good night—music to aid sleep;
(7) A musical boost—music to energize; and

(8) Creativity through music—ideas for making music a regular part of the day.

These strategies have been adapted for even the most cognitively impaired and have been shown to be efficacious in a variety of ways, as described earlier. One indirect outcome of using these techniques has been long-term compliance, as demonstrated by 9-month follow-up maintenance of gains in levels of depression, distress, anxiety, and self-esteem (Hanser & Thompson, 1994). Of course, the supply of music is so vast that there is little satiation, and it is easy and enjoyable to listen, especially when one is feeling the need to change one's mood.

Working From Competence: Musical Performance

Performing music requires mastery of multiple musical skills and can vary from keeping a steady beat or initiating simple percussive sounds to generating polyphonic compositions that necessitate a high level of fine motor coordination and advanced perceptual motor skills. Once a therapist, educator, or coach identifies a person's musical capabilities, mastering successful performance may elicit a great sense of competence. This leads to a positive sense of self-efficacy seldom found in a person's life experience. In some senior centers, healthy older adults enjoy interacting and expressing themselves through activities such as communal drumming (Reuer & Crowe, 1995). As evidenced by Elizabeth R.'s success, it is never too late to learn new musical skills.

Once again, there are so many musical instruments from which to choose, not to mention the voice with its endless potential for development. This means that the opportunity to find a novel creative outlet is great in any individual with the interest to do so. Ensembles and choirs exist in every community, and often, participants find these groups to be tremendous sources of social support. With the explosion of user-friendly music technology and electronic music, untrained musicians can create fully orchestrated melodies and use adaptive switches to explore beautiful combinations of sounds and phrases. Jon Adams' *Switch Ensemble* (1998) is one example of software that enables the gentle touch of an oversized switch to trigger the note of a preprogrammed melody. The program also allows a nonverbal and severely physically challenged individual to perform ready-to-play musical selections in an ensemble of synchronized parts.

Working From Transition: Music at the End of Life

Music may also play a significant part at the end of life. West (1994) refers to the support of a music therapist attending and supporting the death of an individual as akin to a midwife who helps birth a new life. Music therapists in palliative care discuss how an individual near the end of life finds a sense of control when everything else appears uncontrollable (Burns, 1993; Gilbert, 1977; Mandel, 1993; Salmon, 1993; Yamamoto, 1993). Aldridge (1995) and Lee (1995) describe how clinical improvisation allows individuals at the end of life an opportunity to express what words cannot. Guided imagery and music (GIM) offers a unique way to become aware of feelings, express them, and prepare for separation from loved ones (Wylie & Blom, 1986). Songwriting is another technique that provides a legacy for significant others in the form of an original piece of music (Rykov, 1994; O'Callaghan, 1996).

A remarkable study by Boyle and Greer (1983) demonstrates that music, played contingent on movement, may increase responsiveness in comatose patients. Curtis (1986) demonstrates some efficacy for music therapy procedures with terminally ill patients in managing pain.

Individuals who are dying may feel a sense of empowerment when they witness how music changes their emotions. Using the symbolic language of melody, the person and family may select or compose music to express how they feel. In the process, they may become more self-aware and freer to speak about death, loss, and the meaning of their lives.

A FORMAT FOR GROUP MUSIC THERAPY

Given the variety of techniques and the infinite possibilities for engaging in musical experience, it is useful to consider a format for organizing a music session. The first consideration is whether individual or group sessions are most feasible. Because they accommodate the greatest number of individuals, groups are especially popular at nursing homes and in residential and day care facilities. In addition, music therapy functions well in an integrated group therapy process. The following offers one sample format I use in clinical music therapy groups.

The music therapy protocol first calls for a thorough assessment of tastes, preferences, and responsiveness to a variety of musical stimuli. Although interview may be the simplest way to obtain this information in a cognitively competent informant, there is no substitute for actually listening to different musical selections and observing specific effects. Other techniques are then sampled while the therapist observes responses. Musical abilities are also assessed to determine the most appropriate instruments and activities that may be performed successfully. One particularly useful tool is a comprehensive assessment of the musical abilities of individuals with Alzheimer's disease that has been standardized by Elizabeth York (1994).

With these data, the music therapist is able to group individuals by functional abilities and preferences. Observation of typical attention spans will determine the length of sessions, while pretested tasks will define the degree of complexity tolerated. Group size is minimized to individualize the approach and maximize outcome. The following format for group sessions is based on the familiar musical sonata form. It is composed of an introduction, exposition or theme, development, recapitulation, and coda or closing (Hanser, 1987).

Part I.   Introduction

Warm-ups that are success oriented, nonthreatening activities designed to prepare clients for session
    a. introduction of participants, objectives, or materials to be used
    b. information sharing of participants regarding their present state or recent progress
    c. physical or musical exercises to prepare for requirements of activities to be performed later
    d. trust-building exercises to demonstrate supportive environment
    e. assessment of presession feelings/behaviors

Part II. Exposition

Awareness activities that allow participants to explore and become aware of present states

    a. passive music activities that allow for introspection

    b. nonverbal exercises that encourage individual responses to music

    c. projective music experiences that allow the participants to express themselves on an instrument or through a musical recording that relates similar states

    d. a musical problem or choice situation designed as a metaphor for similar problem-solving tests

    e. participation in an active musical experience to generate affective responses

    f. a musical learning situation set up to teach new skills and reinforce social behaviors

Part III. Development

Affective activities that examine responses to awareness activities and express this new understanding in a different dimension

    a. following passive musical activities, active ones to express nonverbal interpretation of the experiences

    b. following nonverbal exercises, verbal or nonverbal activities that use a different musical medium to express reactions to this experience (a musical conversation on two percussion instruments to mirror interaction)

    c. interpretation of a projective music experience by therapist, client, or group, pointing out observations and perceptions of the event

    d. discussion of choices made or problem-solving strategies used in such an activity and opportunities to try out alternatives

    e. further development of affective responses to music through the exploration of contrasting musical stimuli and associated responses

    f. performance of new music skills learned in the session

    g. feedback from therapist, client, or group

Part IV. Recapitulation

Synthesis that attempts to bring together awareness, expression, and nonverbal/verbal and introspective/projective elements of the music experience

    a. an original musical composition to express what transpired in the session

    b. discussion of the meaning of the experience or perceptions at this point

    c. conclusions based on projective information posited for interpretation

    d. an analysis of observed behaviors during session

    e. exploration of affective responses to nonmusical stimuli

    f. evaluation of the musical and nonmusical outcomes of the music learning experience with analogies to other aspects of life

    g. responding to a recording of expressive musical behavior generated during the session

Part V. Coda

Closure

    a. musical or nonmusical summary of the session

    b. description of progress or process at the end of the session

    c. performance of music or musical experience that builds on previously learned music skills or activities

    d. repeat of warm-up activity to highlight differences in behavior as a function of session

    e. assessment of postsession feelings using same technique used at start of session

    f. assignments given to participants to apply new learning to future situations

Within this structure, there is much room for creativity by the therapist and experimentation by the group. Examples of applications for individuals with dementia may be found in Hanser and Clair (1995).

CONCLUSION

Elizabeth R. continues to study piano, is sleeping and eating well, and remaining socially active.

Hyram P. has started voice lessons, which he takes in return for financial planning advice to his teacher. He says he feel competent and alive thanks to the feedback he receives about his voice.

Mrs. K's visits to Dennis have taken on a new perspective. Instead of spending their time in silence, Mrs. K. now sings to Dennis, and they listen together to music that she brings from their home music collection.

This chapter has attempted to acquaint the reader with the field of music therapy and to present an overview that is based on research and clinical work with older adults. I hope that this brief glimpse has enticed the reader to learn more about these applications and observe the effects of music as therapy in daily life.

REFERENCES

Adams, J. (1998). *Switch Ensemble.* Boston, MA: Switch-In-Time.

Aldridge, D. (1989). A phenomenological comparison of the organization of music and the self. *Arts in Psychotherapy, 16,* 91–97.

Aldridge, D. (1995). Spirituality, hope and music therapy in palliative care. *Arts in Psychotherapy, 22,* 103–109.

American Music Therapy Association (1997). *Music therapy as a career.* Silver Spring, MD: Author.

Beatty, W., Zavadil, K., Bailly, R., Rixen, G., Zavadil, L., Farnham, N., & Fisher, l. (1988). Preserved musical skill in a severely demented patient. *International Journal of Clinical Neuropsychology, 10,* 158–164.

Blake, R. L., & Bishop, S. R. (1994). The Bonny method of guided imagery and music (GIM) in the treatment of post-traumatic stress disorder with adults in the psychiatric setting. *Journal of Music Therapy, 12,* 125–129.

Bonny, H. (1994). Twenty-one years later: A GIM update. *Music Therapy Perspectives, 12,* 70–74.

Boyle, M. E., & Greer, R. D. (1983). Operant procedures and the Comatose patient. *Journal of Applied Behavior Analysis, 16,* 3–12.

Brotons, M., Koger, S. M., & Pickett-Cooper, P. (1997). Music and the dementias: A review of literature. *Journal of Music Therapy, 34,* 204–245.

Brotons, M., & Pickett-Cooper, P. (1996). The effects of music therapy intervention on agitation behaviors of Alzheimer's disease patients. *Journal of Music Therapy, 33,* 2–18.

Bruscia, K. (1987). *Improvisational models of music therapy.* Springfield, IL: Charles Thomas.

Burns, S. (1993). In hospice work, music is our great ally. *Pastoral Music, 17,* 11–13.

Carruth, E. K. (1997). The effects of singing and the spaced retrieval technique on improving face-name recognition in nursing home residents. *Journal of Music Therapy, 34,* 165–186.

Casby, J. A., & Holm, M. B. (1994). The effect of music on repetitive disruptive vocalizations of person with dementia. *American Journal of Occupational Therapy, 48,* 883–889.

Christie, M. E. (1992). Music therapy applications in a skilled and intermediate care nursing home facility: A clinical study. *Activities, Adaptation and Aging, 16,* 69–87.

Clair, A. A. (1996a). The effect of singing on alert responses in persons with late stage dementia. *Journal of Music Therapy, 33,* 234–247.

Clair, A. A. (1996b). *Therapeutic uses of music with older adults.* Baltimore: Health Professions Press.

Clair, A. A., & Bernstein, B. (1990). A preliminary study of music therapy programming for severely regressed persons with Alzheimer's type dementia. *Journal of Applied Gerontology, 9,* 299–311.

Clair, A. A., & Bernstein, B. (1994). The effect of no music, stimulative background music and sedative background music on agitation behaviors in persons with severe dementia. *Activities, Adaptation and Aging, 19,* 61–70.

Clair, A. A., Bernstein, B., & Johnson, G. (1995). Rhythm playing characteristics in persons with severe dementia including those with probable Alzheimer's type. *Journal of Music Therapy, 32,* 113–131.

Clarkson, G., & Geller, J. D. (1996). The Bonny method from a psychoanalytical perspective: Insights from working with a psychoanalytic psychotherapist in a guided imagery and music series. *Arts in Psychotherapy, 23,* 311–319.

Cordobes, T. K. (1997). Group songwriting as a method for developing group cohesion for HIV-seropositive adult patients with depression. *Journal of Music Therapy, 34,* 46–67.

Crystal, H. A., Grober, E., & Masur, D. (1989). Preservation of musical memory in Alzheimer's disease. *Journal of Neurology, Neurosurgery, and Psychiatry, 52,* 1415–1416.

Curtis, S. L. (1986). The effect of music on pain relief and relaxation of the terminally ill. *Journal of Music Therapy, 23,* 10–24.

Ficken, T. (1976). The use of songwriting in a psychiatric setting. *Journal of Music Therapy, 13,* 163–172.

Fitzgerald-Cloutier, M. L. (1992). The use of music therapy to decrease wandering: An alternative to restraints. *Music Therapy Perspectives, 11,* 32–36.

Gaebler, H., & Hemsley, D. (1991). The assessment and short-term manipulation of affect in the severely demented. *Behavioural Psychotherapy, 19,* 145–156.

Gerdner, L. A., & Swanson, E. A. (1993). Effects of individualized music on confused and agitated elderly patients. *Archives of Psychiatric Nursing, 7,* 284–291.

Gibbons, A. C. (1988). A review of literature for music development/ education and music therapy with the elderly. *Music Therapy Perspectives, 5,* 33–40.

Gilbert, J. (1977). Music therapy perspectives on death and dying. *Journal of Music Therapy, 14,* 165–171.

Goddaer, J., & Abraham, I. (1994). Effects of relaxing music on agitation during meals among nursing home residents with severe cognitive impairment. *Archives of Psychiatric Nursing, 8,* 150–158.

Groene, R. W. (1993). Effectiveness of music therapy: 1:1 intervention with individuals having senile dementia of the Alzheimer's type. *Journal of Music Therapy, 30,* 138–157.

Hanser, S. B. (1987). *Music therapists handbook.* St. Louis: Warren Green.

Hanser, S. B. (1988). Controversy in music listening/stress eduction research. *Arts in Psychotherapy, 15,* 211–217.

Hanser, S. B. (1996). Music therapy to reduce anxiety, agitation, and depression. *Nursing Home Medicine, 10,* 20–22.

Hanser, S. B., & Clair, A. A. (1995). Retrieving the losses of Alzheimer's disease for patients and caregivers with the aid of music. In T. Wigram, B. Saperston, & R. West (Eds.), *The art and science of music therapy: A handbook* (pp. 342–360). Chur, Switzerland: Harwood Academic Publishers.

Hanser, S. B., & Thompson, L. W. (1994). Effects of a music therapy strategy on depressed older adults. *Journal of Gerontology, 49,* 265–269.

Kovach, C., & Henschel, H. (1996). Behavior and participation during therapeutic activities on special care units. *Activities, Adaptation and Aging, 20,* 35–45.

Lane, D. (1994). *Music as medicine.* Cleveland, OH: Zondervan Publishing.

Lee, C. A. (Ed.). (1995). *Lonely waters.* Oxford: Sobell Publications.

Lee, C. A. (1996). *Music at the edge: The music therapy experiences of a musician with AIDS.* London: Routledge.

Lindenmuth, G. F., Patel, M., & Chang, P. K. (1992). Effects of music on sleep in healthy elderly and subjects with senile dementia of the Alzheimer type. *American Journal of Alzheimer's Disease and Related Disorders and Research, 2,* 13–20.

Lipe, A. (1991). Using music therapy to enhance the quality of life in a client with Alzheimer's dementia: A case study. *Music Therapy Perspectives, 9,* 102–105.

Mandel, S. E. (1993). The role of the music therapist on the hospice/ palliative care team. *Journal of Palliative Care, 9,* 37–39.

Martin, J. A. (Ed.). (1991). *The next step forward: Music therapy with the terminally ill.* Bronx, NY: Calvary Hospital.

McIntosh, G., Thaut, M., Rice, R., Miller, R., Rathbun, J., & Brault, J. (1995). Rhythmic facilitation in gait training of Parkinson's disease. *Annals of Neurology, 38,* 331.

Munro, S. (1984). *Music therapy in palliative/hospice care.* St. Louis: MMB.

Newman, S., & Ward, C. (1993). An observational study of intergenerational activities and behavior change in dementing elders at adult day care centers. *International Journal of Aging and Human Development, 36,* 321–333.

Nolan, P. (1994). The therapeutic response in improvisational music therapy: What goes on inside? *Music Therapy Perspectives, 12,* 84–91.

Norberg, A., Melin, E., & Asplund, K. (1986). Reactions to music, touch, and object presentation in the final stage of dementia: An exploratory study. *International Journal of Nursing Studies, 23,* 315–323.

O'Callaghan, C. C. (1996). Lyrical themes in songs written by palliative care patients. *Journal of Music Therapy, 33,* 74–92.

Olderog-Millard, K. A. O., & Smith, J. M. (1989). The influence of group singing therapy on the behavior of Alzheimer's disease patients. *Journal of Music Therapy, 26,* 58–70.

Pavlicevic, M., Trevarthen, C., & Duncan, J. (1994). Improvisational music therapy and the rehabilitation of persons suffering from chronic schizophrenia. *Journal of Music Therapy, 31,* 86–104.

Pollack, N. J., & Namazi, K. H. (1992). The effect of music participation on the social behavior of Alzheimer's disease patients. *Journal of Music Therapy, 29,* 54–67.

Prickett, C. A., & Moore, R. S. (1991). The use of music to aid memory of Alzheimer's patients. *Journal of Music Therapy, 28,* 101–110.

Rabins, P. V. (1996). Developing treatment guidelines for Alzheimer's disease and other dementias. *Journal of Clinical Psychiatry, 47,* 37–38.

Reuer, B., & Crowe, B. (1995). *Best practice in music therapy: Utilizing group percussion strategies for promoting volunteerism in the well older adult.* St. Louis: MMB.

Riegler, J. (1980). Comparison of a reality orientation program for geriatric patients with and without music. *Journal of Music Therapy, 17,* 26–33.

Rykov, M. (1994). *Last songs: AIDS and the music therapist.* St. Louis: MMB.

Sacks, O., & Tomaino, C. (1991). Music and neurological disorder. *International Journal of Arts Medicine, 1,* 10–12.

Salmon, D. (1993). Music and emotion in palliative care. *Journal of Palliative Care, 9,* 48–52.

Sambandham, M., & Schirm, V. (1995). Music as a nursing intervention for residents with Alzheimer's disease in long-term care. *Geriatric Nursing, 16,* 79–83.

Shaw, J. (1993). *The joy of music in maturity.* St. Louis: MMB.

Shaw, J., & Manthey, C. (1996). Musical bridges: *Intergenerational music programs*. St. Louis: MMB Music.

Shealy, C. N., Cady, R. K., & Cox, R. H. (1995). Pain, stress and depression: Psychoneurophysiology and therapy. *Stress Medicine, 11,* 75–77.

Silber, F., & Hes, J. (1986). The use of songwriting with patients diagnosed with Alzheimer's disease. *Music Therapy Perspectives, 13,* 31–34.

Smith, D. S. (1990). Therapeutic treatment effectiveness as documented in the gerontology literature: Implications for music therapy. *Music Therapy Perspectives, 8,* 36–40.

Smith, G. (1986). A comparison of the effects of three treatment interventions on cognitive functioning of Alzheimer patients. *Music Therapy, 6A,* 41–56.

Smith-Marchese, K. (1994). The effects of participatory music on the reality orientation and sociability of Alzheimer's residents in a long-term care setting. *Activities, Adaptation and Aging, 18,* 41–55.

Swartz, K. P., Hantz, E. C., Crummer, G. C., Walton, J. P., & Frisina, R. D. (1989). Does the melody linger on? Music cognition in Alzheimer's disease. *Seminar in Neurology, 9,* 152–158.

Swartz, K. P., Walton, J., Crummer, G., Hantz, E., & Frisina, R. (1992). P3 event-related potentials and performance of healthy older adults and AD subjects for music perception tasks. *Psychomusicology, 11,* 96–118.

Tabloski, P., McKinnon-Howe, L., & Remington, R. (1995). Effects of calming music on the level of agitation in cognitively impaired nursing home residents. *The American Journal of Alzheimer's Care and Related Disorders and Research, 10,* 10–15.

Tang, W., Yao, X., & Zheng, Z. (1994). Rehabilitative effect of music therapy for residual schizophrenia: A one-month randomised controlled trial in Shanghai. *British Journal of Psychiatry, 165,* 38–44.

Thaut, M., McIntosh, G., Prassas, S., & Rice, R. (1992). Effect of rhythmic auditory cueing on temporal stride parameters and EMG patterns in normal gait. *Journal of Neurological Rehabilitation, 6,* 185–190.

Thaut, M., McIntosh, G., Prassas, S., & Rice, R. (1993). The effect of auditory rhythmic cuing on stride ad EMG patterns in hemiparetic gait of stroke patients. *Journal of Neurological Rehabilitation, 7,* 9–16.

Thomas, D. W., Heitman, R. J., & Alexander, T. (1997). The effects of music on bathing cooperation for residents with dementia. *Journal of Music Therapy, 34,* 246–259.

Ward, C. R., Los Kamp, L., & Newman, S. (1996). The effects of participation in an intergenerational program on the behavior of residents with dementia. *Activities, Adaptation and Aging, 20,* 61–76.

West, T. M. (1994). Psychological issues in hospice music therapy. *Music Therapy Perspectives, 12,* 117–124.

Wylie, M. E., & Blom, R. (1986). Guided imagery and music with hospice patients. *Music Therapy Perspectives, 3,* 25–28.

Yamamoto, K. (1993). Terminal care and music therapy. *Japanese Journal of Psychosomatic Medicine, 22,* 25–28.

York, E. (1994). The development of a quantitative music skills test for patients with Alzheimer's disease. *Journal of Music Therapy, 31,* 280–296.

CHAPTER 6

Family Dynamics and the Flow of Caregiving

Alan J. Lieberman

> "Home is the place where, when you have to go there,
> They have to take you in."
> "I should have called it something you somehow
> haven't to deserve."
> —Robert Frost, *The Death of the Hired Man*

T he dialog, or more accurately, the disagreement over taking in a frail older person in the excerpt from Frost's poem addresses basic issues in family caregiving. The unresolved, or unresolvable, contradiction is between the long-held belief that a member of a family, however tangential, is entitled to care in old age and the less publicly espoused view that that care must be earned and can be refused.

It has become a common-place observation that, in this narcissistic age, the self-serving adult will jettison family responsibilities whenever and wherever it is convenient. Stories appear describing frail, older people abandoned in their wheel chairs, minus identification, a caricature of the baby abandoned on the doorstep. Popular songs extol the importance of paying back bad parents by leaving home at the earliest possible moment and not looking back. And yet there is the ancient tradition that we are all entitled to care from our family, adopted or not, earned or not.

Perhaps we should not be surprised to learn that only about 15% or less of older adults, irrespective of age, live in nursing homes, assisted living, or other kinds of institutional settings (Pruchno, Peters, & Burant, 1995). Where are they? Depending on the age group looked at, the old to the oldest old, many, thanks to modern medicine and public knowledge concerning healthy living, are at home. But many live with chronic illnesses that inexorably drain their vitality and require assistance to maintain a life of relative independence. Who gives this assistance? For the most part, it is the spouse or companion who is well, or at least less disabled (Coward, Horne, & Dwyer, 1992; Merrill, 1993). In many instances, however, it is the adult daughter who makes it possible for the aging parent to live in her own residence, outside of an institution (Pruchno, Dempsey, Carder, & Koropeckyi-Cox, 1993; Pruchno et al., 1995). Some family members, daughters, often at great cost to themselves and their own families, care for their parents.

Is it a problem? It can be. Substantial research indicates that overburdened caregivers are at risk for depression and ill health (George & Gwyther, 1986; Taylor, Ford, & Dunbar, 1995; Tennstedt, Cafferata, & Sullivan, 1992). Family stress may increase to the point where issues of parenting and marital intimacy, which were manageable become unmanageable. New problems in the family, which before could be dealt with effectively, threaten to severely disrupt a fragile equilibrium. Family affiliation may erode to the point that family members are farther apart, not drawn together in a worthy, common effort, depending on how the care is given. The gender bias displayed when care is almost always given by a woman may mean that opportunities that our society has made more available for woman may not be taken (Finley, 1989). But families persist in fulfilling their own and cultural/religious mandates to fulfill what is often referred to as filial piety and filial responsibility (Goodheart & Lansin, 1997; Sung, 1995).

An account of family caregiving cannot, and probably should not, be written without reference to the moral and ethical dimension inherent in giving care to a spouse or aged parent. Often attention is paid only to those families or individuals who shun responsibility. They will be seen as violating a law, a law so basic that it appears embedded in the foundation of civilization itself.

Filial piety has that kind of ubiquity and power. It decrees that a child, often the oldest son, has an absolute obligation to take care of his parents, to make their old age comfortable, that they never want for anything within reason. This ideal, while seemingly, "more honored in the breech than in the observance" still exerts a strong influence on families. We can feel scandalized when someone decides not to be bound by this most ancient of family rules. Or else our cynicism may lead us to nod knowingly as we observe yet another moral verity crash. But we should also abjure dealing on such a superficial level with an entity as complex as a multigenerational family and the way that it defines and implements the responsibilities that family members bear to one another. Rather we might try to understand how the ethics of a family, handed down from previous generations, modified by each, influences the choices made about family caregiving.

The purpose of this chapter is not to advocate for caregiving by family members. That has already been decided by generations of families, in most cultures, through recorded history. Rather I intend to apply the insights of systemic family analysis to describe the multi-generational character of informal family care. I will describe family stress that may accompany such care, methods of helping families to decide whether to give care, and, if they choose to do so, with the choices made about family caregiving. Finally, family caregiving should be looked at from the perspective of care flowing, not only from the younger generation to the older but also in the reverse direction. Two instances will be reviewed, care of an adult child with a chronic, severe disability and extensive care of grandchildren.

RELATIONAL ETHICS IN FAMILY CAREGIVING

Much has been studied and written concerning the family as the primary socializing agency of human civilization. Each of us receives, in the first instance, the precepts of our culture through our earliest family relationships and the experiences that flow from them. Since the days of Freud and his descendants, we are accustomed to view the adult personality and aspects of psychological character as having their roots in the childhood family. We examine closely the way parents act in shaping the emotional life of the child. It is not as usual for us to search for connections between the family culture (as representation of the larger culture in which it is embedded) and the moral and ethical precepts that guide adult behavior, even in the realm of relationships with significant others. We seem to search for those roots in our religious or philosophical traditions, in a generalized way, not looking to see how those values were represented in the interaction between parent and child.

A recent article by Nelson (1998) described the putative decision processes of a man, Robert, who decided to render no care or assistance to his mother when she developed Alzheimer's disease. The author, a professor of philosophy did a very interesting, logical analysis of Robert's likely thought process and the kind of argument which might result if he were challenged to defend his stance. No reference was made to the family history, as though the man's ethical sensibility sprang, de novo, during his adult years.

A student of family relational ethics would consider the possibility that this son, or any other member of a family who shows what appears to be an extreme degree of callous disregard of the needs of a parent and an extreme insensitivity to the needs of siblings may be displaying an ethical stance that is congruent with the family culture and practices. Some families, whether intentionally or not, consistently place the needs of the parents ahead of those of the child. Given the technical term *parentification* by family therapists, it is possible to describe ways in which the child's legitimate, developmental needs are systematically overridden by parental dominance and power. The most egregious examples are those in which the child is exploited, as in incest, but there are many variations on this theme, most of which are less severe and more subtle. It does not seem a big step to consider that a child so treated, now grown to an adult, when again faced with parental neediness, might feel that that parent had already received all that he was entitled to, that further giving on the part of the child would only increase the sense of injustice that was already there.

Interestingly enough, Nelson (1998) concludes his exploration of the ethics of filial duty by proposing an emotional reeducation of Robert, the "selfish" son. Perhaps this is a way of acknowledging, indirectly, that something was missing in Robert's development, a deficit of capacity for empathy, for genuine attachment to the person who gave life and nurture. But is it not incumbent on us to search for a basis of this deficit in the family life of that person? There may be instances where we might agree that the aged parent, deserving as he or she may be at the present time has not earned the right to care owing to the extensive exploitation and deprivation that the child endured. (Of course we might also conclude that he is a selfish man who has turned his back on a good parent and decent siblings.)

EMERGING NEW RELATIONAL ETHICS

The family consultant might go a step further. To simply ratify that Lex Taliones is alive and well may be doing a disservice to this man and to his children. We might agree that he is taking a principled stand: parents who do not give when it is their responsibility to do so are not entitled to receive care when it is needed by them. To do otherwise would be manifestly unfair. But in doing so the adult child is continuing a family tradition that states: Legitimate need for care, whether that of a child who needs nurture and support for healthy growth, or that of an aging parent who, diminished in capacity for self-care by a dementia, needs care to live out the remainder of their life in comfort and dignity, can be denied by a family member because he wants his own needs met and has the power to make that happen. Does Robert want to be responsible for the further propagation of an ethic that marred his own earlier life?

Moreover, not only would he further this ethic in his own life, but, since he now has a wife and children, he would be presenting as an available choice to his children neglect of a parent in need. To be sure, he has his reasons, and they might have considerable merit. Perhaps it would be more useful to point out to him that the decision he makes will have consequences, not only for himself, but for others as it enters the psycho-historic record of his family. It might even be said that he has the ability to change the course of his family history from affirmation of parentification to a new relational ethic based on other values or ethics. Filial responsibility might be one of them.

As with many psychological methods of analysis and intervention, the foregoing could be seen as an example of manipulation to get people to do the "right" thing. While all interventions are likely to have elements of persuasion, the emphasis here is on how decisions are expressed and how they are made. A possible bias on the part of the counselor could be an interest in making what is felt as a purely personal decision part of a family picture. The counselor might feel that he has an ethical problem. Even if she were the therapist for Robert alone, would it be fair to assist him in fulfilling himself by ignoring his mother's needs? Some would say it was not fair, or right, given the larger issues mentioned above not to make these matters part of the therapy context. And, what if Robert deals with his decision by withholding information from his children that might effect them? For example, that their grandmother has a form of Alzheimer's Disease suspected of having a substantial genetic etiology?

Helping one person at the possible expense of others is a therapeutic dilemma that many well-trained and well-intentioned therapists reject as an issue. Some insist that the therapy contract with their patient and the obligation to maintain confidentiality preclude taking into account the welfare of others except with the prospect of imminent harm to them by the patient. Others feel it is part of the therapeutic mission to inform a client about possible unintended adverse consequences of treatment, much as one might advise about the possible side effects of a drug. Some would argue that any focus on matters of ethics or values has no place in a scientifically based and therefore "value-free" therapy.

These concerns regularly arise in connection with decisions about giving care within the family. Those who offer help to individuals or families about giving care should prepare themselves to deal with these matters themselves, if not with clients.

SYSTEMIC FAMILY EVALUATION

A lengthy review of family evaluation and therapy is not possible within the scope of this chapter. However, a brief summary of this large and diverse field will be attempted. The approach to working with families used here is modeled on the work of Ivan Boszormenyi-

Nagy (Boszormenyi-Nagy & Spark, 1973; Boszormenyi & Ulrich, 1981).

Table 6.1 categorizes and lists the major items of information that the family counselor might want to have to begin to understand a family. A family systems approach to families organizes this information so as to allow a conceptual representation of the family as components linked by structural, historical, cultural, psychological, and emotional factors.

The formal structure of the family describes a living system that exists at a particular time to perform the tasks and functions of family life. This structure, however, has extensions of itself that go back into the family past and look forward to the family future. At any given moment, family members may experience themselves as simultaneously in all three domains: past, present, and future. Family coherence and continuity seem a product of multiple factors: oral, written, pictorial, and object histories; residence in specific places, regions, and countries; membership in ethnic, religious, and cultural communities; and the patterning of behavior in relation to developmental stages in the individual and the family. The simultaneity of family being at all points on a continuum of historical time comes about as changes in the lives of individuals overlap with each other

TABLE 6.1 Systemic Family Evaluation

Facts	Family dynamics
Family history	Generational relations
Ethnicity	Coalitions
Culture	Power & hierarchy
Socioeconomic status	Cutoffs
Filial responsibility	Triangulation
	Scapegoating
Individual psychology	Relational ethics
Personality	Fairness/unfairness
Learning style	Loyalty
Goals	Parentification
Psychopathology	Exploitation/abuse

Adapted from Boszormenyi-Nagy, I. & Ulrich, D. (1981). Contexual family therapy. In A. Gurman & D. Kniskern (Eds.), *Handbook of family therapy*. New York: Brunner/Mazel. Reprinted by permission of Taylor & Francis, Inc. Philadelphia, PA.

and with those drawn into the family orbit, starting and stopping at different times, and becoming woven together in the fabric of "our family."

From a child's birth, her features will be compared to aunt this or grandmother that. Giving family names or nicknames, seeing current behavior as reenactments of past accomplishments or failings in older family members, and countless other ways in which the entire family history is made an important part of the present, constantly reinforce the idea that the family contains and gives meaning and direction to the lives of family members. Most family members cannot escape identification with the family, even if they wish to do so.

Efforts to erase the connection to one's family, except for very necessary psychological or cultural reasons, cannot usually happen without negative consequences. Family therapists refer to this phenomenon as family loyalty: a partly theoretical, partly observational construct that calls attention to the fact that most people bestow on their families pride, veneration, obedience, and self-sacrifice. Sometimes family loyalty does not serve the person well, motivating continued attachment even in the face of harm. Whether positively or negatively expressed, family loyalty is a powerful and ubiquitous motive in human behavior.

It is against this backdrop that family caregiving may be viewed. Powerful motivation often exists to take care of one's own. Grandparents, who may have hoped to experience reprieve from a lifetime of hard work and responsibility, will take on the needed care of an adult child or grandchild. Daughters, and sometimes sons, will devote many hours per day, to a parent. An adult daughter, when asked what motivated her and her husband to take her parents into their home said, "We both felt we wanted to give something back for all that we had received growing up."

The realities of family life also include conflict among and between those in differing roles and generations. Coalitions, cliques, triangular relationships, and scapegoating regularly facilitate close relations between some, while causing competitiveness or disconnection for others. When joint effort may be required to reach a family decision, everyone brings these issues to the table, and they become an important, if not the most important, part of the process (Yates, Tennstedt, & Chang, 1999).

Especially important for caregiving is the problem context in which family action may be needed. Very different participation may be called for depending on that context. For our purposes, looking at family caregiving in older age, I will focus on medical crises, chronic illness, and the end of life.

Medical crises are often responded to quickly by families and with a high degree of participation. A sudden heart attack or the need for immediate surgery will bring family members in to give support and help. Other family problems are more easily suppressed during the short time that the emergency is in effect.

Once the issues become more long-term and are combined with diminished awareness or cognitive resources on the part of a parent or spouse, the family involvement will change. The culture may insist that the family make medical decisions instead of the patient, using as a rationale that the patient would be upset by the news of a potentially fatal illness, that information may be withheld. As Fetters (1998) wrote about family medical decision making in Japan, in some instances, the express wishes of a competent patient regarding treatment can be overridden by substitute decision makers from within the family, and those decisions can be accepted by the physician involved. A further reason for this approach can be the acknowledgment that family members will be effected by the outcome of these decisions, especially if the patient were to die.

In present day United States, that kind of family involvement would be unusual. Physicians tend to respect the wishes of the individual, sometimes to the detriment of family members who feel excluded from information and participation. Involvement of the family may be sought at a time when they have already felt excluded and at a disadvantage.

Family decision-making, along the lines of the Japanese model will increasingly be sought as the patient loses his capacity to understand the illness and the treatment options. Health care personnel will increasingly defer to family members since a patient who is no longer competent to agree to treatment represents, to the physician and others, a situation where they can receive future criticism for not obtaining informed consent.

End-of-life decisions are an especially trying but necessary place for family caregiving through making hard decisions. The parent or spouse may reach a stage of an illness were the choices have come down to heroic measures to preserve a semblance of life or, anticipating the imminence of death, administering palliative measures that give relief from pain. Families are asked to give directives as to how to proceed. Families can discuss these options, reach consensus on the basis of what the family member has said about this kind of situation or use their "substitute judgement" about what would have been desired. Many families find that they cannot reach agreement, and sometimes the stress of this situation activates dormant tensions. Recently, while a father lay dying, his brother and a nephew fought so violently over an old grievance that the hospital security officer had to escort them from the building. A mother, after bringing a daughter across the country to help in deciding when to give up active treatment in a terminal situation, openly expressed her resentment as the daughter tried to do what she thought had been asked of her.

TENSION IN DECISION MAKING

The fault lines in families are many, but three are especially likely to show when decisions about care have to be made. First, the relationship among adult siblings is susceptible to fracture under stress of caregiving demands and decisions. Each adult sibling may have developed a life that is complicated and demanding. Not having had to negotiate with each other since childhood, they may be unprepared to express anything except the jealousy and competitiveness that has emerged. Or the oldest daughter, being the responsible one, may try to impose on siblings a concept of family care that they cannot accept. In an example above, the couple who wanted to "give something back" had younger siblings with important roles in their own families. They did not object to the care plan for parents; perhaps they felt they could not. They made promises to help, which they could not keep, creating anger on one side and guilt on the other.

Sibling-like tension may be found in altered form in the extended family, between cousins. A daughter was doing her best to cope with the changing needs of her mother as mother became more and more effected by Alzheimer's Disease. The cousins, who only saw their aunt during well-orchestrated family events, when she was able to look like her old self, accepted her complaint that the daughter was abusive in the way she was trying to run mother's life. When they were helped to see how disabled the aunt really was, how much the aunt needed managing, they became much more supportive of the daughter.

Second, communication among the generations. The most prominent of these, that between the parent(s) and adult children, will be dealt with in a later section on the family life cycle. Next might be the stress aroused when the older person finds it more comfortable to communicate with a grandchild rather than with a son or daughter. Many reasons for this can occur, not the least of which may be the existence of unresolved problems with a son, which do not effect the granddaughter. The mother who finds she must ask her daughter about her own mother may feel humiliated and the victim of a spiteful game. Others will feel relieved that someone else can be the confidante that they have never aspired to be.

Finally, there may be very difficult relationship problems that follow divorce and remarriage. Questions of responsibility, which are clear-cut in the original family, may become clouded when families become "blended." Even though a marriage may have lasted many years, does the ex-wife have a responsibility to her ex-husband's mother? And, if her attachment to the mother has outlasted marriage to son, can she be involved without being in conflict with ex-husband, new wife, or others?

At times serious problems may develop soon after a late, second marriage. The new wife may be able to accept the lack of involvement by the ex-wife but find it hard that the adult children, out of loyalty to their mother, may also refuse to help. When divorce and remarriage happen, family boundaries get redrawn in ways that reflect those changes but can cause confusion and turmoil in family caregiving.

THE FAMILY LIFE-CYCLE AND CAREGIVING

Caregiving for older parents usually comes at a particular moment in the family life-cycle. The children have become adults. They may have children or grandchildren of their own. If the lives of these adult children have turned out well, and they have established good adult relationships with siblings, taking on the responsibility for support of parents may just be one more task that is added to the ones that are already performed with competence and energy. Faced with the mounting evidence that their beloved, respected father with Alzheimer's Disease could no longer operate the power tools in his home workshop, the family devised a plan to slowly dismantle the shop by "borrowing" the tools and not returning them. Telling lies to ease necessary losses for someone with Alzheimer's Disease is often a good strategy that is possible when family members communicate openly and can agree that a desirable goal may justify undesirable means.

However, families may have developmental problems that place the adult child in a position of considerable stress. Called by some the "sandwich generation," a mother or father may find himself or herself dealing not only with the problems of parents but with those of his or her own family. A son or daughter may be dealing with substance abuse, a failing marriage or divorce, or other problems. A child's marriage, needing time and effort to adapt to the ending of parenting, may not get attention when the mother or father needs recurrent crisis management. In these situations, the stress may be cumulative, increasing insidiously until one more problem is added. A caregiver, at that time, can develop a severe stress reaction, which may include depression, anxiety, and physical illness. It may seem a sudden breakdown, not in proportion to an ostensible cause because it is only the most recent of the many stressors that have been building up.

Given that taking responsibility for one's parents, whether mandated by filial responsibility or any other cultural/religious values, can be a difficult and stressful endeavor, can families benefit from doing it? Is there a developmental task that families need to complete that might be facilitated by the effort to care for parents?

The answer may lie in reexamining how families perpetuate themselves. The most obvious way is to have children, but that alone will not preserve the family as a vital organism that can instill pride of membership and motivate succeeding generations to remain connected to one another. We are all familiar with families that seemed unable to pass on to the next generation an ability to lead, to communicate directly, to resolve conflict and to organize the family rituals that mark birth, marriage, and death. Dealing with the care of older parents may provide that possibility. While parents are vital and active, few adult children may feel concern for the future of the family. It is easy to assume that the parents will continue to take that responsibility as they and others in their generation have in the past. When parents start to fail, physically or mentally, it can be seen as a signal that the future of the family may not continue to be managed by them. When adult children can come together to make good decisions for the care of the parents they have taken an important step in creating the framework around which the future of their family may take place.

For example, most of the adult children in a family, finding that they were having difficulty coming together to help their mother in her struggles with memory loss, arranged for family counseling. They realized, in trying to talk with one another, that numerous conflicts, unresolved trust issues, and other scars from earlier family experiences were getting in the way. As they continued to meet to deal with reorganizing the family for mother's benefit, they also talked to one another about themselves. They discovered how little they really knew about each other's lives and the problems that each had faced. They discovered that they wanted to know more, and, at the conclusion of the counseling, they resolved to hold regular meetings to continue the work. They began to look like a family that would continue.

Family continuity is one task made more possible, but there are others. A related issue is one termed by Williamson and Bray (1991) the growth of *personal authority*. In their view, personal growth in adulthood may be slowed or halted out of excessive concern by a son or daughter that their appropriate efforts to be themselves and to make the decisions about their own lives that are needed will lead to a loss of love and relationship with the parents. Typically they see themselves as sabotaging their own efforts to have a different, more mature relationship with parents and siblings. Often they experience the parents as unwilling or unable to enter with them in efforts at change. Williamson and Bray offer a program of therapy that enables the adult son or daughter to renegotiate, with a willing parent, the parent-child relationship. The goal of this therapy is to transform that relationship to an adult-adult one and to remain connected as family. When the adult children of a family take on, in a serious and respectful manner, the responsibility of giving care to their parents, they are, in effect creating personal authority and transforming their role from child to adult.

PSYCHOLOGY OF CAREGIVING

Specific factors that influence the nature and quality of caregiving include: characteristics of the caregiver; relationship to the recipient of care; the nature and degree of impairment of the care recipient; the health and other resources available to the care giver; and the degree of conflict, connectedness, and communication in the nuclear family of the care giver and the extended family.

Care has almost always been the province of the female spouse or daughter. While there are many examples of devoted attendance to an invalid spouse by her husband, the demographics of gender longevity and the socialization of women to be caretakers has, until the present time, virtually guaranteed that a daughter will fill this role for her father. When the care is given to an aging parent, it is almost always the daughter (usually the oldest). Much has been studied concerning depression, burn-out, increased vulnerability to physical illness, and problems with marriage and parenting that may occur in care givers who become overextended. An older wife, trying to care for a much larger and heavier husband with severe mobility restrictions, would be an obvious candidate for physical and emotional stress. But, many kinds of stress are not obvious, either to a caregiver or to the larger family group of which she is a member.

For example, more impairment in the care-recipient generally means more difficulty in the caregiving task, but the correlation is far from perfect. Caregiving with a severely impaired spouse or parent may become doable with support and respite help from the nuclear and extended family. Functional limitations tend to cause less stress in the caregiver than cognitive loss. Especially if the relationship with the loved one has been important and valued, the loss of personhood that follows progressive dementia may become unbearable even when there are few significant physical problems. Moreover, cognitive impairment may increase significantly interpersonal conflict and turbulence. A woman with Alzheimer's Disease, cared for by her spouse, persistently split him into two distinct people with the same name. He never knew when he would be seen as the good Bud or the bad Bud. He might find himself given a warm welcome or treated with suspicion and distrust. He never knew what to expect by a wife he adored through many years of marriage. The stress of this situation, as well as other problems in caring for her seemed to be causative factors in his subsequent severe stroke.

Not all of the effects of caregiving are negative. Studies suggest that for some caregivers, who are mostly women, there may be a significant increase in feelings of mastery and competence. A wife expressed pride in herself for the 11 years she had devoted to her husband from the time he developed Alzheimer's Disease until his death. Other caregivers find that as a disease progresses, they lose a sense of competence. The problems of giving care seem to multiply, and despite their knowledge that they are fighting a losing battle, they feel that they are losing the war.

Caregiving may become very stressful for the adult who feels called on to care for a parent who has abused them. The worst of these situations are those in which a woman who was sexually abused is expected to give physical care to her father. Some women find that they cannot do it. Moreover, in dealing with the feelings which are stimulated by the necessary refusal, a daughter may come upon the unwelcome and very disturbing knowledge of sexual abuse about which she had been unaware. Or, if it has not been possible to disclose known abuse to spouse or siblings, there may be no way to avoid looking uncaring. Not understanding what is involved, a spouse or siblings may be very unsupportive and pressure the victim. Most of the stress of the foregoing has to do with giving physical care. If touching is not necessary, or can be done by others, caregiving may still be possible. Many such adult children are in conflict: their adult selves want to carry out filial responsibility, but their anger and hurt over childhood abuse demands expression as well.

FAMILY COUNSELING

Counseling families concerning problems associated with aging and the family relationship issues that come along with that focus has been mentioned previously in this chapter. Here I will give a more technical description of the process.

All family counseling and therapy begins with the joining process. During this beginning phase, the counselor is approached by someone, not necessarily a member of the family, who feels that there is problem that helping the family might alleviate. The task for the counselor is to be accepted by a family member as a source of help. If the family member is trusted and respected, she can act as a "gatekeeper" and admit the counselor into the private space of the family.

The counselor may then be able to hear the family definition of the problem, often noting that it may bear little resemblance to the description given by the referrer. As the information listed in Table 6.1 is gathered, a picture of this family begins to emerge. In an internal process similar to that of the anthropologist, the counselor tries to indicate her interest and respect for the family culture, making an effort to understand the family and its problem on their terms. She may learn that those outside of the family have misunderstood family concerns, seeing them as unwillingness to cooperate or expressing some form of psychopathology. Often that is a paradigm for dysfunctional interaction between a family and complex systems of health care, social welfare, or law. For example, in traditional, paternalistic families, a woman doctor may have a difficult time communicating with a family if she insists on talking only to a woman family member who is not a gatekeeper.

The counselor's task, at the outset, may be to act as interpreter between the family and the larger systems with which the family must interact. Having learned the language of the family, it may become possible to tell the family what they have been asked to do and to inform the outsiders how to frame their requests in a form that may result in it being heard. Often, the counselor may find himself acting as an advocate for the family, losing sight of his role as an extension of the outside and not as an agent of the family. The counselor then works at the boundary between the family and its surround.

At this point, there is little to differentiate this family counseling from others. Differences emerge in what follows. Counseling of families dealing with problems of aging most closely resembles what has been termed *medical family therapy* (MFT) (McDaniel, Hepworth, & Doherty, 1995; McDaniel, Hepworth, & Doherty, 1992). In MFT, the goals are to promote the capacity to manage a difficult situation or illness, often over the long term. And to "attend to the communication and emotional bonds that can be frayed by the challenges of pain and illness." Note that the counselor tries to make it possible to *externalize* the problem. This is the mirror image of behavioral family counseling, which tries to have the family *internalize* a behavioral problem that can be linked to the family's interaction patterns. In MFT, the counselor tries to discourage the family from taking inappropriate responsibility for problems not of their own making, directing attention outward to help devise better methods of coping with father's failing strength or mother's terminal illness. In behavioral family counseling, encouragement is given to look inward, to take as much responsibility as possible for ways in which the family relationships have created the circumstances for vulnerability and dysfunction.

The MFT approach is particularly suited to problems that arise at different stages of Alzheimer's Disease. We will focus on the first signs of the disease. In the earliest stage, it is very possible to attribute the changes in the afflicted family member to a variety of causes. Especially since a substantial portion of people who turn out later to have Alzheimer's Disease first present with personality and behavior changes that can be very troubling. A man noted for his equanimity becomes morose and nasty. A woman known as fastidious and cool becomes untidy, impulsive, and emotional. It is not unusual for these changes to be attributed to psychological or psychiatric causes. The family may feel blamed, not only by the family member, but in subtle ways by health care personnel.

When enough indication has appeared to suggest Alzheimer's or some related form of dementia, it is advisable to get a professional evaluation and a diagnosis. It is usually vital to have an evaluation so that members of the family can become convinced that it is a disease that has caused the changes. The accepted reality of a disease makes it much easier to see the problems not as part of normal aging and not susceptible to remediation by acts of will. The family often becomes active at this time, having become increasingly concerned about the changes in father and worried about the increasing stress on mother as she tries to conceal the problems and cope with them at the same time. This is when long-term issues between parent and adult child, between siblings or the extended family can be seen facilitating or blocking action. Many of the issues of relational ethics and of family structure can be seen quite clearly. Long-established family roles that have prescribed who is in and who is out, who is smart and who is not, who is competent and who is flaky can make their appearance (Globerman, 1995). This may be the first opportunity for the family to hear and realize that their own view of their family may be based so much on the past that dealing with the current problem is much more difficult than it could be. This may also be a time to begin to understand the family relational ethics and where they are with respect to filial responsibility.

The focus, however, is on making it possible to find out if this is a case of Alzheimer's Disease and to help the family to take concerted action that is consistent with their own manner of communication and their family culture so that they can use the experience not only to give care but for individual and family growth.

REFERENCES

Boszormenyi-Nagy, I., & Spark, G. M. (1973). *Invisible loyalties*. Hagerstown, MD: Harper & Row.

Boszormenyi-Nagy, I., & Ulrich, D. (1981). Contextual family therapy. In A. Gurman & D. Kniskern (Eds.), *Handbook of family therapy* (pp. 159–186). New York: Brunner/Mazel.

Coward, R. T., Horne, C., & Dwyer, J. W. (1992). Demographic perspectives on gender and family caregiving. In J. W. Dwyer & R. T. Coward (Ed.), *Gender and family care of the elderly* (pp. 18–33). Newbury Park, CA: Sage.

Fetters, M. D. (1998). The family in medical decision making: Japanese perspectives. *Journal of Clinical Ethics, 2,* 132–146.

Finley, N. (1989). Theories of family labor as applied to gender differences in caregiving for elderly parents. *Journal of Marriage and the Family, 51,* 79–86.

George, L. K., & Gwyther, L. P. (1986). Caregivers' well-being: A multidimensional examination of family caregivers of demented adults. *The Gerontologist, 26,* 253–259.

Globerman, J. (1995). Unencumbered child: Family reputations and responsibilities in the care of relatives with Alzheimer's Disease. *Family Process, 34,* 87–99.

Goodheart, C. D., & Lansing, M. H. (1997). *Treating people with chronic disease. The family and chronic illness* (pp. 141–154). Washington, DC: American Psychological Association.

McDaniel, S. H., Hepworth, J., & Doherty, W. J. (1995). Commentary: Medical family therapy with somaticizing patients: The co-creation of therapeutic stories. *Family Process, 34,* 349–361.

McDaniel, S. H., Hepworth, J., & Doherty, W. J. (1992). *Medical family therapy: A biopsychosocial approach to families with health problems.* New York: Basic Books.

Merrill, D. M. (1993). Daughters-in-law as caregivers to the elderly. *Research on Aging, 15,* 70–91.

Nelson, J. L. (1998). Reasons and Feeling, Duty and Dementia. *Journal of Clinical Ethics, 2,* 58–65.

Pruchno, R. A., Dempsey, N. P., Carder, P., & Koropeckyi-Cox, T. (1993). Multigenerational households of caregiving families: Negotiating shared space. *Environment and Behavior, 25,* 349–366.

Pruchno, R. A., Peters, N. D., & Burant, C. J. (1995). Mental health of coresident family caregivers: Examination of a two-factor model. *Journal of Gerontology, 50,* 247–256.

Sung, K. (1995). Measures and dimensions of filial piety in Korea. *The Gerontologist, 35,* 240–247.

Taylor, R., Ford, G., & Dunbar, M. (1995). The effects of caring on health: A community-based longitudinal study. *Social Science and Medicine, 40,* 1407–1415.

Tennstedt, S., Cafferata, G. L., & Sullivan, L. (1992). Depression among caregivers of impaired elders. *Journal of Aging and Health, 4,* 58–76.

Williamson, D. S., & Bray, J. H. (1991). Family development and change across the generations: An intergenerational perspective. In C. J. Falicov (Ed.), *Family transitions, continuity, and change over the life cycle* (pp. 357–384). New York: Guilford.

Yates, M. E., Tennstedt, S., & Chang, B. (1999). Contributors to and mediators of psychological well-being for informal caregivers. *Journal of Gerontology, 54,* 12–22.

PART II

Sociological Understandings of Aging

CHAPTER 7

Women's Issues in Aging

Diana Laskin Siegal

The 80-plus age group is the fastest growing age group, especially women. Currently every tenth person is an old woman. Getting old is a social concept, and our feelings about it may only be slightly related to the biological process of aging. By the year 2025 every seventh person will be an old woman. By the year 2040, 13 million people living in the United States will be over the age of 85, about 2.6 women to each man (Campion, 1994). Though the gap has closed slightly, women continue to live longer than men. These facts about the future number of old women must be considered by all policy and program makers.

WOMEN'S LONGEVITY

Why do women live so long? Speculations include the fact that women are less likely than men to engage in health endangering or life-shortening behaviors such as smoking, drinking excessive alcohol, fighting, and other aggressive behaviors. Some credit women's hormones with offering protection up until the time of menopause, but poor sanitation spreading communicable diseases and deaths in childbirth were the causes of young women dying before the twentieth century. Women who lived until menopause then lived long lives.

Anthropologists have begun to speculate about why women live so long past menopause. One theory proposed is that humans mature so slowly that they need a long-lived mother. Support for this theory is found in the fact that except for one species of whale, humans are the only female mammals who live a significant period of time past their ability to reproduce. Like the human child, the young of this type of whale does not attain maturity for many years and therefore requires many years of care.

Other speculations about why human females live so long past menopause include the need to transmit to later generations the accumulated knowledge on how to survive. In the past, for example, the ability of long-lived female food gatherers to sustain the population with a more dependable food source than provided by the male hunters continued past menopause (Angier, 1997; Raymo, 1998).

SEXISM PLUS AGEISM

Whatever the reasons for the longevity of women, modern United States society does not respect the aged person as much as other cultures do. So the sexism old women faced all their lives plus the additional barriers of ageism leave old women invisible and in need. These attitudes have also been rampant in the medical care system, which is, after all, part of and therefore influenced by the general society.

Fortunately, some changes have been made. After being excluded for many years, women were finally added to long-term studies such as the Baltimore Longitudinal Study on Aging and the Framingham Heart Study. At last, some consideration is being given to what the differences in female and male patterns can contribute to general knowledge about aging and to the special issues of each gender.

POVERTY

One major difference between old women and old men is that the women are more likely to be poor. Women make up nearly three quarters of the elderly poor. One quarter of all women over the age of 65 (including Hispanics) live in poverty, and the figure rises to 38% for African-American women. Half of all women collecting Social Security rely on it for at least 90% of their income compared with 29% for men (Doress-Worters & Siegal, 1994).

Women still earn only 71.1 cents to every dollar earned by men (Health and Medicine Policy Research Group, 1997). Also, twice as many women as men work part-time jobs, and only 15% of part-time employees pay into any pension system (Kaprielian, 1998). So the three-legged stool of savings, pensions, and Social Security, which was intended as security for retired persons, is very wobbly for women. The proposed fourth leg of retirement security is individual private investment. This option will be of no use to women who must use all their income merely to survive.

The major health problem of old women is poverty. While women have traditionally been adept at "stretching the dollar," they need more financial resources. In addition, women need assistance in financial planning for retirement. This is true even for younger and more affluent women (The National Center on Women and Aging, 1998).

ALONE OR LONELY—NOT THE SAME

Women are rich in one resource that encourages a long life—their relationships and attachments to the others. Contrary to the stereotype, women who have never married are as embedded in relationships and social networks as women who are presently or have been married. As women age, however, they are increasingly alone. The average age of widowhood in the United States is 56, and the average widow lives for 18 years after her husband's death. Overall, 46.3% of American women over age 65 were widows in 1997, down from 54.4% in 1970 (Schmid, 1998). The change occurred as men began living longer and as more couples divorced. In 1970, just 2.3% of elderly women were divorced; that figure is now 7.4%. The share of women over the age of 65 still living with their husbands has risen from 34 to 40% (Schmid, 1998) but among the very oldest group, only 10% live with husbands (Campion, 1994).

As women age, they still not only outlive their spouses, partners, and friends, but sometimes even their children. Senior housing, senior centers, and senior clubs are predominantly filled with women. Many of these women, according to the lyrics of an old song, "Make new friends and keep the old; One is silver and the other gold." By so doing, they support, help, and enrich each other's lives. Those who are unable or refuse to participate in such activities may become isolated in their homes. Even these women are often linked by frequent and long telephone calls to friends and family. In some towns, telephone lines are often busy on stormy or cold days as elderly persons chat to each other from the security of their homes.

MYTH OF FAMILY DESERTION

Contrary to myth, families have not abandoned elders. Middle-aged women, in particular, often care for elder family members in addition to their responsibilities for family, household work, and labor force participation. Thirty-seven percent of women over the age of 18 will care for elders and 31% will care for both children and elders at some point in their lives (Doress-Worters, 1994). Nationally, the value of time spent providing care to elderly parents has been estimated at $7 billion annually (Doress-Worters, 1996).

MYTH OF DEPENDENCY

Another common myth of aging is that old people are dependent on others because of their disabilities. In fact, the very elderly are staying free of serious disability to an older and older age. Some 70% of elderly widows lived by themselves in 1997, up from 56% in 1970. During the same period, the share of widowers living by themselves increased from 53% to 60% (Schmid, 1998). Women who are 85 years of age can expect that two thirds of their remaining years will be free of serious disability. However, nearly a third of the very elderly have some degree of dementia (Campion, 1994), so because there are more old women than men, more women than men will be afflicted with dementia.

When old women do need help, they depend on themselves, their children, their friends among other old women, and the network of social service agencies and health care facilities. Most of the employees of these services are other old women and new immigrant women paid low wages, thus perpetuating the cycles of poverty. Women are the primary users of long-term care services (Doress-Worters & Siegal, 1994).

WOMEN'S USE OF LONG-TERM CARE SERVICES

As budgets are cut and cost containment measures increased, many old women are losing services and do have not enough money to pay for needed services themselves. Shorter lengths of stay in hospitals, cuts in hospital discharge planning services and in home care services, and restrictions in nursing home placements to contain rising Medicaid costs are endangering frail elderly persons who are most vulnerable. Because so many women are alone, 13% of women will reside in nursing homes for 5 years or more, compared with 4% of men (Agency for Health Care Policy and Research [AHCPR], 1998). One quarter of all women over the age of 84 live in nursing homes compared to only 15% of men in that age group (Campion, 1994). As the number of old women increases, the needs for services will increase also.

HEALTH PROBLEMS OF OLD WOMEN

The leading cause of death for women under age 75 remains cancer, with heart disease second. In spite of new reports casting more doubt on their effectiveness to prevent heart disease (Reuters, 1998), drug companies continue to promote hormones to women in their forties and fifties on the grounds that heart disease is the number one killer without reference to age.

Past the age of 75, heart disease is the leading cause at a rate almost 2.5 times that of cancer. Stroke is the third cause in both groups. Some research suggests a link between strokes and Alzheimer's Disease (The Boston Women's Health Book Collective, 1998). Methods to prevent or reduce the incidence of heart disease and stroke are known but not necessarily prescribed or even encouraged by physicians; namely reducing smoking, high blood pressure, high blood cholesterol, diabetes, obesity, and physical inactivity. These risk factors are interrelated. Women who are very overweight are at greater risk for developing high blood pressure (Doress-Worters & Siegal, 1994).

Women are more likely to die of heart attacks and after bypass surgery and angioplasty than men even when women's older ages than men at the time of illness are considered. In one large study that matched women and men with identical risk factors, more women died, sometimes twice as often as men (AHCPR, 1998; Associated Press, 1998).

Other serious and often overlooked causes of death and disability include hip fractures in White women over the age of 85 and death from residential fires among persons over the age of 65. In both instances, lifelong education about injury prevention, safety measures, and the importance of lifestyle factors such as smoking and healthful nutrition and activity will reduce deaths and injuries.

AGEISM AND SEXISM IN THE MEDICAL CARE SYSTEM

The difficulties in changing physician behaviors are illustrated by one large study in which the interventions designed to change behaviors failed. These interventions, including semiannual reports to the physicians of their behaviors and even financial incentives, did not increase physicians' compliance with cancer screening guidelines and for older women in a Medicaid HMO (AHCPR, 1998). One is forced to conclude that age, gender, class, and racial stereotypes prevailed over recommended medical behavior.

Though elderly persons are supposed to be included in studies of new drugs, the distinctions between old women and old men are still not always made. Complaints from past years about the high rate of inappropriate psychoactive prescription drugs given to women persist. A recent study reported that 11% of women over the age of 59 are addicted to such drugs and concluded that half the prescriptions for tranquilizers and sleeping pills should not have been given (The National Center for Addictions and Substance Abuse at Columbia University [CASA], 1998). These drugs also contribute to falls, leading to hip fractures among old women.

Mental health and substance abuse problems are often overlooked among elderly persons. Eighty percent of the physicians in the same study reported above diagnosed symptoms of alcohol abuse as depression (CASA, 1998). Appropriate treatment for depression among elderly persons is not always available or utilized. Staff in mental health centers and psychiatric services may not be trained to assist elderly persons.

Data collection, though improved, continues to reflect the ageist and sexist views of society. For example, though possibly available, data was not distributed at a major women's health conference on condom use at last sexual intercourse in females past age 44 or on rape and attempted rape of women past age 34, and no breakdowns were given by age groups for data on domestic violence against women reported at emergency room visits (Center for Disease Control [CDC]/National Center for Health Statistics [NCHS], 1998). Their omission reinforces the inaccurate myths that older women are not sexually active and are not victims of abuse and violence. The lack of these statistics also hides the sexually transmitted disease rates (including HIV/AIDS) among older women (Siegal, 1996; Siegal & Burke, 1997).

RECENT PROGRESS

The major discovery of the past two decades has been understanding the importance of lifelong physical activity and fitness, especially continuing or even starting in the later years. This is important news for women now in old age who were not generally encouraged to be physically active in their younger years. Many women who are now old were brought up believing that "ladies don't sweat" and need encouragement to try new activities. A balanced program including flexibility, postural improvement, aerobic, and muscle-strengthening activities will improve both quantity and quality of life (Doress-Worters & Siegal, 1994).

While we do see instances of overexercising in some young women, generally the trend to encourage activity is a very positive one, with benefits including strong muscles and bones, healthy hearts, and reduced likelihood of diabetes (Doress-Worters & Siegal, 1994). Women need strength to continue their personal and household care and the activities that give them pleasure. In designing fitness programs, the differences between women's and men's bodies must, however, be taken into consideration to avoid injury.

NEED FOR KNOWLEDGE ABOUT AGING

Knowledge and training about elderly persons in general and old women in particular are needed in many professional fields. The number of gerontologists and geriatricians is increasing, though not fast enough to meet the needs of the aging population. Even among gerontologists and geriatricians, many authors of books and journal articles lump all the aged together without making distinctions between women and men or among various racial, ethnic, or economic groups or different stages of aging. The United States is becoming more diverse, and such diversity must be considered in establishing appropriate policies, programs, and training. For example, by the year 2030, half the women in the United States will be women of color, who are poorer and receive medical care later in the course of their diseases than the average (CDC/NCHS, 1998).

WOMEN AS ADVOCATES FOR THEMSELVES

While elder advocacy groups continue to be a powerful and active voice for elderly persons in general, women are increasingly effective in advocating for their needs. Many women's organizations continue to confront income disparities, and breast cancer advocacy groups have succeeded in increasing funds for research, detection, and treatment of this disease.

OWL, The Voice of Midlife and Older Women, was organized because older women faced greater challenges and problems than older men. OWL has effectively changed pension rights for women, raised consciousness on many issues including violence against older women, and continues to issue an invaluable Mother's Day Report on an important topic each year.

A chapter on women and aging must highlight the strengths of old women as well as reciting the problems they face. Old women have seen and survived much. They often shake off many of the restrictions society imposed in the past and the many that continue today. They often become more confident and outspoken than they were when they were young.

Examples of activity and creativity of old women abound. Readers should look, for example, for "Crossing the Threshold," an exhibit of 31 women artists ages 70 to 105 who are or have worked throughout the twentieth century. This exhibit, organized by the Steinbaum Krauss Gallery in New York, is touring the United States from December 1997 to December 2000.

REFERENCES

Agency for Health Care Policy and Research (1998). *Women's health highlights (Newsletter), February 4,* p. 12.

Angier, N. (1997, September 16). Theorists see evolutionary advantages in menopause. *The New York Times,* pp. C1, C8.

Associated Press (1998, July 30). Heart bypass surgery risk found greater for women. *The Boston Globe,* p. A3.

The Boston Women's Health Book Collective (1998). *Our bodies ourselves for the new century.* New York: Simon & Schuster.

Campion, E. W. (1994). The Oldest Old. *New England Journal of Medicine, 330,* 1819–1820.

Center for Disease Control/National Center for Health Statistics. (1998, May 20). Data distributed at the conference on Healthy People 2000: Women's Health Progress Review, Boston, MA.

Doress-Worters, P. B. (1994). Adding elder care to women's multiple roles: A critical review of the caregiver stress and multiple roles literature. *Sex Roles, 31,* 597–616.

Doress-Worters, P. B. (1996). Choices and chances: How a profit-driven health care system discriminates against middle-aged women. In M. B. Lykes (Ed.), *Myths about the powerless: Contesting social inequalities* (pp. 201–218). Philadelphia: Temple University Press.

Doress-Worters, P. B., & Siegal, D. L. (1994). *The new ourselves, growing older: Women aging with knowledge and power.* New York: Simon & Schuster.

Health and Medicine Policy Research Group (1997). *Women's health: A New England profile.* U.S. Department of Health and Human Services. Washington, DC.

Kaprielian, R. (1998, July 16). Women are more likely than men to face poverty in retirement. *The Boston Globe*, p. A19.

The National Center on Women and Aging (1998). *Financial challenges for mature women: Creating financial plans and evaluating financial planners.* Waltham, MA: Heller Graduate School, Brandeis University.

The National Center on Addiction and Substance Abuse at Columbia University. (1998). *Under the rug: Substance abuse and the mature woman.* Washington, DC: The National Council on Patient Information and Education (NCPIE).

Raymo, C. (1998, June 22). Whatever are grandmothers for? *The Boston Globe*, pp. D2.

Reuters (1998, August 19). Hormone hopes dashed: No benefit Found for heart attacks. *The Boston Globe*, p. A15.

Schmid, R. E., (1998, August 27). Older women staying independent longer. (Figures quoted from the Census Bureau) *Marital status and living arrangements, Senior Advocate (Newsletter), 24,* p. 4.

Siegal, D. L. (1996). This could save your life: What all midlife and older women need to know about HIV/AIDS. *Women's initiative fact sheet.* Washington, DC: American Association of Retired Persons.

Siegal, D. L., & Burke, C. (1997). Midlife and older women and HIV/AIDS: My (grand) mother wouldn't do that. In N. Goldstein & J. L. Marlowe (Eds.), *The gender politics of HIV/AIDS in women: Perspectives on the pandemic in the United States* (pp. 155–167). New York: New York University Press.

CHAPTER 8

Understanding and Planning for Retirement

Raymond Bossé

W hy do we need to understand and plan for retirement? Because after death and taxes, retirement is a life event most adults in industrialized nations are likely to experience. In fact, during the twentieth century the trend has been toward increasingly earlier withdrawal from the workforce on the part of men, while workforce participation on the part of women has remained fairly constant. In 1890, for instance, 73.8% of men aged 65+ were in the workforce and 8.3% of women of that age. Forty years later, in 1930, at the outset of the great depression, the percentages had dropped to 58.3% for men and remained at 8.0% for women. By 1960, the percentage of men remaining in the workforce at age 65+ declined to 30.6%, to 16.4% by 1990, and is projected to decline to 14.4% by the year 2005. The number of retirement-age women working during those same years was 10.4% in 1960, 8.7% in 1990, and is projected at 8.8% for 2005 (Jacobs, Kohli, & Rein, 1991; U.S. Bureau of Labor Statistics, 1995). Considering that roughly 85% of men and 90% of women aged 65+ are currently out of the workforce, it is safe to say that retirement is a life event experienced by the vast majority in later life.

UNDERSTANDING RETIREMENT

Defining Retirement

As simple and straightforward as defining retirement may seem, there is no unanimously accepted definition. Any one or a combination of five criteria have been used to identify someone as retired:

1. Having separated from one's "career";
2. Exited the labor force;
3. Receiving a pension;
4. Giving a reduced effort;
5. Considering oneself retired.

Theoretically, although a person who ascribes to one or several of the above may be viewed as retired by some, the concrete reality may be more complex and subject to considerable debate. Consider the person who leaves a lifelong career, receives a pension, and returns to a full-time job. This person could be 70 or older and also receive Social Security benefits. It has been reported that 20% of retirees receiving a pension or Social Security also work part-time for 40 to 52 hours per week. Some retirement experts define someone as retired when they receive a pension, have a reduced work effort, and consider themselves retired (Ekerdt & DeViney, 1990).

Reasons for Retirement

Equally important to understanding retirement is the reason why someone retired. The success or failure of the retirement experience begins with its circumstances, what motivated or initiated the event (Bossé, Spiro, & Kressin, 1996). There is a tendency for people to think that workers retire simply because they have reached the retirement age of 62, 65, or 70. As with defining retirement, the reason why someone retires may be considerably more complex than the stereotypic view that people retire because they have reached retirement age. Nevertheless, it is important to understand the reason someone retired because whether a retiree is stressed, unhappy, delighted, healthy, or sick may depend to a great extent on what led to the retirement. In their study of retirement among some

2000 men participating in the Normative Aging Study (NAS), a longitudinal study of aging at the Veterans Administration (VA) Outpatient Clinic, Boston, I and my colleagues specifically researched the reasons for retirement. (For a description of the NAS see Bossé, Ekerdt, & Silbert, 1984). Participants in the study were asked to indicate in their own words the principal reason they retired. The hundreds of reasons indicated were summarized into 39 specific reasons grouped into subsets under three major reasons: health, negative reasons, and positive reasons as shown in Figure 8.1.

It should be added that although specific reasons for retirement have been enumerated, individuals may retire for several reasons simultaneously, both positive and negative. As will be seen later, it became very important in the course of the NAS research program at the VA to know the reason for retirement. The success or failure of retirement is not only a financial matter as many believe. Equally important is how people view the retirement, how they plan for it, and why they retire. All aspects of a retiree's life, physical, and emotional health as well as marital and family relations, may be affected by the reason he or she retired (Bossé et al., 1996). In subsequent research, the reason for retirement became one of the principal factors explaining whether the retirement was stressful and consequently if the retiree was found to be physically and emotionally healthy.

PLANNING FOR RETIREMENT

Two issues will be raised in this section. Part A deals with the importance of planning for retirement, including issues most relevant to plan for and a list of specific dos and don'ts. Part B reviews mostly published results of the NAS research relative to retirement such as: Do people plan for retirement? How accurate are people's plans? How do preretirement plans for activities in retirement match up with reality after retirement?

Theoretical Perspective

The popular tendency is to think that planning for retirement has to do with finances. There is no doubt that finances may well be

124   *Sociological Understandings*

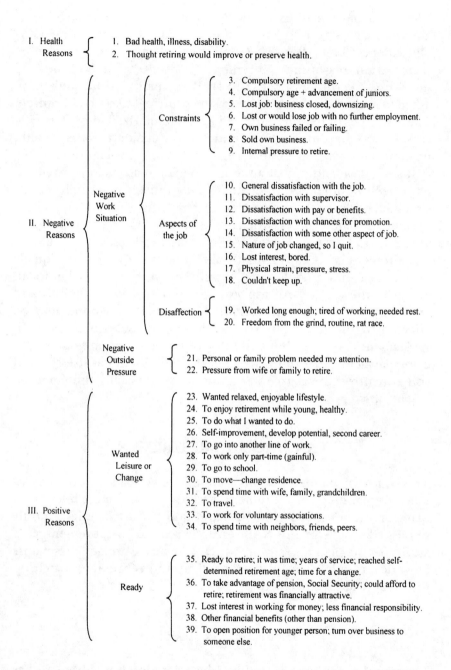

FIGURE 8.1.

the most important issue in planning for a successful retirement. However, even with the best possible financial planning, other factors can sour the experience if not attended to.

Of the many factors one should pay attention to, 10 are of particular significance and should be viewed as musts in the planning process. Of course the opposite of each must is a mistake to be avoided:

1. Begin planning at least a year before the event.
2. Attend a preretirement seminar.
3. Keep your retirement plans confidential. This allows you to change your mind if plans change.
4. Discuss your plans with your spouse so both of your interests can be preserved in your new lifestyle.
5. Learn the facts of the possible retirement options in your company.
6. Review your life and health insurance needs and figure the costs as you decide which policies to take with you into retirement if applicable.
7. Do not relocate for at least a year after retirement. This helps to make a wise decision. It also helps to visit or vacation in any new location before finalizing plans.
8. Take advantage of the various savings plans available to you. Save the maximum you can even if only for a year or less.
9. Take a financial inventory and budget for unexpected expenses like increasing college tuition for your children or for medical expenses.
10. Take advantage of all the retirement information provided by your employer.

Hopefully the preceding list helps to illustrate the fact that there is more to retirement planning than finances. Although it is important to underscore that fact, it is just as important not to neglect financial planning as is also apparent from the number of items that refer to finances in the 10 musts list.

The Reality

How well do people plan? Having examined the various aspects of retirement planning, it has been very informative to explore just how well and how accurate people are about their plans and expectations for retirement. This is a domain that has been studied to a certain extent in retirement research.

Preferred, Expected, and Actual Age of Retirement

In the opening paragraph of this chapter it was shown that there has been a tendency for workers in the United States to retire at earlier and earlier ages. This is a fascinating phenomenon when compared with workers' responses to questions about preferred and expected age of retirement and with the actual age of retirement on the part of retirees.

Ekerdt, Bossé, and Mogey (1980) asked a panel of over 900 men who ranged in age from 35 to 64 "On a realistic basis, at what age to you expect to retire?" Then they were asked, "At what age would you prefer to retire?" Ten years later the same respondents were asked the same questions. The youngest cohort aged 35 to 39 at time 1 and 45 to 49 at time 2 preferred to retire at the youngest age of all cohorts (about 57) at both times. In all of the other cohorts the respondents increased or retarded the age at which they would prefer to retire as they got older. The wishful thinking of the youngest ages turned to realism at older ages so that the two oldest cohorts realistically preferred to retire between 63 and 68 at time 2.

When the researchers examined the age at which cohorts expected to retire, they found the two youngest cohorts expected to retire earlier over time, the oldest cohort expected to retire later, and the two middle cohorts showed no change. Again the younger workers may be idealistic and the oldest realistic. Interestingly, when the preferred and expected retirement ages were plotted together they drew closer and closer together from the youngest to the oldest cohort. So even though the men in the study generally preferred to retire sooner than they planned to, preferences were revised upward over time and tended to converge with the expected age for withdrawal from work. The data appear to suggest that as men drew nearer to retirement their preferences tended to converge with the expected age for withdrawal from work, and thereby, to coincide with the normative expectations of society.

To examine this question more specifically, Ekerdt, Vinick, and Bossé (1989) examined whether men really know when they will retire. The respondents were asked in 1978, 1981, and 1984 to give the year and month they planned or expected to retire. Some were retired by 1981, others by 1984. Over the course of the study, 66% of the workers accurately predicted their retirement date to within 1 year; 40% were accurate to within 3 months; one third were very inaccurate by retiring much earlier, later, or not at all.

Having 66% predict accurately appears impressive at first glance because of the span of time between the prediction and the actual event. However, retirement is seen as a normative life cycle event occurring at the specific ages of 62, 65, or 70. In that regard, the predictability of retirement based on this study leaves much to be desired. From a practical perspective, this can cause problems for institutions, agencies, or groups attempting to target specific populations with preretirement information, efficient planning for employee replacements, pension withdrawals, or even to identify potential candidates for pre- and postretirement studies.

Evidence of Preparation for Retirement

Retirement has traditionally been thought of as a process that includes pre- and postretirement socialization (Rosow, 1974). Very little research has been undertaken, however, into the preretirement process. Evans, Ekerdt, and Bossé (1985) did test the hypothesis that retirement-oriented activities increase with proximity to retirement. They addressed two research questions: (1) What is the relationship between retirement proximity and preretirement involvement behaviors? and (2) How might retirement involvement levels be further affected by attitude toward retirement, job characteristics, and personal resources?

They found a consistent rise in retirement-oriented behavior as retirement drew nearer. This behavior included reading about retirement and talking about it with wife, relatives, friends and coworkers. Chronological age, by contrast, was not found to be significantly related to preretirement involvement. Interestingly, the increase in preretirement involvement was found to apply whether respondents looked forward to retirement or not, were satisfied or dissatisfied with their job, and whether or not a friend preceded them into retirement. Clearly the findings confirm the hypothesis that a process of anticipating retirement in underway among older male workers as much as 15 years before retirement.

In a follow-up study, Ekerdt and DeViney (1993) explored the hypothesis that men's attitudes toward their job would become progressively more negative as they approached retirement. They used four waves of data extending over 9 years (1978–1987) in a panel of 1365 nonretired workers aged 50 to 69. Results of the study showed that, having controlled for age, as the men approached retirement they evaluated their jobs as more burdensome and reported feeling more nervous and tired at the end of a working day. As workers remain on the job they gain experience, competence, skills, greater knowledge of procedures, increased pay, and other rewards. Nevertheless, anticipated "time-left" in the labor force adds a new dimension to a worker's perspective, influenced by others who are also aware of the impending approach of retirement.

The shift in consciousness from time-in-state to time-left is seen as further support for a preretirement process. In this case, proximity to retirement, a generally normative and even mandatory life event, prompts a reappraisal of work. In a work-oriented society, a life of leisure as is anticipated for retirement can prompt feelings of guilt. Possibly one way these guilt feelings are being handled is through what has been labeled the "busy ethic" of many retirees who report never finding enough time to do all the things that need to be done on a daily basis (Ekerdt, 1986). Still another way of calming feelings of guilt in our strong "Protestant Work Ethic" society may be in the expressed conviction of workers close to retirement that withdrawal from the workforce became necessary due to the fatigue, stress, burdensomeness of work, and its impending ill effect on physical and emotional health.

Planning for Leisure Activities in Retirement

With the approach of retirement, workers have been found to be optimistic about the time they will spend on leisure activities (Bossé & Ekerdt, 1981). In their plans for retirement, workers within 3 years of retirement significantly overestimated their levels of physical, social, and cultural activities in retirement. Only the level of solitary activities was correctly estimated based on responses to actual levels of these activities after the respondents had retired. Probably the most outstanding longitudinal finding in this study of change in leisure activities with retirement was continuity. In short, when the workers had retired their levels of social, solitary, physical, and cultural activities tended to resemble their preretirement levels.

Possibly as we grow older along with reaching retirement age, we feel more secure and comfortable with what have been lifelong preferences. One may wonder, therefore, how retirees use the 40 or more hours a week that used to be work time. Although this may be somewhat speculative, there is considerable evidence to suggest that the time is used in what are called "maintenance" activities, that is, all those projects that were postponed due to prior work demands (Kabanoff, 1980). This "busyness," which on the one hand is real and reasonable, may also fulfill the suggested need to ease the sense of guilt and provide justification for a life of leisure in our work-oriented society.

Phases in Adaptation to Retirement

The research just reviewed provided support for a preretirement process. The question arises as to a continuing process into retirement. In answering that question, Atchley (1976) offered a theoretical framework that included several phases of retirement adaptation. The initial phase hypothesized by Atchley was a busy, euphoric, honeymoon phase, perhaps followed by a letdown or disenchantment phase, and eventually a stability phase with the settling into a satisfying routine. Though no evidence was provided, Atchley's scheme provided an incentive for research. Although many other studies have explored Atchley's proposed model, there have been no consistent findings. And certainly no findings resembling Atchley's model. Ekerdt, Bossé, and Levkoff (1985) thought that an answer to the issue of postretirement phases would be beneficial to retirees, retirement counselors, and others engaged in issues related to the retirement years.

Using retirees from the NAS described earlier, the authors compared level of life satisfaction and of leisure activities across a 6-month time interval within the first 3 years of retirement. Findings showed that recent retires, 0 to 6 months, showed greater optimism, life satisfaction, and future orientation than men retired 13 to 18 months, who, in addition, also reported lesser amounts of involvement in physical activities. The pattern varied again for men retired 19 months or more.

Though the findings cannot be seen as confirming Atchley's broad, sweeping model, it may be seen as providing partial support for an early euphoric state followed by a temporary letdown or dysphoria during the second year of retirement. It should be noted that the Ekerdt, Bosse, and Levkoff study was cross-sectional. Given possible cohort or generational differences in retirement adaptation, these findings would need to be confirmed by longitudinal analyses in the same or other populations.

CONCLUSION

The two components of this chapter, understanding and planning for retirement, are two very distinct entities. To understand retirement it is necessary to consider its various complexities. The first complexity is the fact that retirement itself means something so different for different retirees that it is almost impossible to define retirement. There are many combinations of full-time and part-time work after retirement, a great variety of private and public pensions, many different reasons why people retired to begin with, a diversity of retirement ages, and hence a plethora of lifestyles or ways of experiencing retirement. Nevertheless, recognizing the complexities of retirement is a first step toward understanding it, and we can only hope that the first part of this chapter accomplished that.

Much attention is directed today to the issue of planning for retirement. The vast majority of the literature concerns financial planning, with an infinite number of ideas about 401K plans, annuities, and individual retirement accounts. This is all quite positive and may even be partly responsible for the observations made in this chapter to the effect that people approaching retirement give ample evidence of thinking about the impending event.

This was seen in the fact that respondents to retirement questionnaires give evidence of having definite ideas about their preferred and expected ages for retirement, about the specific date when they plan to retire, and about planned leisure activities in retirement. It was also shown that as workers approached retirement they reported thinking, reading, and talking more about it. The evidence in the second part of this chapter suggested that since the mid-1930s, when Social Security was initiated, retirement became not only a financial possibility but an expected life event. Within the next few years, workers began retiring not only when they reached mandatory retirement age, but as soon as possible. Now it appears that retirement is clearly a normative life event. We should, therefore, not be surprised to learn that as workers approach retirement there is increased evidence of their planning for it. We can only expect that planning for the inevitable event will even increase in the near future as we are constantly reminded of the disastrous impact the baby boom generation is predicted to have on the Social Security system when it reaches retirement age unless Congress takes action to modify the system.

The reader may have noticed the absence of gender differences in this chapter. One reason for this is that for many sections of the chapter there are no anticipated gender differences, as in the need to plan for retirement, Social Security Earnings Test and others. On the other hand, clear differences could be expected in research findings relative to preferred and expected age for retirement, plans for leisure activities, and phases of retirement adaptation. Retirement research, however, has only recently begun to focus on women as well as men. The main reason for this may be historic in that women tended not to have had a continuous work experience. They entered the labor force after their schooling, withdrew during child bearing and rearing years, then sometimes reentered after the empty nest. Since the 1950s, however, women began to maintain their workforce participation. Now retirement research is reflecting this in increasing numbers of studies that focus on women as well as men. Much of this recent research may be found in Szinovacz (1986–1987), in Szinovacz, Ekerdt, and Vinick (1992), and in Szinovacz (1993).

REFERENCES

Atchley, R. D. (1976). *The sociology of retirement.* New York: Halsted Press.

Bossé, R., & Ekerdt, D. J. (1981). Change in self-perception of leisure activities with retirement. *The Gerontologist, 21,* 650–654.

Bossé, R., Ekerdt, D. J., & Silbert, J. E. (1984). The Veterans Administration Normative Aging Study. In S. A. Mednick, M. Harway, & K. M. Finello (Eds.), *Handbook of longitudinal research: Teenage and adult cohorts* (pp. 273–283). New York: Praeger.

Bossé, R., Spiro, A. III, & Kressin, N. R. (1996). The psychology of retirement. In R. T. Woods (Ed.), *Handbook of the clinical psychology of aging* (pp. 141–157). London: John Wiley & Sons.

Ekerdt, D. J. (1986). The busy ethic: Moral continuity between work and retirement. *The Gerontologist, 26,* 239–244.

Ekerdt, D. J., Bossé, R., & Levkoff, S. (1985). An empirical test for phases of retirement: Findings from the Normative Aging Study. *Journal of Gerontology, 40,* 95–101.

Ekerdt, D. J., Bossé, R., & Mogey, J. M. (1980). Concurrent change in planned and preferred age for retirement. *Journal of Gerontology, 35,* 232–240.

Ekerdt, D. J., & DeViney, S. (1990). On defining persons as retired. *Journal of Aging Studies, 4,* 211–229.

Ekerdt, D. J., & DeViney, S. (1993). Evidence for a pre-retirement process among older male workers. *Journal of Gerontology, 48,* 35–43.

Ekerdt, D. J., Vinick, B. H., & Bossé, R. (1989). Orderly endings: Do men know when they will retire? *Journal of Gerontology, 44,* 28–35.

Evans, L., Ekerdt, D. J., & Bossé, R. (1985). Proximity to retirement and anticipatory involvement: Findings from the Normative Aging Study. *Journal of Gerontology, 40,* 368–374.

Jacobs, K., Kohli, M., & Rein, M. (1991). The evolution of early exit: A comparative analysis of labor force participation patterns. In M. Kohli, M. Rein, A. M. Guillemard, & H. VanGunsteren (Eds.), *Time for retirement* (pp. 36–66). New York: Cambridge University Press.

Kabanoff, B. (1980). Work and non-work: A review of models, methods, and findings. *Psychological Bulletin, 88,* 60–77.

Rosow, I. (1974). *Socialization to old age.* Berkeley, CA: University of California Press.

Szinovacz, M. E. (1986–1987). Preferred retirement timing and retirement satisfaction in women. *International Journal of Aging and Human Development, 24,* 301–317.

Szinovacz, M. (1993). *Couples' work/retirement patterns and marital relationships.* Summary of findings of a project funded by the American Association of Retired Persons [AARP]—Andrus Foundation. Washington, DC.

Szinovacz, M. E., Ekerdt, D. J., & Vinick, B. H. (1992). *Families in retirement.* Newbury Park, CA: Sage.

U.S. Bureau of Labor Statistics, *Bulletin 2307* (1995).

CHAPTER 9

Issues in Rural Aging

Patricia Flynn Weitzman, Yeon Kyung Chee, and Sue E. Levkoff

A pproximately one in four older persons in America lives in a small town or rural community (Clifford & Lilley, 1993). With the aging of the baby boomers, this number will grow (although by a smaller percentage than it will for nonrural elders). The prototypical rural elder is a married, White female who possesses less than a twelfth-grade education, and lives in substandard housing (Scheidt & Norris-Baker, 1990). Rural elders are, on average, more likely to be poor than their nonrural counterparts, with roughly 27% living in poverty compared to 19% of nonrural elders (cf. Clifford & Lilley, 1993). Greater awareness on the part of gerontologists and health service providers of the dramatic ways in which context can affect health and aging has simultaneously raised awareness of the special health needs of rural elders.

Key issues with regard to the health of rural elders fall into four broad categories: physical and mental health, social support, housing, and service delivery. Although these issues are similar to those that shape the health of nonrural elders, rural status impacts them in unique ways. In this chapter, we present an overview of the interplay of rural status with each of these issues, and outline some of the solutions that have been called for by health services providers and researchers to deal with attendant problems.

PHYSICAL AND MENTAL HEALTH

Although we know of no studies that suggest that there are major differences between the types of illnesses prevalent among rural elders and nonrural elders, several studies do suggest that there may be differences in the course that illness takes for rural elders. To start with, individuals residing in rural areas enter old age with relatively poorer health than nonrural individuals, and this difference holds across all racial and gender categories (Clifford & Lilley, 1993). Rural elders have more chronic conditions than do nonrural elders and are more likely to die prematurely from those conditions (Sennott-Miller, May, & Miller, 1998). They are also more likely to suffer from nutritional deficiencies due to meal skipping, which puts them at greater risk for complications arising from diabetes and hypertension, and can weaken immune system responses (Lee, Templeton, & Wang, 1995). A significantly higher rate of alcoholism is seen in rural elders (Richardson, 1988) which not only creates its own set of symptoms, but also affects the course of concurrent chronic illnesses.

Studies of depression in rural populations show conflicting findings, with some suggesting higher rates of depression among rural elderly persons (Chalifoux, Neese, Buckwalter, & Litwak, 1996; Johnson & Booth, 1990) and other studies finding no differences (Johnson et al., 1988; Ortega, Metroka, & Johnson, 1993). It is clear that all elderly persons are particularly vulnerable to secondary depressions, whose etiologies include chronic and terminal old-age illnesses such as cancer and stroke (Buckwalter, Smith, & Caston, 1994). This fact would suggest that rural elders are, indeed, more likely to experience higher rates of depression due to the evidence that rural elders have higher morbidity rates in general.

Furthermore, social support in old age is a key to good mental health (Antonucci, Fuhrer, & Dartigues, 1997). Hessler and his colleagues have shown that participation in formal social networks may be closely linked to mortality in rural elders, with those who access formal social supports having lower mortality rates (Hessler, Jia,

Madsen, & Pazaki, 1995). Most of the current generation of rural young adults flee to more populated areas offering greater job opportunities. The result of this flight is that the adult children of the current generation of rural elders are likely to live far from their parents and are thus less able to provide social and tangible support to their parents than the adult children of nonrural elders (Clifford & Lilley, 1993). Furthermore, as we will discuss later, a cultural value of self-reliance that is common in rural areas can cause elders to resist support services (Smith & Buckwalter, 1993), as can transportation barriers. Taken together, these factors would suggest that rural elders are, indeed, more likely than nonrural elders to suffer from depression. Conflicting research findings with regard to depression might be explained by differing sensitivity of measurement instruments, and differences between farm family and nonfarm family elders such that farm family elders report their physical and mental health to be better than nonfarm family elders (Ortega et al., 1993). It may be important to distinguish differing characteristics of rural elders, farm versus nonfarm, and those residing in rural towns versus those residing in more isolated areas, to better understand the epidemiology of depression in rural areas.

SOCIAL SUPPORT

Geographic distance between rural elders and their family members and between rural elders and other members of their communities is a major factor in the quality of their social support. Even for African-American rural elders, who generally have a larger, more diverse group of family members on whom they can call for support than White rural elders (Kivett, 1993), there is a decrease in intergenerational exchanges as geographic distance increases (Kivett, 1991). More than 50% of Native Americans live in rural areas, even though they constitute the smallest rural elder minority group (cf. Kivett, 1993). Like other groups of rural young adults, Native American young adults have begun to move away from rural areas, which has diminished the family-based social supports traditionally available to older Native Americans (John, 1985). Asian and Latino rural elders, groups which are relatively small in number compared to White and African-American rural elders, have similarly been affected by migration patterns of young adults. A further complication to the access of social support for minority rural elders is a lack of ethnically based social services, which are more widely available to nonrural minority elders, especially those living in the inner-cities. In general, community support services for rural elders are rare relative to nonrural elders (Russell, Cutrona, de la Mora, & Wallace, 1997), and may be a significant predictor of higher mortality rates (Hessler et al., 1995). Cooperation among churches, county extension agencies, area agencies on aging, area health education centers, and other local organizations can help remove barriers to support services for rural elders.

Another factor that may affect the efficacy of social support networks for rural elders has to do with reciprocity. In a study of social relationships and health of rural elders, Craig (1994) showed that reciprocity was key to the acceptance by rural elders of social and material support from nonfamily sources, that is, the community at large. In other words, as long as elders felt that they were able to offer something back to the community in exchange for the support they were to receive, they were more likely to accept it.

An alternative aspect of the social support deficit picture is the fact that rural elders are more likely to have a marital partner than their same-age nonrural peers (Coward, Lee, & Dwyer, 1993). From 59 to 70% of rural elders are married, compared to 53 to 56% of urban/suburban elders, and 48% of elders living in the inner-city (Coward, Cutler, & Schmidt, 1988). A recent study of the impact of marriage on the health of elders shows that marriage improves the odds that elders will engage in positive health behaviors, such as eating breakfast, wearing seat belts, and not smoking (Schone & Weinick, 1998). Dugan and Kivett (1994) studied the social supports of rural elders and found that emotional isolation (e.g., the lack of a confidant or spouse) was significantly associated with loneliness and depression, whereas social isolation (e.g., infrequent visits and phone conversations with friends and family) was not. These studies collectively suggest that, as a result of their married status, rural elders may have an advantage over nonrural elders, either directly through the better health behaviors that marriage may engender or indirectly through improved emotional support. It should be noted, however, that rural women may benefit most from the advantages brought by marriage because there are fewer rural/urban differences between the percentages of older men who are married compared to the large rural/urban differences between percentages of older women who are married (Coward et al., 1993).

HOUSING

As stated in the introduction, about 27% of rural elders live in poverty, compared to 19% of nonrural elders. For minority elders living in rural areas, poverty rates may be even higher than for their nonminority neighbors (Belden, 1993; Ralston, 1993). For example, according to the 1990 census, African-American elderly women living alone in a rural area had a poverty rate of 70%, which is the highest rate for any population subgroup (cf. Belden, 1993). A direct result of the impoverished status of most rural elders is that they live in poorer quality housing than nonrural elders. One reason for this is that there are fewer alternative housing options available to them, such as apartments, housing projects, or intermediate care facilities. Aging in place, while generally viewed as a desirable option by elders and gerontologists, may, for some rural elders who would like to relocate, be a burden rather than a choice. The flight of young adults from rural areas means there is less demand for housing, which provides rural elders with less opportunity to sell their homes so they can relocate. Relocating to more elder-friendly accommodations may simply not be an option for many rural elders because of insufficient income to move, the out-migration of younger citizens, or a lack of alternative housing in their area.

Belden (1993) reports that funding in 1992 for all federal rural housing programs was only at about one third of the constant dollar levels of 1980. While programs such as the Farmers Home Administration finance rural elder housing and repair programs, they are of limited value because they have fewer federal dollars to lend out. State housing programs also exist that attempt to help rural elders find and develop shared living arrangements, but many rural elders prefer to live in a manner that allows for privacy and independence (Scheidt & Norris-Baker, 1990). Housing assistance programs are also widely recognized as having lengthy and complicated application processes that may pose barriers to many, particularly those who are poorly educated, as are most rural elders. Residential care, provided vis a vis nursing homes, extended rehabilitation centers, acute care centers, and adult day care are less available to rural elders (Havens & Kyle, 1993; Scheidt & Norris-Baker, 1990). Thus, the key for health service providers in rural areas may be to transform aging in place from a negative experience for those who do not have other options into one that enhances overall well being.

Overcoming distance barriers to home health services, respite care, and other ancillary services is central to the ability of rural elders to thrive while remaining in their homes. Havens and Kyle (1993) point out that delivery of services to rural elders, either directly at home or on-site at agencies (which provide transportation) costs less than providing acute and long-term care. Service networks, while beginning to emerge, unfortunately are still not widely available in rural areas. Rural elders who would otherwise prefer to live independently can end up being admitted to nursing homes prematurely because of lack of preventive care or social supports, such that nursing home admission becomes a social admission, the solution to loneliness (Liu, McBride, & Coughlin, 1994; Russell et al., 1997). Furthermore, since adult daughters often provide caregiving to demented or physically disabled elderly parents (Guberman, Maheu, & Maille, 1992), the out-migration of adult children may mean that rural elders have less access to in-home family caregiving, which may add to the problem of premature nursing home admission.

SERVICE DELIVERY

At the heart of practically every social and health-related issue affecting rural elder outcomes is the issue of service delivery. Research on the threat that geographic distance places on the receipt of services for rural elders is mixed, with some studies showing it accounting for a large portion of service delivery problems (Coward & Cutler, 1989; Nelson, 1994; Parks, 1988), and others showing it not to be a barrier for rural elders any more than for urban elders (Blazer, Landerman, Fillenbaum, & Horner, 1995; Krout, 1994). Regional variation in weather conditions may underlie these contradictory findings such that distance barriers are more easily overcome for elders and service providers residing in more temperate climates (e.g., the Southeast or Southwest) and less so for elders in harsher climates (e.g., the Midwest, Northeast, and Alaska). Loss of the ability to drive, while significant for many nonrural elders, may be even more so for rural elders because of a lack of public transportation. Rural husbands often do most of the driving. Elderly rural women are less likely to drive than nonrural women, and many of those who do drive hesitate to do so in the winter. Thus, a husband's death can lead to sharply curtailed health and social supports for rural women (Stoller & Lee, 1994).

Another factor that may affect service use and delivery is a cultural one. Rural elders from diverse ethnic groups seem to share a strong cultural belief in self reliance, which can lead to an avoidance of service use, particularly mental health services (Ralston, 1993; Smith & Buckwalter, 1993). As noted above, building in opportunities for reciprocity by rural elders may help overcome this cultural barrier. Models that emphasize innovative and culturally appropriate services and cooperation between service providers, volunteers, clergy, and other community agencies have been proposed (e.g., Ralston, 1993; Snustad, Thompson-Heisterman, Neese, & Abraham, 1993). Cost-efficiency has been emphasized in these models because of the limited resources of both community members and rural county and state treasuries in general. Cost may be the single greatest barrier to care among rural elders themselves, much more so than for nonrural elders (Blazer et al., 1995). One study has shown that participation by rural elders in health-promoting programs may hinge largely on Medicare reimbursement (Lave, Ives, Traven, & Kuller, 1995). An integrated service approach, in which decision making, staffing, and physical space is shared among several provider organizations may not only provide better continuity of care, but can keep costs down (Buckwalter et al., 1994). Greater federal financial incentives for rural providers, especially those who can provide psychiatric care (of which there is a particular lack in rural areas), are needed (Chalifoux et al., 1996; Roybal, 1988). Telemedicine offers the opportunity for rural elders to receive medical care from nonlocal providers, particularly specialists, through the use of interactive televideo. Since Congress has passed legislation requiring Medicare to cover telemedical care (*APA Monitor*, November, 1997), it may become a feasible and more widely available option for rural elders. Ease of access to telemedical facilities, as well as the nature of the particular medical complaint (e.g., rural elders may prefer consultations for oncology to be face-to-face), however, can affect elders' satisfaction with telemedicine (Allen & Hayes, 1994).

Aside from issues of cost efficiency, an important and necessary feature of coordinated services is a clear mechanism for communication among participating member agencies. Collaboration may fail miserably when there are poor working relationships within and especially between member agencies (Buckwalter et al., 1994). Whichever model is adopted by rural service providers, it is important that built into it is a component that allows for community-building between members. Another key to the success of service delivery models for rural elders is avoiding a simple adaptation of models from urban or even other rural areas to a given locale. Needs assessments are critical to determine the unique cultural factors of the elderly individuals and the community at large, which may affect service delivery, and to determine what resources are available and how to link them to other resources. Included in those assessments should be information on the availability of rural work forces, especially with respect to paraprofessional home health aides, chore aides, and personal care aides (Nelson, 1994). If, for example, it is found that there is an undersupply of individuals who can provide home health care services, then alternative home care systems may need to be developed, such as adult foster care (Fetterman & Chamberlain, 1994).

CONCLUSION

Although this chapter focuses on the challenges to aging in a rural community, it should not be assumed that life for elderly persons living in a rural area is bleak. On the contrary, rural elders are believed to generally benefit from a more salubrious natural environment in which to live (Ortega et al., 1993), and some research shows them to have a more positive outlook than nonrural elders, which may bring health benefits (Clayton et al., 1994). Furthermore, more individuals from rural areas have a marriage companion with whom they can grow old, thus possibly staving off loneliness and depression. It is also possible that lifelong habits of physical activity of rural farm elders may offer some protection against obesity and osteoporosis, although we know of no studies that have examined this relationship.

Many elders living in nonrural areas, particularly those in urban and inner-city areas, are stressed daily by fears relating to crime (Levkoff, Levy, & Weitzman, 1999). Presumably rural elders are less plagued by such fears. Furthermore, due to the cultural emphasis placed on self-reliance, rural elders may be particularly adept at handling everyday problems. Research on the health advantages of aging in a rural environment is virtually nonexistent and is important to our theoretical understanding of the interplay of context and aging. Such information could also be useful to intervention and service programs for rural elders.

As to the challenges to successful aging in a rural area, we have outlined some potential solutions above. Additional solutions to the various challenges are also worth noting. For example, a solution to the problem of isolation and loneliness may be drawn from the work of Heller and his colleagues, who tested a social support intervention program designed to help lonely older women (Heller et al., 1991). Participants were randomly matched with other lonely women, with whom they engaged in frequent telephone contact for several months. Participants did not report feeling less lonely at the end of the intervention. The failure of this intervention, however, highlights the importance of matching individuals with similar backgrounds and interests (which was not done) or focusing on improvement in qualitative aspects of the existing relationships of lonely elders such as communication skills and trust, rather than quantitative aspects such as the frequency of contact (e.g., Dugan & Kivett, 1994). This empirical information should be considered when designing psychosocial interventions to address loneliness. Additional solutions to geographic and access barriers might come through transportation lending programs, in which vans are accessed by area agencies on aging or area health education centers and lent to community agencies on a regular basis. Home health care and other home service groups might also pool transportation resources with other agencies to bring services to elders. Emerging volunteer driver systems have shown some success in rural areas (Kihl, 1993). Solutions to the problems of rural housing might be drawn from the successful Habitat for Humanity program, which uses volunteers to build and rehabilitate housing for low income families. Rural housing programs might be able to capitalize on local skilled labor pools of farmers and retired farmers for volunteer housing rehabilitation efforts. Solutions to the problems of medical care might come by strengthening loan repayment programs to draw more medical professionals to rural areas. And while Medicare may reimburse telemedical treatment, federal subsidization of telemedical hardware is still needed to make it more widely available. Finally, programs to develop rural elders as child care providers, foster grandparents, and telephone tutors could not only provide the necessary opportunities for reciprocity shown to be important to them, but also prevent the diminution in feelings of self-worth to which all elders, rural and nonrural alike, can be subject (Rubinstein, 1989).

REFERENCES

Allen, A., & Hayes, J. (1994). Patient satisfaction with telemedicine in a rural clinic. *American Journal of Public Health, 84,* 1693.

Antonucci, T. C., Fuhrer, R., & Dartigues, J. (1997). Social relations and depressive symptomatology in a sample of community-dwelling French older adults. *Psychology and Aging, 12,* 189–195.

APA Monitor (November 1997). *Medicare to reimburse providers who deliver care from a distance.* Washington, DC: American Psychological Association.

Belden, J. N. (1993). Housing for America's rural elderly. In C. N. Bull (Ed.), *Aging in rural America* (pp. 71–83). Newbury Park, CA: Sage.

Blazer, D. G., Landerman, L. R., Fillenbaum, G., & Horner, R. (1995). Health service access and use among older adults in North Carolina: Urban vs. rural residents. *American Journal of Public Health, 85,* 1384–1390.

Buckwalter, K. C., Smith, M., & Caston, C. (1994). Mental and social health of the rural elderly. In R. T. Coward & C. N. Bull (Eds.), *Health services for rural elders* (pp. 203–232). New York: Springer.

Chalifoux, Z., Neese, J. B., Buckwalter, K. C., & Litwak, E. (1996). Mental health services for rural elderly: Innovative service strategies. *Community Mental Health Journal, 32,* 463–480.

Clayton, G. M., Dudley, W. N., Patterson, W. D., Lawhorn, L. A., Poon, L. W., Johnson, M. A., & Martin, P. (1994). The influence of rural/urban residence on health in the oldest-old. *International Journal of Aging & Human Development, 38,* 65–89.

Clifford, W. B., & Lilley, S. C. (1993). Rural elderly: Their demographic characteristics. In C. N. Bull (Ed.), *Aging in rural America* (pp. 3–17). Newbury Park, CA: Sage.

Coward, R. T., & Cutler, S. J. (1989). Informal and formal health care systems for the rural elderly. *Health Services Research, 23,* 785–806.

Coward, R. T., Cutler, S. J., & Schmidt, F. E. (1988). Residential differences in marital status and household type among the elderly. In R. Martoz-Baden, C. B. Hennon, & T. H. Brubaker (Eds.), *Families in rural America: Stress, adaptation, and revitalization* (pp. 104–115). St. Paul, MN: The National Council on Family Relations.

Coward, R. T., Lee, G. R., & Dwyer, J. W. (1993). Family relations of rural elders. In C. N. Bull (Ed.), *Aging in rural America* (pp. 216–231). Newbury Park, CA: Sage.

Craig, C. (1994). Community determinants of health for rural elderly. *Public Health Nursing, 11,* 242–246.

Dugan, E., & Kivett, V. R. (1994). The importance of emotional and social isolation to loneliness among very old rural adults. *The Gerontologist, 34,* 340–346.

Fetterman, E., & Chamberlain, V. (1994). Adult foster care: An economic and social alternative to institutionalization for some elders and other adults. *Adult Residential Care Journal, 8,* 91–102.

Guberman, N., Maheu, P., & Maille, C. (1992). Women as family caregivers: Why do they care? *The Gerontologist, 32,* 607–617.

Havens, B., & Kyle, B. (1993). Formal long-term care: Case examples. In C. N. Bull (Ed.), *Aging in rural America* (pp. 173–188). Newbury Park, CA: Sage.

Heller, K., Thompson, M. G., Trueba, P. E., Hogg, J. R., & Vlachos-Weber, I. (1991). Peer support telephone dyads for elderly women: Was this the wrong intervention? *American Journal of Community Psychology, 19,* 53–74.

Hessler, R. M., Jia, S., Madsen, R., & Pazaki, H. (1995). Gender, social networks, and survival time: A 20-year study of the rural elderly. *Archives of Gerontology and Geriatrics, 21,* 291–306.

John, R. (1985). Service needs and support networks of elderly Native Americans: Family, friends, and social service agencies. In W. A. Peterson & J. Quadano (Eds.), *Social bonds in later life* (pp. 229–247). Newbury Park, CA: Sage.

Johnson, D. R., & Booth, A. (1990). Rural economic decline and marital quality: A panel study of farm marriages. *Family Relations, 39,* 159–165.

Johnson, T. P., Hendricks, J., Turner, H. B., Stallones, L., Marx, M. B., & Garrity, T. F. (1988). Social networks and depression among the elderly: Metropolitan/nonmetropolitan comparisons. *Journal of Rural Health, 4,* 71–81.

Kihl, M. R. (1993). The need for transportation alternatives for the rural elderly. In C. N. Bull (Ed.), *Aging in rural America* (pp. 84–100). Newbury Park, CA: Sage.

Kivett, V. R. (1991). Centrality of the grandfather role among older black and white males. *Journal of Gerontology, 46*, S250–258.

Kivett, V. R. (1993). Informal supports among older rural minorities. In C. N. Bull (Ed.), *Aging in rural America* (pp. 204–215). Newbury Park, CA: Sage.

Krout, J. A. (1994). Rural aging community-based services. In R. T. Coward & C. N. Bull (Eds.), *Health services for rural elders* (pp. 84–107). New York: Springer.

Lave, J. R., Ives, D. G., Traven, N. D., & Kuller, L. H. (1995). Participation in health promotion programs by rural elderly. *American Journal of Preventive Medicine, 11*, 46–53.

Lee, C. J., Templeton, S., & Wang, C. (1995). Meal skipping patterns and nutrient intakes of rural southern elderly. *Journal of Nutrition for the Elderly, 15*, 1–14.

Levkoff, S. E., Levy, B., & Weitzman, P. F. (1999). The roles of ethnicity and religion in the help seeking of family caregivers. *Journal of Cross-Cultural Gerontology, 14*, 335–356.

Liu, K., McBride, T., & Coughlin, T. (1994). Risk of entering nursing homes for long versus short stays. *Medical Care, 32*, 315–327.

Nelson, G. M. (1994). In-home services for rural elders. In R. T. Coward & C. N. Bull (Eds.), *Health services for rural elders* (pp. 65–183). New York: Springer.

Ortega, S. T., Metroka, M. J., & Johnson, D. R. (1993). In sickness and in health: Age, social support, and psychological consequences of physical health among rural and urban residents. In C. N. Bull (Ed.), *Aging in rural America* (pp. 101–116). Newbury Park, CA: Sage.

Parks, A. G. (1988). *Black elderly in rural America*. Bristol, IN: Wyndham.

Ralston, P. A. (1993). Health promotion for rural black elderly: A comprehensive review. *Journal of Gerontological Social Work, 20*, 53–78.

Richardson, H. (1988). The health plight of rural women. *Women and Health, 12*, 41–54.

Roybal, E. R. (1988). Mental health and aging: The need for expanded federal response. *American Psychologist, 43*, 189–194.

Rubenstein, R. L. (1989). Temporality and affect: The personal meaning of well-being. In L. E. Thomas (Ed.), *Research on adulthood and aging*. (pp. 201–215). Albany, NY: State University of New York.

Russell, D. W., Cutrona, C. E., de la Mora, A., & Wallace, R. B. (1997). Loneliness and nursing home admission among rural older adults. *Psychology and Aging, 12*, 574–589.

Scheidt, R. J., & Norris-Baker, C. (1990). A transactional approach to environmental stress among older residents of rural communities. *Journal of Rural Community Psychology, 2*, 5–30.

Schone, B. S., & Weinick, R. M. (1998). Health-related behaviors and the benefits of marriage for elderly persons. *The Gerontologist, 38,* 618–627.

Sennott-Miller, L., May, K. M., & Miller, J. (1998). Demographic and health status indicators to guide health promotion for Hispanic and Anglo rural elderly. *Patient Education and Counseling, 53,* 13–23.

Smith, M., & Buckwalter, K. C. (1993). Mental health care for rural seniors. *Health Progress, 74,* 52–56.

Snustad, D. G., Thompson-Heisterman, A., Neese, J. B., & Abraham, I. L. (1993). Mental health outreach to rural elderly: Service delivery to a forgotten risk group. *Clinical Gerontologist, 14,* 95–111.

Stoller, E., & Lee, G. R. (1994). Informal care of rural elders. In R. T. Coward & C. N. Bull (Eds.), *Health services for rural elders* (pp. 33–64). New York: Springer.

CHAPTER 10

Elder Abuse

Rosalie S. Wolf

CASE #2104

The client has returned to her residential hotel and pretty much taken up her old routine: volunteering part time in a religious bookstore and attending church regularly. She states that every time her phone rings or someone knocks on her door, she is in a panic for fear it might be her son. Since the client's son (perpetrator) has been quasi-dependent financially on his mother for most of his adult life, it is likely that he will return when his funds again run out. He is her only child. His father, her husband, has died. There are no other known family members. According to the mother, the son has a history of lost opportunities in money-making ventures, whereas the client has lived rather frugally and presently has a good retirement income. There is evidence that there may never have been an emotionally supportive relationship between mother and son. All of these factors mitigate against a final resolution of this situation (Case reassessment, worker's notes).

CASE #3025

The client is more depressed than at time of initial assessment. Can't see her way out of abusive situation. Sees abuse as her fate; for her, this is life. Does not see that she has the power to change, despite the fact that she is financially secure in her own right. Husband continues to psychologically abuse her in the same manner as always. His physical frailty has put an end to his physically abusive acts. He still controls her coming and going to do certain things, such as meeting with her volunteer advocate or going to . . . She must wait until he is busy with TV and then escape. At the present, it appears that the abuse will continue until the husband dies. The client does not appear to be waiting for this, but she is aware of his impending decline. (Case reassessment, worker's notes).

Sorrowfully, successful and productive aging is an unrealistic goal for tens of thousands of older persons each year who are the victims of elder mistreatment in their own homes. Although little research has been done on the consequences of elder mistreatment, the finding that the mortality rate of abused/neglected elders is three times that of nonabused/neglected seniors (Lachs, 1996) confirms what common sense predicts: that abuse, neglect, and exploitation have a deleterious effect on the well-being of older persons. Studies have shown an increased prevalence of depression among abused elders compared to nonabused persons (Bristowe & Collins, 1989; Pillemer & Prescott, 1989; Phillips, 1983; Straus & Gelles, 1990). Case records have documented their helplessness, alienation, and withdrawal, as well as symptoms of posttraumatic stress syndrome. What kinds of services are available to these elders? How successful are the services in reducing or eliminating the abuse? Can victims hope to gain their self-esteem and rid themselves of the guilt, shame, fear, and denial so they can achieve a better quality of life?

This chapter describes the service system operated by the states for mistreated elders, presents several program examples, and ends with a discussion of issues related to service delivery and aging in good health. Elder abuse in this presentation is limited to domestic settings. It is defined as:

> aggressive or invasive behavior/action(s), or threats of same, inflicted on an older adult within the context of a relationship connoting trust, and of sufficient intensity and/or frequency to produce harmful physical, psychological, social and/or financial effects of unnecessary suffering, injury, pain, loss, and/or violation of human rights and poorer quality of life for the older adult. (Hudson, 1991, p. 145)

ADULT PROTECTIVE SERVICES

The adult protective services (APS) program in the 50 states and District of Columbia is responsible for responding to cases of elder abuse, neglect, and exploitation. The precursor to the present day APS system was established with the passage of the 1962 public welfare amendments to the Social Security Act. This legislation allocated funds to the states for the purpose of providing an array of services (known as protective services) to meet the social, psychological, medical, and legal needs of persons who, because of physical or mental limitations, were unable to act in their own behalf or were neglected, exploited, or living in unsafe conditions. Initially carried out by the states on a voluntary basis, protective services became a mandatory federal program in 1974 for all adults 18 years and older without regard for income. Within a few years, most states had established APS units in their public welfare (human services) departments or contracted with other public or private entities to provide the services.

Shortly thereafter, following a series of Congressional hearings and investigations (U.S. Select Committee on Aging, 1979, 1981), the nation was alerted to the "new" problem of elder abuse. Since cases involving neglected and exploited adults were already the responsibility of the APS programs, there was no need to create a new elder abuse service system. Some states did pass specific elder abuse legislation; others amended their adult protection law to reflect the new emphasis on elder abuse.

Today, if an APS program operates under adult protective services legislation, it is more apt to be limited to "incapacitated" or "dependent" adults 18 years and older, letting other agencies such as the law enforcement, legal services, and the criminal justice system deal with the more competent older victims. On the other hand, programs authorized under elder abuse legislation usually apply to any person 60 years and older who is at risk of abuse, neglect, or exploitation; responsibility for the 18- to 59-year-old adults is assigned to other agencies. Most APS units restrict their cases to persons living in their own homes.

In 42 states, protective services legislation mandates certain categories of workers to report suspected cases of elder abuse. As many as 50 different occupations are specified by the states, but the most often listed ones are social workers, physicians, nurses, and police (Tatara, 1995). A few states mandate "any person" who suspects that abuse has occurred to file a report. The remaining states use a voluntary reporting system buttressed by professional education and public awareness campaigns.

The state systems also vary in their administrative structure. Most are state administered with local (county/regional) offices (e.g., Tennessee, Texas). A smaller number of APS programs are state-supervised but locally administered with the responsibilities for service delivery carried out by county employees or in some instances contracted to private agencies (e.g., California, Ohio, South Carolina). Several other state-administered programs contract with nonprofit local case management agencies to conduct their elder abuse work (e.g., Illinois, Massachusetts).

Various funding sources are used to support APS programs: federal dollars that come to the states as part of the social services block grant (SSBG), and, most recently, as Medicaid payments that can be used for case management expenses of eligible individuals; state appropriations; and county/local tax revenue. The level of support received from these sources ranges from a totally state-funded program in a few states to complete dependence on the federal SSBG in a larger number of states; the rest use funds from several sources. The more highly developed APS programs have state or county support.

When a call is made to an adult protective services office, it is screened for potential seriousness. If mistreatment is suspected or the safety of an individual is threatened, an investigation is conducted by a caseworker. Should the situation be an emergency, the investigation must be done within a few hours. On the basis of a comprehensive assessment that includes physical, psychological, social, environmental, and financial components, a care plan is developed and, if agreeable to the individuals involved, the services are provided. For example, the Illinois Department on Aging (1995) reported that about one quarter of the victims in 1994 received home care, such as chore and homemaker services; one in five, mental health counseling and substance abuse services; and a somewhat smaller proportion, legal services. In most other states, once the abuse or neglect situation has been addressed, the case is turned over to other community agencies for ongoing case management and service delivery if needed.

If the mistreatment is thought to be mainly a result of caregiving stress, the focus of the intervention in on helping the caregivers: bringing into the home skilled nursing, homemaker assistance, personal care, meals-on-wheels, and chore services; providing respite care; or placing the victim in adult day care. When it is advisable to remove the victims from the home temporarily, emergency shelters are used. It also may be necessary to initiate guardianship proceedings if the victims lack the capacity to make decisions about their care. In cases of abusive adult children who are dependent on their victims, services to encourage independence, such as housing and financial assistance, job training, and substance abuse and mental health counseling may be appropriate. Legal instruments, such as protective orders or temporary commitment papers may be necessary in cases when the victim and abuser must be separated or when a medical or psychiatric assessment must be carried. Increasingly, law enforcement and the criminal justice system are becoming involved because these cases often involve criminal or civil offenses that are prosecutable.

Over the years, the number of reports of suspected domestic abuse, neglect, and exploitation received by APS programs has increased dramatically. In 1986, 117,000 reports were received nationwide. By 1996, the total was 293,000, of which about half were self-neglect cases (Tatara, Kusmeskas, & Duckhorn, 1997). Because of the variation in criteria for reporting and definitions among the states, these totals can only be considered as approximations. It is estimated that about one million elders became victims of various types of mistreatment in 1996 (excluding self-neglect). The median age of reported cases was 78 years. Fifty-five percent involved neglect; 14.6%, physical abuse; 12.3%, financial exploitation; 7.7%, psychological abuse; 0.3%, sexual abuse; and 10.1%, unknown or other. Two thirds of the victims were female. Adult children were the most frequent abusers, 36.7%; spouses, 12.6%; other family members, 10.8%.

It is important to keep in mind that these numbers are based on incidence reports made to official agencies. They do not represent the amount of elder abuse in the community. The only prevalence study conducted in the United States took place in the metropolitan Boston area (Pillemer & Finkelhor, 1988). It found that spouse abuse was more prevalent than abuse by adult children, the proportion of victims was roughly equally divided between males and females, and economic status and age were not related to the risk of abuse, results that contrast markedly with agency reports. Based on this survey and others carried out in Canada (Podnieks, 1992), Finland (Kivelä, Köngäs-Saviaro, Kesti, Pahkala, Ijäs, 1992), and Great Britain (Ogg & Bennett, 1992), a 4 to 6% prevalence rate is estimated.

MULTIDISCIPLINARY TEAMS

Because of the complexity of elder abuse cases, often involving medical, legal, psychological, social, environmental, and ethical issues, coordination with other agencies has come to be regarded as crucial to case resolution. Many communities have responded by establishing multidisciplinary teams, called together by the APS program either on a regular basis or when a particularly difficult case requires more skills, expertise, or resources than one worker or one agency can supply. Members of a team might include representatives from a variety of disciplines including case management, family counseling, mental health, geriatric medicine, civil and criminal law, financial management, and APS. Several states require teams as part of the APS system.

Supported by a federal grant, the protective services unit of the Illinois Department of Aging (1990) carried out a study comparing paid and voluntary teams in rural and urban settings. The authors of the study concluded that public awareness of abuse was enhanced and team members benefitted from the networking, but the teams had little impact on case success. Payment for the members' services was irrelevant. However, because the advice and support from the team participants were found to be helpful to the APS case managers and supervisors, teams became a requirement of the APS system for those local elder abuse programs whose service area included 7500 or more older residents. Under state law, the team is to include representatives from medical, legal, law enforcement, mental health, religious, and financial institutions.

The newest version of the multidisciplinary team is the fiduciary abuse specialist team (FAST), which focuses on financial matters. Organized first in Los Angeles County, it has been replicated in several California counties and other cities in the United States. Representatives from law enforcement, the district attorney's office, legal services, probate court, mental health services, public guardian's office, private conservatorship agencies, and financial and real estate experts (e.g., bankers, stock brokers, insurance agents, and realtors) meet on a regular basis to discuss cases involved with property and asset exploitation referred by APS. Not only has the team been successful in prosecuting offenders and recovering estates, but the participants have developed special expertise in these matters, particularly in understanding aging issues and how to work with older victims. Further, they have used the experience to advocate for changes in legislation (Aziz, 1994).

MENTAL HEALTH SERVICES

It is obvious from the list of psychosocial issues associated with elder abuse, with regard to both victims and perpetrators, that the mental health field has a major role to play. To what degree this is happening is not clear. The APS program may make a referral to the mental health system, but the response depends on the availability of services. In a survey of the Massachusetts protective services program (Wolf & Hathaway 1996), only half of the supervisors of the 27 local APS programs reported that community-based mental health services were available, and, depending on the type of service, only one half to one fifth of the programs could access home-based mental health services.

Several models linking the mental health system and protective services can be found across the country. The multidisciplinary team is one approach, where the mental health professional serves as a consultant to the APS program or other agencies dealing with abused elders. One California APS program conducts its investigations jointly with a psychiatric nurse from the county's geriatric mental health service if the report to the APS program suggests that a serious mental health situation is involved. Should a mental health admission be needed, it can be done without bureaucratic red tape. A nonprofit geriatric center in Ohio has the contract from the state to provide protective services in its county. The extensive mental health resources of the center, including therapists, paraprofessionals, and consultants, are available for the abuse and neglect cases. Unlike most APS programs, this model allows the agency to remain involved with the clients beyond the problem identification and crisis intervention stages. Still another model is found in Massachusetts. One of the local protective services programs, which generally are located within nonprofit case management agencies, is housed in a community mental health center, enabling the protective service workers to call on an array of mental health services without the administrative delays that often occur when working across systems.

VICTIM SUPPORT GROUPS

Support groups for older victims of family violence are still a relatively new and rare program as revealed in a nationwide survey (Wolf, 1998). Patterned after the battered women's shelter programs, they are intended to help older persons cope with the myriad of problems that they face when leaving (or remaining in) an abusive relationship. Some are under the auspices of domestic violence programs (e.g., shelters), some are sponsored by aging programs (e.g., Area Agencies on Aging), and some are cosponsored by both or other health and social service agencies. Although the sample was small (30 groups), the survey disclosed among the group leaders a high level of enthusiasm for their work, strong belief in the concept, and ongoing commitment to the group members. For some of the leaders, the support group is an extra program for which they do not receive compensation or operating funds. For many of the coleaders it is a volunteer undertaking. The survey findings showed a close resemblance between groups sponsored by aging services and domestic violence programs in organizational structure and function despite a philosophical difference about the nature of abuse and the role of the perpetrator. Both types of sponsors viewed the programs most successful in improving self-esteem, increasing awareness of abuse, and fostering feelings of personal growth. As the leader of one support group has written (Seaver, 1996, p. 19):

> The women who have made it to the program have been able to get past the barriers of fear, shame, and isolation that keep many women captive.

ISSUES IN THE ASSESSMENT OF PROGRAM OUTCOMES

Although directors of elder abuse projects, such as the group leaders cited above, and even APS workers are confidant about the value of their programs, few have undergone rigorous evaluation. The assessment of these interventions has been hampered by the difficulties in dealing with the multiple factors, complex interpersonal relationships, and ethical issues. Case outcome is often approached in terms of case resolution, defined as the elimination or alleviation of the abuse/neglect and based on the clinical judgment of the case worker and supervisor. It may mean a decrease in the number of manifestations of mistreatment and their severity, a reduction in the level of threat they posed for the victim, diminution in the degree of dependency of the perpetrator or victim, or improvement in the quality of the relationship.

In studies involving four elder abuse projects, about one quarter of the cases were rated as either "not resolved" or "resolved a little" (Wolf & Pillemer, 1997) with project staff selecting "change in living/social situation of the victim and interdependency of perpetrator and victim" as having the most positive impact on case resolution. Resolved cases were more apt to include intentional neglect and perpetrators who were arrested or hospitalized for mental problems. Nonresolved cases in comparison were more likely to include mistreatment of a more serious and frequent nature, particularly psychological abuse; victims who were a source of stress to the perpetrators; and perpetrators who were a source of stress to the victims.

Sometimes cases are administratively closed before the abusive/neglectful situation is completely resolved. The victims may have become resigned to their fate, do not want to destroy the ties to the perpetrator, lack any other companionship, or fear moving into unknown or new situations, especially a nursing home. Almost one quarter of Massachusetts cases over the years (Massachusetts Executive Office of Elder Affairs, 1990, 1991–1992, 1994, 1997) have refused services. The emphasis on client safety over client autonomy, which characterized protective services a quarter of a century ago, is no longer the rule. Today, the client's right to self-determination is paramount. When a competent, abused, neglected, or exploited person refuses services, the APS worker has to withdraw from the case, often to the dismay of family, friends, neighbors, and other professionals who believe that the health and property of the person are in danger. If a case involves an incompetent individual, court action may be required, often resulting in the client losing all rights.

Following the lead of child protective services, some state APS programs have instituted forms that monitor the risk of future abuse. A survey of APS programs found that 28 of the 44 responding states used a risk assessment instrument but differed in how often and when it was used: during the initial assessment or at the substantiation decision point; at case intake or case closure. The system utilized by the Illinois Department on Aging is probably the most advanced among the states (Neale, Hwalek, Goodrich, & Quinn, 1996). A numeric score of risk is assigned by the caseworker to the client based on a risk factor matrix. The risk factors are scored low (i.e., the situation is alleviated with low likelihood of recurring or escalating), medium (i.e., potential exists for the situation to continue and possibly escalate), or high risk (i.e., very likely the situation will continue and probably escalate in the future) based on prescribed behaviors and conditions. Analyzing 552 Illinois APS clients, researchers found 19% in the high risk category, of which a little more than half moved into a lower risk category after intervention.

PREVENTION

For some victims who choose not to separate from their abusers or not to accept services, successful and productive aging may be elusive. The fact that many cases remain at risk even after intervention from a wide array of service providers indicates the need for a stronger commitment to primary elder abuse prevention. Even though researchers are still searching for clues to the nature of the problem and its causes, enough information about case types and circumstances is available to suggest a number of preventive strategies. Adequate, available, and accessible medical and social services are essential for all older people but especially for those at risk of being victimized: physically or mentally dependent older persons, Alzheimer's Disease patients, older parents with adult children who have emotional or substance abuse problems, caregivers, and elderly couples with marital difficulties. Mental health services for vulnerable families should be a high priority, including close monitoring of discharged mental hospital patients who return home to live with elderly parents, better utilization of family-oriented therapy to strengthen family function, improved linkage between the aging and mental health networks, and more training for caregivers about the risk of abuse, management of stress and anger, and community resources. Although the relationship between substance abuse and violence is not clear, alcohol is present in a large proportion of cases, enough to suggest that greater attention to this problem in at-risk families is needed. Educational programs on healthy or successful aging with a focus on building self-esteem and self-confidence should be available through senior centers or church groups. However, the greatest strides in preventing elder abuse may depend on educating young people in the ways to resolve conflicts without violence.

REFERENCES

Aziz, S. (1994). *Multidisciplinary fiduciary abuse consultation team.* Santa Monica, CA: WISE Senior Services.

Bristowe, E., & Collins, J. B. (1989). Family mediated abuse of non-institutionalized elder men and women living in British Columbia. *Journal of Elder Abuse and Neglect, 1,* 45–54.

Hudson, M. (1991). Elder mistreatment: A taxonomy with definitions by Delphi. *Journal of Elder Abuse and Neglect, 3,* 1–20.

Illinois Department on Aging. (1990). *Elder abuse and neglect program: Multidisciplinary team member handbook.* Springfield, IL: Author.

Illinois Department on Aging. (1995). *Elder abuse and neglect program: FY 1994 final report.* Springfield, IL: Author.

Kivelä, S. L., Köngäs-Saviaro, P., Kesti, E., Pahkala, K., & Ijäs, M. (1992). Abuse in old age: Epidemiological data from Finland. *Journal of Elder Abuse and Neglect, 4,* 1–18.

Lachs, M. (1996). *The Paul Beeson physician faculty scholars in aging research program.* New York: American Federation for Aging Research.

Massachusetts Executive Office of Elder Affairs. (1990, 1991–1992, 1994, 1997). *Elder protective services program report.* Boston, MA: Author.

Neale, A. V., Hwalek, M. A., Goodrich, C. S., & Quinn, K. M. (1996). The Illinois abuse system: Program description and administrative findings. *The Gerontologist, 36,* 502–511.

Ogg, J., & Bennett, G. (1992). Elder abuse in Britain. *British Medical Journal, 305,* 998–999.

Phillips, L. R. (1983). Abuse and neglect of the frail elderly at home: An exploration of theoretical relationships. *Advanced Nursing, 8,* 379–392.

Pillemer, K. A., & Finkelhor, D. (1988). The prevalence of elder abuse: A random sample survey. *The Gerontologist, 28,* 51–57.

Pillemer, K. A., & Prescott, O. (1989). Psychological effects of elder abuse: A research note. *Journal of Elder Abuse and Neglect, 1,* 65–74.

Podnieks, E. (1992). National survey on the abuse of the elderly in Canada. *Journal of Elder Abuse and Neglect, 4,* 5–58.

Seaver, C. (1996). Muted lives: Older battered women. *Journal of Elder Abuse and Neglect, 8,* 3–21.

Straus, M., & Gelles, R. J. (1990). *Physical violence in American families.* New Brunswick, NJ: Transaction.

Tatara, T. (1995). *An analysis of state laws addressing elder abuse, neglect, and exploitation.* Washington, DC: National Center on Elder Abuse.

Tatara, T., Kusmeskas, L., & Duckhorn, E. (1997). *Elder abuse information series 1-3.* Washington, DC: National Center on Elder Abuse.

U.S. House of Representatives, Select Committee on Aging (1979). *Elder abuse: The hidden problem.* Washington, DC: U.S. Government Printing Office.

U.S. House of Representatives, Select Committee on Aging (1981). *Elder abuse: An examination of a hidden problem.* Washington, DC: U.S. Government Printing Office.

Wolf, R. S. (1998). *Survey of support groups for older victims of domestic violence: Sponsors and programs.* Worcester, MA: National Committee for the Prevention of Elder Abuse.

Wolf, R. S., & Hathaway, J. (1996). *Report of the Massachusetts Elder Protective services Program Evaluation.* Worcester, MA: National Committee for the Prevention of Elder Abuse.

Wolf, R. S., & Pillemer, K. A. (1989). *Helping elderly victims: The reality of elder abuse.* New York: Columbia University Press.

Wolf, R. S., & Pillemer, K. A. (1997). *Elder abuse case resolution: What does it mean?* A paper presented at the Annual Meetings of the International Family Violence Research Conference, June, Durham, NH.

PART III

Biomedical Understandings of Aging

CHAPTER 11

Medication Use in Older Individuals

Jerry H. Gurwitz and Paula A. Rochon

D rug therapy for individuals of any age is difficult, but prescribing for older patients offers special challenges. Older people take about three times as many prescription medications as younger individuals do, mainly because of an increased prevalence of chronic medical conditions (Chrischilles et al., 1992). However, taking several drugs together substantially increases the risk of drug interactions, redundant drug effects, and adverse reactions. Many medications need to be used with special caution because of age-related changes in pharmacokinetics and pharmacodynamics.

PHARMACOKINETICS

Pharmacokinetics is defined as what the body does to a drug. Of the traditional components of pharmacokinetics—absorption distribution, and clearance (drug removal from the body)—only absorption appears to be unaffected by age. For certain medications, drug distribution can vary importantly in the elderly. An age-related increase in body fat at the expense of muscle leads to a greater volume of distribution for lipid-soluble medications (e.g., many of the benzodiazepines) (Greenblatt, Sellers, & Shader, 1982). Additionally, important pathways of drug metabolism in the liver and drug excretion by the kidney may be impaired in elderly patients. Such age-related changes in pharmacokinetics can have important implications for dosing of medications in this population.

The liver represents the major site of metabolism for many drugs. Hepatic biotransformation of drugs is categorized into phase I (preparative) and phase II (synthetic) reactions. Phase I reactions lead to intermediate products (often with their own drug effects) that then undergo transformation to pharmacologically inactive, polar, water-soluble metabolites by phase II reactions. Phase I reactions include oxidation, reduction, and hydrolysis. Phase II reactions involve conjugation reactions (glucuronidation, acetylation, and sulfation). The efficiency of phase I reactions is reduced somewhat with advancing age, while aging has little impact on phase II metabolic pathways.

An increase in the volume of distribution or a reduction in clearance will cause a prolongation of elimination half-life, which might prolong the duration of action of a single dose of a drug. Selected agents in the benzodiazepine class show the impact of aging on drug elimination half-life. Because diazepam is very fat soluble, it has an increased volume of distribution in older patients. It is metabolized initially by phase I reactions in the liver. The elimination half-life of diazepam in a young person is approximately 24 hours compared with 75 hours in the elderly. In contrast, oxazepam is substantially less fat soluble than diazepam and is metabolized through a single phase II reaction. The elimination half-life of oxazepam is unchanged with advancing patient age (approximately 7 hours).

It is frequently assumed that the duration of clinical action of a drug is related to its half-life. Under this assumption, a long elimination half-life implies a long duration of action, and a short elimination half-life implies a short duration of action. This is not always a correct interpretation, but epidemiologic data do support an association between the use of agents with a long elimination half-life and the occurrence of drug side-effects in the elderly (Hemmelgarn, Suissa, Huang, Boivin, & Pinard, 1997).

PHARMACODYNAMICS

In elderly persons, the clinical response to a drug may be enhanced due to higher drug concentrations and increased accumulation after repeated dosing (i.e., an age-related pharmacokinetic change). Alternatively, older patients may be intrinsically more sensitive to a medication. Therefore, at any particular serum concentration, the clinical response may be greater than in younger patients (i.e., an age-related pharmacodynamic change).

Pharmacodynamics is defined as what a drug does to the body. Pharmacodynamic changes with aging have been more challenging to describe than pharmacokinetic changes. One of the first studies describing age-related changes in pharmacodynamics involved a group of patients between the ages of 30 and 90 years of age undergoing elective cardioversion who were medicated with intravenous diazepam. The clinical endpoint used was the patient's inability to respond to vocal stimuli, with preservation of response to a painful stimulus. The serum level of diazepam at which this central nervous system effect occurred was significantly lower in elderly patients (Reidenberg et al., 1978).

Similar findings have emerged from other studies involving benzodiazepines and the opioids. Various studies have also suggested that increasing patient age is associated with an increased sensitivity to the effects of warfarin therapy (Gurwitz, Avorn, Ross-Degnan, Choodnovskiy, & Ansell, 1992). By contrast, the elderly have been shown to be less sensitive to the effects of some medications, including beta-adrenergic agonists and antagonists.

Be careful when drawing conclusions from the results of studies examining age-related changes in pharmacodynamics and applying these findings to clinical practice. For example, while older patients have been shown to be more sensitive to the effects of opioid analgesics, such as morphine, this research finding should never limit the provision of adequate analgesic therapy to treat an elderly patient in pain. While older persons may be less sensitive to the effects of beta-adrenergic antagonists, do not use this observation to formulate general dosing guidelines for beta-blocker therapy in elderly patients. However, age-related changes in pharmacokinetics or pharmacodynamics of some benzodiazepine sedatives and hypnotics do suggest a need to reduce dosage in elderly persons. Furthermore, the increased sensitivity to warfarin therapy in elderly persons may indicate a need to intensify monitoring of anticoagulant therapy.

ADVERSE DRUG EFFECTS

Avoidable adverse drug effects are the most serious consequences of inappropriate drug prescribing in elderly persons. Indeed, misinterpretation of an adverse reaction as another medical condition may lead to the prescription of additional medications with their own potential to cause side-effects (Stephen & Williamson, 1984). For example, a patient started on a high potency antipsychotic medication such as haloperidol may develop extrapyramidal side-effects. These may be misdiagnosed as a new medical condition (Parkinson's disease) so that the patient is inappropriately put on antiparkinsonian medication. He or she is now susceptible to the adverse effects of the newly prescribed treatment. It would have been better to try reducing the dose of haloperidol or to select an antipsychotic drug with less propensity to cause parkinsonian symptoms at low doses such as thioridazine, recognizing that thioridazine itself has other adverse effects (e.g., it is more sedating than haloperidol and has more striking anticholinergic effects) (Salzman, 1992).

High dose nonsteroidal anti-inflammatory drug (NSAID) therapy may cause an increase in blood pressure that is modest but still beyond the threshold that prompts the prescription of or intensification of antihypertensive treatment (Gurwitz et al., 1994). A further example is constipation in a patient on a strongly anticholinergic antidepressant such as amitriptyline; as a result, the patient may become dependent on laxatives (Monane, Avorn, Beers, & Everitt, 1993). By careful drug selection within a class, by starting at the lowest feasible dose, with carefully monitored increments, and by considering any new symptoms and signs as possible drug side-effects, both the risk of adverse reactions and the need for further therapy to counteract them can be reduced (Rochon & Gurwitz, 1995, 1997).

REVIEWING A PATIENT'S MEDICATION

Periodic evaluation of the drugs a patient is taking is an essential component of the medical care of elderly persons. This may indicate the need for changes—discontinuation of a therapy prescribed for an indication that no longer exists, substitution of a required therapy with a potentially safer agent, reduction in dosage of a drug that the patient still needs to take, or an increase in dose or even addition of a new medication. Information in medical records or provided by the patient will often be inaccurate or incomplete, and the physician may have to ask patients to display all the bottles of pills that they are using. Over-the-counter products that the patient may not consider the domain of the physician should be included, as should skin products, vitamins, herbals, nutritional supplements, and all ophthalmic preparations.

COMPLIANCE

The failure of a patient to adhere to a thoughtfully prescribed therapeutic regimen is discouraging to every physician. The effects of noncompliance may be obvious, but often they are not fully appreciated. The worsening of a chronic condition that results from failure to take a prescribed medication may lead to the prescription of a larger dose or a more potent agent. This in turn can lead to serious toxicity should the patient begin taking the medication as prescribed. When noncompliance leads to unnecessary morbidity and mortality, the physician is left to consider what factors contributed to these adverse consequences and what strategies might have prevented their occurrence.

The problem of noncompliance with prescribed medical therapies is certainly not restricted to elderly patients, and is probably not increased in elderly patients relative to the young if the number of prescribed drugs is taken into account. Across various patient age groups, compliance with long-term medication regimens has been found to be approximately 50% (Sackett & Snow, 1979). However, for a number of reasons, including greater use of both prescription and nonprescription medications, impaired homeostasis related to age-related decrements in many physiologic parameters, an increased prevalence of multiple coexisting chronic disease states, and the financial burden of substantial out-of-pocket costs in the face of fixed incomes, the compliance issue demands special attention in the geriatric population.

There are many types of noncompliant behavior associated with prescribed pharmacotherapy (Simonson, 1984). The most common type of noncompliance is simply the failure of the patient to take a medication. Other categories of noncompliance include the premature discontinuation of a medication, its use at the wrong time, excessive consumption ("If one pill is good, then two must be better"), and the use of medications not currently prescribed. This last category includes the inappropriate use of over-the-counter medications and the use of medications shared by family members and friends (Hammarlund, Ostrom, & Kethley, 1985; Ostrom, Hammarlund, Christensen, Plein, & Kethley, 1985).

Although problems with visual impairment, functional disability, and cognitive dysfunction have been frequently assumed to be the prime contributors to noncompliance in elderly patients, the results of a number of studies have confirmed that the major factor predicting compliance with a medication regimen is the total number of concurrently prescribed medications: the more prescriptions, the lower the compliance (Darnell, Murray, Martz, & Weinberger, 1986; German, Klein, McPhee, & Smith, 1982; Gurwitz et al., 1993; Kendrick & Bayne, 1982). Other factors contributing to noncompliance in elderly persons include poor labeling instructions, difficulty in opening childproof containers, and misunderstanding of verbal instructions (Simonson, 1984). In addition, confusion may lead to noncompliance when multiple drugs of similar appearance are prescribed for the same patient (Mazzullo, 1972).

A variety of strategies have been proposed for improving patient compliance with medication regimens (Sackett & Snow, 1979; Simonson, 1984). Since the prescription of multiple concurrent medications reduces compliance, a primary strategy in improving compliance is to limit prescribing to the smallest possible number of medications and to make dosing instructions as simple as possible. Tailoring the regimen to the patient's schedule, such as mealtimes or other regularly scheduled activities, can be helpful. Compliance aids, such as commercially prepared or home-made pill boxes and medication calendars, may also be helpful. Family members and friends can be enlisted as support networks to supervise and encourage compliance, and this can be crucial to maintaining compliance with both long- and short-term therapies. A regular reminder telephone call by a family member or other caregiver may be all that is required to complete an important course of therapy.

CASE EXAMPLE

Mr. P. is an 83-year-old man who was transferred to a nursing home following a hospital admission for exacerbation of congestive heart failure. His past medical history is significant for degenerative joint disease involving the knees and hips and open-angle glaucoma. Reasons for nursing home admission include increasing functional difficulties and the need for increased supervision with prescribed cardiovascular medications. Prescribed medications as summarized in the hospital discharge summary include: digoxin 0.25 mg; furosemide, 40 mg; and potassium chloride, 20 mEq (each taken orally every day); ibuprofen, 600 mg orally four times a day; misoprostol, 200 mcg four times a day; timolol, 0.25% one drop to each eye twice a day; oxazepam, 15 mg orally every night; and dioctyl sodium sulfosuccinate, 100 mg orally twice a day. Careful questioning of the patient indicates that he is receiving many more medications than he had ever taken in the past. Before hospitalization, he was receiving only digoxin, furosemide, potassium choride, ibuprofen, and the timolol eye drops. He reports no history of peptic ulcer disease. He has had recent difficulties with sleeping and loose stools, but did not experience these problems before hospitalization. When asked about his glaucoma therapy, Mr. P. stated that he often instilled two to three drops in each eye once a day to avoid the inconvenience of twice daily administrations.

The case of Mr. P. makes several important points regarding pharmacotherapy in older persons. It is not uncommon for elderly patients to accumulate many new drug treatments during the course of an acute hospitalization. At the time of nursing home admission, one must carefully scrutinize the treatment plan with a goal of simplification whenever possible. Based on Mr. P.'s history and the complaint of loose stools in the absence of fecal impaction, it is obvious that he does not require a stool softener and this treatment can be discontinued. In addition, another medication in this resident's drug regimen (misoprostol) may be contributing to this complaint.

Although the choice of oxazepam (a short elimination half-life benzodiazepine) as a hypnotic is a good choice for an elderly patient due to its favorable pharmacokinetic profile, one should avoid long-term use of any hypnotic therapy and try nonpharmacologic approaches to improve sleep before resorting to drug therapy. A program to promote good sleep hygiene should include the limitation of daytime napping and maintenance of regular bedtimes. Environmental strategies include the use of a bed only for sleeping and a comfortable bedroom temperature. Other nonpharmacologic strategies include the omission of caffeine-containing beverages after midday, gentle exercise, and a light evening snack.

When drug therapy is deemed absolutely necessary, there are sometimes safer alternatives to the medications that a newly admitted resident has been receiving. Mr. P. has been treated with chronic nonsteroidal anti-inflammatory drug therapy (ibuprofen). In some patients, NSAID therapy can produce damage to the gastric mucosa ranging from superficial erosions to ulcer craters and severe hemorrhage. Many have topical irritative effects on the mucosa, but their ulcerogenic effects are more likely the result of inhibition of prostaglandin production. Elderly persons may be at a particularly increased risk for the development of gastrointestinal toxicity following NSAID therapy. The inhibition of renal prostaglandin synthesis by NSAIDs can also place patients at risk for impairment of renal function and exacerbation of congestive heart failure.

Because of the iatrogenic nature of these disorders, the most prudent approach is to limit NSAID therapy to those clinical situations in which it is absolutely required and to prescribe the lowest feasible dose for the shortest time necessary to achieve the desired therapeutic effect. Alternative safer analgesic therapies are available and effective for many. These include acetaminophen and nonacetylated salicylates.

For older persons entering a nursing home from the community, a potential problem exists in that as many as half have not adhered to medication regimens as prescribed. Mr. P.'s history indicates a problem with nonadherence in relation to the topical beta blocker therapy prescribed for treatment of glaucoma (timolol). Glaucoma is an insidious and disabling disease that affects over 4% of persons 80 years of age or older. (Prevalence is probably even higher in the nursing home population.) Used properly, topical therapy reduces

TABLE 11.1   Guidelines for Prescribing Drugs to Elderly Patients

- Take a careful drug history, including any use of over-the-counter medications
- Become familiar with the effects of age on the pharmacology of the drugs prescribed
- Strive to make a diagnosis before treatment
- In general, use smaller initial doses in the elderly
- Adjust the dose according to the patient's response
- Review the drugs in the medication regimen regularly and simplify the therapeutic regimen whenever possible
- Be alert to the possibility of drug-induced illness and interactions between disease states and drugs

---

intraocular pressure and reduces the risk of visual impairment and eventual blindness. Although topical agents used to treat glaucoma are used for their local effect on the eye, considerable systemic absorption may occur with consequent systemic side-effects. The drug enters the systemic circulation by drainage into the lacrimal ducts with subsequent absorption through the vascular mucosa of the nasopharynx.

Systemic absorption of ophthalmic beta blockers affects the cardio-vascular system through beta-1 blockade. Such blockade can lead to a reduction in cardiac contractility and potentially an exacerbation of congestive heart failure. The risk of such adverse effects is reduced by using the medication according to the prescribed dosage and by occluding the lacrimal puncta with gentle finger pressure for 3 to 5 minutes after application of the drug to limit systemic absorption. Table 11.1 summarizes guidelines for use of medications in elderly patients.

REFERENCES

Chrischilles, E. A., Foley, D. J., Wallace, R. B., Lemke, J. H., Semla, T. P., Hanlon, J. T., Glynn, R. J., & Ostfeld, M. A. (1992). Use of medications by persons 65 and over: Data from the established populations for epidemiologic studies of the elderly. *Journal of Gerontology, 47,* 137–144.

Darnell, J. C., Murray, M. D., Martz, B. L., & Weinberger, M. (1986). Medication use by ambulatory elderly: An in-home survey. *Journal of the American Geriatrics Society, 34,* 1–4.

German, P. S., Klein, L. E., McPhee, S. J., & Smith, C. R. (1982). Knowledge of and compliance with drug regimens in the elderly. *Journal of the American Geriatrics Society, 30,* 568–571.

Greenblatt, D. J., Sellers, E. M., & Shader, R. I. (1982). Drug disposition in old age. *New England Journal of Medicine, 306,* 1081–1088.

Gurwitz, J. H., Avorn, J., Ross-Degnan, D., Choodnovskiy, I., & Ansell, J. (1992). Aging and the anticoagulant response to warfarin therapy. *Annals of Internal Medicine, 116,* 901–904.

Gurwitz, J. H., Avorn, J., Bohn, R. L., Glynn, R. J., Monane, M., & Mogun, H. (1994). Initiation of antihypertensive treatment during nonsteroidal anti-inflammatory drug therapy. *Journal of the American Medical Association, 272,* 781–786.

Gurwitz, J. H., Glynn, R. J., & Monane, M., Everitte, D. E., Gilden, D., Smith, N., & Avorn, J. (1993). Treatment for glaucoma: Adherence by the elderly. *American Journal of Public Health, 83,* 711–716.

Hammarlund, E. R., Ostrom, J. R., & Kethley, A. J. (1985). The effects of drug counseling and other educational strategies on drug utilization of the elderly. *Medical Care, 23,* 165–170.

Hemmelgarn, B., Suissa, S., Huang, A., Boivin, J. F., & Pinard, G. (1997). Benzodiazepine use and the risk of motor vehicle crash in the elderly. *Journal of the American Medical Association, 278,* 27–31.

Kendrick, R., & Bayne, J. R. D. (1982). Compliance with prescribed medication by elderly patients. *Canadian Medical Association Journal, 127,* 961–962.

Mazzullo, J. (1972). The nonpharmacologic basis of therapeutics. *Clinical Pharmacology and Therapeutics, 13,* 157–158.

Monane, M., Avorn, J., Beers, M. H., & Everitt, D. E. (1993). Anticholinergic drug use and bowel function in nursing home patients. *Archives of Internal Medicine, 153,* 633–638.

Ostrom, J. R., Hammarlund, E. R., Christensen, D. B., Plein, J. B., & Kethley, A. J. (1985). Medication usage in the elderly population. *Medical Care, 23,* 157–164.

Reidenberg, M. M., Levy, M., Warner, H., Coutinho, C. G., Schwartz, M. A., Yu, G., & Cheripko, J. (1978). Relationship between diazepam dose, plasma level, age, and central nervous system depression. *Clinical Pharmacology and Therapeutics, 23,* 371–374.

Rochon, P. A., & Gurwitz, J. H. (1995). Drug therapy. *Lancet, 346,* 32–36.

Rochon, P. A., & Gurwitz, J. H. (1997). Optimising drug treatment for elderly people: The prescribing cascade. *British Medical Journal, 315,* 1096–1099.

Sackett, D. L., & Snow, J. C. (1979). The magnitude of compliance and noncompliance. In R. B. Haynes, D. W. Taylor, & D. L. Sackett (Eds.),

Compliance in health care (pp. 11–12). Baltimore: The Johns Hopkins University Press.

Salzman, C. (1992). *Clinical geriatric psychopharmacology* (2nd ed.). Baltimore: Williams & Wilkins.

Simonson, W. (1984). *Medications and the elderly: A guide for promoting proper use.* Rockville, MD: Aspen Systems Corporation.

Stephen, P. J., & Williamson, J. (1984). Drug-induced Parkinsonism in the elderly. *Lancet, ii,* 1082–1083.

CHAPTER 12

Nutritional Issues in Geriatrics

Naomi K. Fukagawa and Amy E. H. Prue

People over the age of 65 are the fastest growing segment of the U.S. population, and it is estimated that by the year 2030, 21% will be over the age of 64 (Schlenker, 1993). Similar numbers are expected for other industrialized countries. With advancing age comes an increased incidence of chronic diseases such as atherosclerosis, diabetes mellitus, arthritis, and heart disease. There is increasing evidence that nutritional status and nutrient intake play an important role in the occurrence and susceptibility to many diseases, making it imperative to include nutritional assessment and recommendations as integral to patient management.

The aging process per se can have a profound effect on the nutritional status of elderly persons, which is also influenced by social, psychological, and economic factors. As we grow older, many of these aspects of our lives change, leading to changes in the selection, preparation, and consumption of food. Twice as many older adults live in poverty compared to younger adults as a result of decreases in income and increases in living costs such as medication, specialized aides (hearing, walking), and so forth. Socioeconomic status can contribute significantly to an elder's risk for malnutrition. Elders on a limited budget may not have the financial resources to buy the food that they need to help them remain healthy. The expense of smaller packaging and high quality, perishable food can strain an elder's limited budget. In addition, transportation difficulties may influence selection of foodstuffs. Decreased mobility due to illness or disease can limit an elder's ability to get out and shop for food. Older persons who can no longer drive or does not feel comfortable driving in heavy, city traffic may depend on relatives or friends to drive them to go food shopping. Psychological factors may also play a significant role in influencing nutritional status. Cognitive deficits may affect an individual's ability to prepare food or even to recognize hunger. Dementia is seen in several age-related diseases and illnesses including Alzheimer's Disease, stroke, or other cerebrovascular incidents. An elder who experiences dementia may forget to eat or have difficulty differentiating between meals and may only rely on certain foods. Stressful life events such as an illness or death of a family member can also influence nutritional status. The loss of a spouse is also the loss of an eating partner, which can cause depression and loss of appetite for the remaining spouse. Depression and loneliness often lead to decreased appetite and interest in food. Combined with changes in living situations, social roles, and support networks, all of these factors can predispose elders to nutritional deficits (Chernoff, 1991; Schlenker, 1993).

Numerous biochemical and physiologic changes with potential impact on nutritional status occur with aging. At the molecular, subcellular, and cellular levels, alterations include changes in DNA concentration and gene dosage of ribosomal RNA in various tissues, ultrastructural changes in the mitochondria and in the degree of cross-linking in collagen, and tissue accumulation of pigmented inclusion bodies, all of which may affect nutrient utilization or storage. The composition of cell and subcellular membrane changes during senescence and includes alterations in the binding sites for hormones and in the activities of enzymes. In some organs, such as the kidney and central nervous system, the number of cells is reduced with advancing age (Finch & Hayflick, 1977). In this chapter, we will focus on some of the changes in physiologic function and body composition that have an impact on an elder's nutritional status. We will also discuss risk factors for malnutrition in the older population and discuss ways to promote good nutritional health.

BIOLOGICAL CHANGES WITH NUTRITIONAL CONSEQUENCES

Aging is accompanied by progressive functional declines in many organ systems that may ultimately result in altered absorption, transport, metabolism, and excretion of nutrients (Chernoff, 1991). Age-associated changes in the oral cavity and gastrointestinal tract may have a significant effect on nutritional status. For example, age-related decreases in gastric acid and enzyme production may reduce absorption of vitamin B12, iron, folic acid, and possibly zinc as well as calcium. Altered gastrointestinal motility may contribute to constipation resulting in poor appetite. Changes in olfactory and taste acuity may affect food intake. Decreased saliva production, tooth loss, or ill-fitting dentures may make it difficult to chew certain foods such as raw vegetables and meat. The incidence of chronic diseases, which also increases with advancing age, can impair mobility and appetite, thus affecting food intake and consequently nutritional status. In addition, the medications frequently used in the treatment of chronic diseases may alter the digestion, absorption, and utilization of nutrients as well as affect appetite, taste, and smell and cause gastrointestinal upset.

One of the major changes associated with advancing age is a loss of lean body mass and concomitant decline in body protein stores. Studies indicate that this equates to a decline in skeletal muscle with relative preservation of nonmuscle lean tissue (Korenchevsky, 1961). In the young adult, skeletal muscle accounts for about 45% of total body weight. However, by the age of 70, skeletal muscle only accounts for approximately 27% of total body weight (Carter, 1991). Loss of lean tissue implies a loss of body protein, and protein nutriture is an important factor in an individual's response to injury and stress (Kinney, 1995; Kinney & Elwyn, 1983). The mechanisms responsible for these changes are numerous, and ways to reverse the trend are the focus of a number of studies (Dutta, 1997). Concern about the maintenance of body protein status in elderly persons must therefore be addressed. Inadequate protein intake may be an important factor in the age-related loss of fat-free mass (FFM) (Evans & Cyr-Campbell, 1997). Castaneda et al. have reported that low protein intakes in elderly women are associated with a loss in lean body mass and impaired immune function and muscle strength (Castaneda, Charnley, Evans, & Crim, 1995). It has been suggested that the decline in physical activity may be of causal significance and studies have shown that strength training in elderly adults, including frail nursing home residents, has stopped or reversed sarcopenia (Fiatarone et al., 1990). High intensity strength training exercises have been shown to counteract some of the effects of age by increasing skeletal muscle mass and decreasing body fat mass with a concomitant rise in resting metabolic rate (Fielding, 1995). Preservation or an increase in muscle may be associated with greater insulin sensitivity and may prevent the reduced consumption of calories by elderly persons that is related to lowered metabolic rate.

With the decline in FFM, which influences estimates of protein requirements, also comes a decline in resting metabolic rate (RMR). Basal metabolism directly reflects the lean, metabolizing portion of body mass. RMR reflects the total amount of energy needed for all the metabolic processes involved in maintaining cell function in the resting state and accounts for 60 to 80% of one's total daily energy requirements. Synthetic processes (protein, nucleic acid, lipid, and urea synthesis and gluconeogenesis), transport processes (including the pumping of ions to maintain ion gradients within cells and organelles), and mechanical processes (involving muscular activity) all require energy inputs. These are obtained from high-energy phosphate compounds such as adenosine triphosphatase and guanosine triphosphate that are generated during the oxidation of energy-yielding substrates. Various nutritional, physiologic, and pathologic factors alter the activities of these processes and the types and sources of substrate used for supplying their energy needs. With a decline in energy intake, a reduction in micronutrient intake may also occur, leading to deficiency states. Since body weight changes very little or increases with advancing age, the loss of FFM implies a rise in total adipose tissue (Schlenker, 1993). Many older individuals are classified as obese when the standard criterion of an increase of more than 20% over ideal body mass is applied. Standards of ideal body mass have been developed utilizing data obtained from young or middle-aged adults (Mohs, 1994). These cannot be applied accurately to the elderly population because of the significant differences in muscle mass when compared to younger individuals. The need for standards to be developed specifically for the elderly population is clear.

Age-related changes in the metabolism of energy-yielding substrates can also have an impact on nutritional status. Advancing age is known to be associated with an increased prevalence of impaired glucose tolerance as well as diabetes mellitus. It is estimated that approximately 20 to 30% of older adults have impaired glucose tolerance and 10 to 35% have diabetes mellitus (Schlenker, 1993). Insulin resistance together with body compositional changes predispose the older patient to greater risk for cardiovascular disease. Moreover, food selection may become complicated as carbohydrates provide a major portion of dietary energy intake. Lipids or fat also contribute to a significant proportion of the total dietary intake. Little data has been collected in older humans regarding lipid metabolism, although studies have been conducted in animals. Human studies are often difficult to interpret, even longitudinal data can pose problems with interpretation because of the continued change in diet and exercise that has occurred in the past few decades. Presently available data indicate that the circulating levels of low-density lipoproteins, which are associated with increased risk of atherosclerosis, increase with age; whereas levels of high-density lipoproteins, which appear to offer increased protection against atherosclerosis, do not change with age. Generally, elderly individuals consume a higher percentage of their food intake as fat (42.8% for males and 38.1% for females) than is recommended by the Food and Nutrition Board (Food and Nutrition Board, 1989). How this may affect mortality and morbidity in elderly persons has not been explored. Further work needs to be done to ascertain the optimal fat intake for elderly individuals.

Bone density, or total body calcium, decreases with age. Women are at higher risk than men and typically lose approximately 40% of total skeletal calcium over their lifetime, with half of that being lost within 5 years postmenopause (Rosenberg, 1994). During this period, prevention of calcium depletion is not possible with supplementation alone, although older, postmenopausal women with low calcium intake have been shown to benefit from calcium supplementation. Insufficient vitamin D intake can lead to bone loss and an increased risk for osteoporosis. Levels of 25-hydroxyvitamin D, a clinical indicator of vitamin D status, are known to fluctuate with the seasons (increase in summer and decrease in winter). Possible reasons for a seasonal decline in 25-hydroxyvitamin D include seasonal changes in exercise, nutrition, and blood levels of hormones.

In addition to the seasonal decline of 25-hydroxyvitamin D, there is also an age-related reduction that may be the result of a decline in intake, a decrease in sun exposure, and less efficient skin synthesis of vitamin D (Webb, Kline, & Holick, 1988). Studies have reported that vitamin D supplementation in women with seasonal bone changes is associated with significant gain in bone density, especially in the spine (Dawson-Hughes et al., 1991).

Another age-related phenomenon is a reduction in immune tissue and associated decline in immune function, which depends heavily on adequate macro- and micronutrient nutrition (protein, vitamins, and minerals). The age-related increase in susceptibility to infection and certain types of cancer may be related to the decline in immune function, and it has been argued that this decline could be prevented with careful attention to the effects of diet and nutrition on immune function (Rosenberg, 1994). Mediators of immune function such as cytokines, eicosanoids, prostaglandins, and leukotrienes are dependent on dietary sources of its precursors (proteins, lipids), vitamins and minerals. Chandra has shown that a daily multivitamin/mineral supplement can improve in vitro tests of lymphocyte function (Chandra, 1992). In fact, it has been argued that much of the age-related decline in immune function that could be prevented by vigorous attention to the effects of diet and nutrition (Rosenberg, 1994).

Health status differs from one individual to another that can impact an individual's nutritional requirements. With the onset of an acute illness or chronic disease, dietary requirements may change greatly not only due to the disease itself but to the medications that are used in its management and treatment. Persons over 60 years of age represent 17% of the population but receive 39% of all prescription drugs, and this number will increase as the elderly population grows (Lamy, 1994). Therefore, the elderly population is at the highest risk for potential drug-nutrient interactions. Medications can interfere with nutritional status in four ways: (a) suppression or stimulation of appetite; (b) alteration of nutrient digestion and absorption; (c) alteration of metabolism or utilization of a nutrient; and (d) alteration of excretion of a nutrient (Lamy, 1994). The most frequent type of drug-nutrient interaction is alteration of nutrient absorption affecting a particular or whole class of nutrients. Elderly adults are often prescribed multiple medications for long periods of time that require numerous doses per day, making them more apt to encounter adverse drug-nutrient interactions. It is estimated that older adults take 4–5 medications on average at any given time, including both prescription drugs and over-the-counter medications (Schwartz, 1999). Overuse of laxatives, for example, can cause malabsorption of essential nutrients, including calcium, potassium, and vitamin D. Laxative abuse can result in the development of osteomalacia. Antacids can cause proximal limb muscle weakness, malaise, paresthesias, anorexia, and osteomalacia in elderly individuals, as well as diminish the absorption of riboflavin, copper, and iron. Anti-inflammatory drugs, such as aspirin, can produce multiple small hemorrhages of the mucosa in the intestines, which leads to iron deficiency, and impair the absorption of vitamin C (Blumberg & Suter, 1991).

Many other nonphysiological factors (dietary, individual, and environmental) influence the nutritional status and nutrient requirement of elderly individuals. The way food is processed or prepared can greatly affect an individual's dietary needs. Processed or prepackaged food may not be adequate in providing essential nutrients that fresh food, of the same amount, can provide. Environmental factors such as unsuitable housing or poor sanitary conditions can also alter an elder's nutritional status and requirements.

NUTRITIONAL RISK

Although not all elderly people are malnourished, they belong to a group that is at risk for malnutrition. Those that are hospitalized or institutionalized are at the highest risk. Many hospitalized individuals show signs of malnutrition upon admission or develop it during their stay, leading to higher morbidity and mortality rates. Studies have shown that recovery time can be reduced with presurgery nutritional supplementation in those identified as being severely malnourished (Rolandelli & Ullrich, 1994). Preoperative parenteral nutrition is not possible in emergency surgeries but postoperative parenteral or enteral feeding may still be beneficial in rehabilitating elderly patients.

Approximately 5% of the elderly population in the United States reside in institutions and represent another group at high risk for malnutrition (Schlenker, 1993). Surveys conducted at nursing homes have found malnutrition to be as high as 52% and 85% of their residents (Rolandelli & Ullrich, 1994). Many of these patients have difficulty swallowing or feeding themselves, and 70% have chronic brain disease, which can be accompanied by dementia. Malnutrition is commonly found in nursing home patients with severe dementia. Although long-term care patients suffer from the same illnesses and diseases as free-living elders, long-term care residents are among the heaviest prescription drug users. Consideration of a hospitalized or institutionalized elder's nutrient intake is obviously an important part of the provision of health care.

NUTRITIONAL RECOMMENDATIONS

Optimal intake of macronutrients (protein and energy) and proper exercise are vital in the maintenance of health and function at all ages. A summary of some of the recommendations for specific nutrients by the Food and Nutrition Board of the National Academy of Sciences is found in Table 12.1. The recommendations for the B vitamins and choline were recently updated (Food and Nutrition Board, 1999) whereas the others were published in 1989.

Protein accounts for approximately 10 to 15% of total daily energy intake. Although earlier studies suggested that the protein requirement of older individuals might be less than that of the young, more recent studies indicate that the protein requirement per kg of body weight does not decline with age (Fereday, Gibson, Cox, Pacy, & Millward, 1997; Millward, Fereday, Gibson, & Pacy, 1997). In contrast, Campbell et al. suggested that older persons required more than the present Food and Agriculture Organization of the United Nations/ World Health Organization/United Nations University (FAO/ WHO/UNU) recommendations for safe protein intakes for adults (Campbell, Crim, Dallal, Young, & Evans, 1994). The issue of the essential amino acids (EAA) intake is beyond the scope of this chapter, but it is important to note that there is no information about EAA requirements in the elderly population. However, studies suggest that approximately 30% of dietary protein intake should provide an appropriate mixture of the EAA. When necessary, protein intake must be increased to satisfy the demands of certain diseases and to replenish protein stores.

TABLE 12.1 Recommended Levels for Individual Intake of Selected Vitamin and Minerals, 1998

	1989 recommendations			
	Males		Females	
	25–50 yrs	51+ yrs	25–50 yrs	51+ yrs
Vitamin A (μg RE)[a]	1000	1000	800	800
Vitamin D (μg)[b]	5	5	5	5
Vitamin E (mg α-TE)[c]	10	10	8	8
Ascorbic Acid (vit C, mg)	60	60	60	60
Vitamin K (μg)	80	80	65	65
Calcium (mg)	800	800	800	800
Iron (mg)	10	10	15	10
Selenium (μg)	70	70	55	55
Zinc (mg)	15	15	12	12

	1998 recommendations			
	Males		Females	
	31–50 yrs	51+ yrs	31–50 yrs	51+ yrs
Vitamin B_6 (mg/d)	1.3	1.7	1.3	1.5
Folic Acid (μg/d)	400	400	400	400
Thiamin (mg/d)	1.2	1.2	1.1	1.1
Vitamin B_{12} (μg/d)	2.4	2.4	2.4	2.4
Riboflavin (mg/d)	1.3	1.3	1.1	1.1
Niacin (mg/d)	16	16	14	14
Pantothenic Acid (mg/d)	5	5	5	5
Biotin (μg/d)	30	30	30	30
Choline (mg/d)	550	550	425	425

[a]Retinol equivalent 1 RE = 1 μg retinol or 6 μg β-carotene.
[b]As cholecalciferol, 10 μg cholecalciferol = 400 IU of Vitamin D.
[c]α-Tocopherol equivalents. 1 mg d-α tocopherol = 1 α-TE.

Adapted from Food and Nutrition Board, Institute of Medicine, National Academy of Science (1999). Dietary preference intakes: Recommended intakes for individuals. In *Dietary reference intakes for thiamin, riboflavin, niacin, vitamin B6, folate, vitamin B12, pantothenic acid, brotin, and choline.* Reprinted by courtesy of National Academy Press, Washington, D.C.

Energy intake and requirements decline with advancing age. Since energy requirements are intimately related to FFM, efforts to maintain FFM in elderly persons will inevitably lead to an increase in energy intake and requirements. Numerous studies have been conducted to determine ways to estimate energy requirements, and the FAO/WHO/UNU Expert Group calculated regression equations relating basal metabolic rate to body weight for three adult age groups as presented in Table 12.2. Total energy intake can then be estimated by multiplying the basal or resting metabolic rate by factors accounting for the energy cost of physical activity and thermic effect of food.

A prudent diet for elders does not differ significantly from that for the young. Dietary carbohydrates, whose major purpose is to provide energy, should be about 55 to 60% of dietary energy intake. A lack of carbohydrates in the diet can lead to the incomplete metabolism of fatty acids, leading to ketosis, which can cause lethargy and depression (Carter, 1991). Older individuals are encouraged to eat generous amounts of foods high in fiber. Foods high in fiber have been associated with proper serum lipoprotein patterns and a lower incidence of cardiovascular disease (Schlenker, 1993). Appropriate intake of fiber contributes to better bowel function and a decreased incidence of constipation, which is common in elderly individuals. Some fibers such as guar, pectin, and oat bran and high-fiber foods including cereals, starchy vegetables, and beans have been reported to lower serum lipids, decrease total cholesterol, low-density lipoprotein cholesterol, and triglycerides (Carter, 1991). It is recommended that fiber intake be 25 to 35 g per day to ensure

TABLE 12.2 Basal Metabolic Rate Estimates (kcal) According to Age and Gender

Age range (Years)	Men	Women
18–30	$15.3 \, W^* + 679$	$14.7 \, W + 496$
30–60	$11.6 \, W + 879$	$8.7 \, W + 829$
60+	$13.5 \, W + 487$	$10.5 \, W + 596$

$^*W$ = body weight in kilograms.

Adapted from Food and Nutrition Board and National Research Council, *Recommended Dietary Allowances (10th Ed.)*, 1989. Reprinted by courtesy of National Academy Press, Washington, D.C.

the above benefits. Fiber supplements are not necessary and can, if taken excessively, contribute to bowel dysfunction and interrupt the absorption of important minerals.

In general, intake of fat, another major energy source in the diet, does not differ between healthy younger and older adults. The average American diet includes 40% of total energy intake as fat, and contains a higher proportion of saturated fat and cholesterol than is desired for optimal health. To retard atherosclerosis, the American Heart Association recommends total daily fat intake less than 30% with saturated fat 10 to 15% and cholesterol under 300 mg a day.

Water is often not thought of as a "nutrient" but is important in any diet. Requirements of water intake do not differ greatly between young and elderly persons, although older persons seem to be more prone to insufficient fluid intake. In many cases, mental or physical incapabilities can prevent elders from recognizing their thirst. Medications that are prescribed to individuals with illness or disease may affect the ability to detect thirst. Elderly individuals should be consuming about 2 liters of water per day to avoid dehydration (Carter, 1991).

With the exception of calcium, limited information is available regarding mineral requirements for elderly individuals. Wood et al. report that the current recommended value of calcium as 800 mg per day is too low for the elderly population and suggest a higher daily intake because of age-related calcium loss (Wood, Suter, & Russell, 1995). Daily intake of iron is suggested to be 10 mg for men and 15 mg for women. Given the uncertainty of age-related iron accumulation, more research is needed in the area of iron nutrition in the elderly population. Zinc daily intake is currently 15 mg per day for men and 12 mg per day for women, which reflects average sex differences in body weight. More information is needed regarding daily mineral intake for the elderly population and whether these requirements may differ at various stages of senescence.

Currently, there is great interest in the role of nutrition in increasing longevity. Caloric restriction of at least 20% less than animals would eat ad libtum has been shown to increase longevity and reduce mortality in rodents. Mechanisms for the positive effects of caloric restriction have not yet been defined, but studies in humans are necessary and timely.

CONCLUSION

Although the majority of elderly persons are not malnourished, they represent a vulnerable segment of the population. Their nutritional balance can be easily disturbed by illness, decreased mobility, or increased economic hardship. Hence, it is essential that health care providers pay attention to assessing the nutritional status of older individuals. If we are to reduce morbidity in the aged, thereby achieving associated reductions in recurrent hospitalization and institutionalization, it is essential to pay attention to nutritional needs.

REFERENCES

Blumberg, J., & Suter, P. (1991). Pharmacology, nutrition, and The elderly: Interactions and implications. In R. Chernoff (Ed.), *Geriatric nutrition: The health professional's handbook.* Gaithersburg, MD: Aspen.

Campbell, W. W., Crim, M., Dallal, G., Young, V., & Evans, W. (1994). Increased protein requirements in elderly people: New data and retrospective reassessments. *American Journal of Clinical Nutrition, 60,* 501–509.

Carter, W. (1991). Macronutrient requirements for elderly persons. In R. Chernoff (Ed.), *Geriatric nutrition: The health professional's handbook.* Gaithersburg, MD: Aspen.

Castaneda, C., Charnley, J. M., Evans, W. J., & Crim, M. C. (1995). Elderly women accommodate to a low-protein diet with losses of body cell mass, muscle function, and immune response. *American Journal of Clinical Nutrition, 62,* 30–39.

Chandra, R. (1992). Effect of vitamin and trace-element supplementation on immune responses and infection in elderly subjects. *Lancet, 340,* 1124–1127.

Chernoff, R. (1991). *Geriatric nutrition: The health professional's handbook.* Gaithersburg, MD: Aspen.

Dawson-Hughes, B., Dallal, G., Krall, E., Harris, S., Sokoll, L., & Falconer, G. (1991). Effect of vitamin D supplementation on wintertime and overall bone loss in healthy postmenopausal women. *Annals of Internal Medicine, 115,* 505–512.

Dutta, C. (1997). Significance of sarcopenia in the elderly. *Journal of Nutrition, 127,* 992–993.

Evans, W., & Cyr-Campbell, D. (1997). Nutrition, exercise, and healthy aging. *Journal of the American Dietary Association, 97,* 632–638.

Fereday, A., Gibson, N., Cox, M., Pacy, P., & Millward, D. (1997). Protein requirements and aging: metabolic demand and efficiency of utilization. *British Journal of Nutrition, 77*, 685–702.

Fiatarone, M., Marks, E., Ryan, N., Meredith, C., Lipsitz, L., & Evans, W. (1990). High-intensity strength training in nonagenarians: Effects on skeletal muscle. *Journal of the American Medical Association, 263*, 3029–3034.

Fielding, R. (1995). Effects of exercise training in the elderly: Impact of progressive-resistance training on skeletal muscle and whole-body protein metabolism. *Proceedings of Nutrition Society, 54*, 665–675.

Finch, C., & Hayflick, L. (1977). *Handbook of the biology of aging.* New York: Van Nostrand Reinhold.

Food and Nutrition Board and National Research Council (1989). *Recommended dietary allowances* (10th ed.). Washington, DC: National Academy Press.

Food and Nutrition Board, Institute of Medicare, National Academy of Science. (1999). *Dietary reference intakes for thiamin, riboflavin, niacin, vitamin B6, folate, vitamin B12, pantothenic acid, biotin, and choline.* Washington, DC: National Academy Press.

Kinney, J. (1995). Metabolic responses of the critically ill patient. *Critical Care Clinics, 11*, 569–585.

Kinney, J. M., & Elwyn, D. H. (1983). Protein metabolism and injury. *Annual Review of Nutrition, 3*, 433–466.

Korenchevsky, V. (1961). *Physiological and pathological aging.* Basal, Switzerland: Karger.

Lamy, P. (1994). Drug-nutrient interactions in the aged. In R. Watson (Ed.), *Handbook of nutrition in the aged.* Boca Raton, FL: CRC Press.

Millward, D., Fereday, A., Gibson, N., & Pacy, P. (1997). Aging, protein requirements, and protein turnover. *American Journal of Clinical Nutrition, 66*, 774–786.

Mohs, M. (1994). Assessment of nutritional status in the aged. In R. Watson (Ed.), *Handbook of nutrition in the aged.* Boca Raton, FL: CRC Press.

Rolandelli, R., & Ullrich, J. (1994). Nutritional support in the frail elderly surgical patient. *Surgical Clinics North America, 74*, 79–92.

Rosenberg, I. (1994). Nutrition and ging. In W. Hazzard, E. Bierman, J. Blass, W. Ettinger, & J. Halter (Eds.), *Principles of geriatric medicine and gerontology.* New York: McGraw-Hill.

Schlenker, E. (1993). *Nutrition in aging* (2nd ed.). St. Louis, MO: Mosby.

Schwartz, J. B. (1999). Clinical pharmacology. In W. R. Hazzard, J. P. Blass, W. H. Ettinger, J. B. Halter, & J. G. Ouslander (Eds.), *Principles of geriatric medicine and gerontology* (4th ed.) (pp. 303–332). New York: McGraw-Hill.

Webb, A., Kline, L., & Holick, M. (1988). Influence of season and latitude on the cutaneous synthesis of vitamin D3: Exposure to winter sunlight in Boston and Edmonton will not promote vitamin D3 synthesis in human skin. *Journal of Clinical Endocrinology and Metabolism, 67,* 373–378.

Wood, R., Suter, P., & Russell, R. (1995). Mineral requirements of elderly people. *American Journal of Clinical Nutrition, 62,* 493–505.

CHAPTER 13

The Integration of Exercise and Nutrition in Geriatric Medicine

Maria A. Fiatarone Singh

In this chapter, we will consider the interaction of habitual physical activity, nutritional status, and chronic disease expression in the older adult, with an aim to identify the intersection of these fields as they relate to both prevention and treatment of common geriatric syndromes. It is clear that the optimum approach to successful aging or to health care in the older adult cannot ignore the overlap of these areas. In some cases, exercise can be used to avert "age-related" decrements in physiologic function and thereby optimize function and quality of life in elderly persons. On the other hand, the combination of exercise and nutrition, particularly in relation to favorable alterations in body composition, will have numerous important effects on risk factors for chronic disease as well as the disability that accompanies such conditions. Therefore, understanding the basics of the exercise prescription in the older adult, including its specific utility in nutritional and medical diseases, is critical for health care practitioners and gerontologists.

BIOLOGICAL CHANGES OF AGING
IMPAIR EXERCISE CAPACITY

One of the major goals of gerontological research over the past several decades has been to separate the true physiologic changes of aging from changes due to disease or environmental factors, including disuse or underuse. However, since most people in modern urban societies become increasingly inactive with age, it is difficult to pinpoint the degree to which an individual's regular level of physical activity influences the way in which he or she ages. Nevertheless, numerous studies point out the superior physical condition of those who exercise regularly compared to their more sedentary peers (Bortz, 1989). On the other hand, research indicates that years of physiologic aging of diverse organ systems and metabolic functions can be mimicked by short periods of enforced inactivity such as bed rest, casting, denervation, or loss of gravitational forces. These two types of studies have led to a theory of disuse and aging that suggests that aging as we now know it in modern society is, in many ways, an exercise deficiency syndrome (Bortz, 1989), implying that we may have far more control over the rate and extent of the aging process than we previously thought.

Table 13.1 summarizes the major physiologic changes that relate to exercise capacity in elderly persons and whether they can be modified by higher habitual physical activity levels. As can be seen, with the exception of maximal heart rate, pulmonary flow rates, and possibly loss of alpha motor neurons in the spinal cord and other central and peripheral nervous system control of movement, all of the other changes are minimized by exercise, and therefore probably caused to some degree by inactivity, rather than representative of immutable biological processes.

Musculoskeletal function (strength, power, muscle endurance) is dictated largely by the size of the muscle mass that is contracting, and to a lessor extent by changes in surrounding connective tissue in the joint (cartilage, tendons, and ligaments) and neural recruitment, conduction velocities, and fatigue patterns. Sedentary individuals lose large amounts of muscle mass over the course of adult life (20–50%), and this loss plays a major role in the similar losses in muscle strength observed in both cross-sectional and longitudinal studies (Asmussen & Heeboll-Nielsen, 1961; Frontera, Hughes,

TABLE 13.1   Age-related Changes in Physiologic Function that Influence Nutrient Needs or Intake

Decreased energy requirement	Increased protein requirement	Increased micronutrient and other requirements	Potential for micronutrient toxicity	Decreased nutrient intake
Muscle mass decreases, lowering basal metabolic rate	Decreased protein synthesis rate	Decreased immune function partially corrected with vitamin E, zinc, and other antioxidants	Peripheral tissues take up fat soluble vitamins at slower rates, resulting in higher circulating levels of vitamin A	Loss of olfactory and taste sensations
Fewer calories are used in physical activity	Decreased nitrogen retention in the face of low energy intakes	Intestinal absorption of calcium declines	Increased adipose tissue mass increases total body stores of fat soluble vitamins (A, D, E, and K)	Altered neuropeptides controlling food intake (appetite and satiety)
Thermic effect of meal reduced as food intake is reduced		Skin synthesis of vitamin D diminishes	Decreased thirst sensation may lead to intravascular volume depletion, mineral, electrolyte imbalances	Functional difficulties in food procurement, preparation, and ingestion
		Renal hydroxylation to 1,25 dihydroxy vitamin D decreases		Changes in dentition
		Metabolic utilization of vitamin B6 is less efficient		Decrease in salivary gland function

(continued)

TABLE 13.1   *(continued)*

Decreased energy requirement	Increased protein requirement	Increased micronutrient and other requirements	Potential for micronutrient toxicity	Decreased nutrient intake
		Diminished stomach acid (atrophic gastritis) impairs absorption of vitamin B12, calcium, iron, folic acid, and zinc		
		Loss of estrogen increases the needs for calcium and vitamin D		
		Decrease in gut motility and impaired thirst sensation predispose to constipation which may respond to increased insoluble fiber in diet		

Lutz, & Evans, 1991; Larsson, Grimby, & Karlsson, 1979). However, unlike many other changes that impact on exercise capacity, muscle mass cannot be maintained into old age, even with habitual aerobic activities in either individuals with average activity levels (Pollack et al., 1971) or master athletes (Pollock, Foster, Knapp, Rod, & Schmidt, 1987). Only loading of muscle with weight-lifting exercise (resistance training) has been shown to avert losses of muscle mass (and also strength) in older individuals (Klitgaard et al., 1990). In this study,

Klitgaard and colleagues found that elderly men who swam or ran had similar measures of muscle size and strength as their sedentary peers, whereas the muscle of older men who had been weight lifting for 12 to 17 years was almost indistinguishable, and even superior in some aspects, from healthy men 40 to 50 years younger than them. Appropriate progressive resistance training programs of 3 to 6 months in duration can be shown to increase muscle strength by an average of 40 to 150%, depending on the subject characteristics and intensity of the program, and to increase total body muscle mass by several kilograms (Cartee, 1994; Charette et al., 1991; Fiatarone et al., 1994; McCartney, Hicks, Martin, & Webber, 1995; Pyka, Taaffe, & Marcus, 1994; Skelton, Young, Greig, & Malbut, 1995). Thus, even if some of the neural control of muscle and absolute number of motor units remaining is not maintained by exercise, the adaptation to muscle loading, even in very old age causes neural and structural changes in muscle that can completely compensate for the biological changes of aging. It is not at all unusual to see elderly individuals after training who are stronger than they have ever been, even in their youth, and stronger than their untrained sons and daughters.

Cardiovascular endurance capacity, or aerobic capacity, is dependent primarily on cardiac output (stroke volume × heart rate), capillary density, oxygen carrying capacity of the blood, pulmonary function, extraction of oxygen by the working muscles, and oxidative capacity of the muscle fibers, including oxidative enzyme content, mitochondrial density, proportion of Type I (slow-twitch) fibers, and storage of glycogen for fuel. In healthy older individuals without chronic pulmonary disease, pulmonary airflow rates and oxygen carrying capacity in the blood are not limiting factors in exercise tolerance. The major reason for reduced maximal aerobic capacity with aging is the diminished maximal heart rate in response to exercise, which appears to be limited by an age-related decreased sensitivity of the myocardium to beta-adrenergic stimulation (Heath, Hagberg, Ehsani, & Holloszy, 1981; Lehmann, Schmid, & Keul, 1984). This observation was used to estimate maximal heart rate as "220 − age of subject," 220 being the approximate maximal heart rate achievable by healthy young individuals challenged with increasing exercise loads. Therefore, the approximate maximal heart rate of an 80-year old can be estimated as 140 beats/min. This insensitivity to sympathomimetic stimulation has not been shown to be altered by lifestyle factors such as habitual activity (Panton et al., 1995; Stratton et al., 1992), and therefore stands as a primary biological aging factor for which there is no known remedy. However, although peak workload achievable is therefore always lower in aged individuals, the cardiovascular and musculoskeletal adaptations to chronic aerobic exercise (Mazzeo, Brooks, & Horvath, 1984; Meredith, Zackin, Frontera, & Evans, 1987; Meredith, Frontera, Fisher, & Hughes, 1989; Poulin, Paterson, Govindasamy, & Cunningham, 1992; Rogers, Hagberg, Ehsani, & Holloszy, 1990; Seals, Hagberg, Hurley, Ehsani, & Holloszy, 1984) enable the trained individual to sustain higher submaximal workloads with less of a cardiorespiratory response (heart rate, blood pressure, dyspnea), as well as less overall and musculoskeletal fatigue. In addition to maximal heart rate, muscle mass is an important contributant to maximal aerobic capacity in older persons. Therefore, resistive exercise which maintains or increases muscle mass will also preserve or improve aerobic capacity (Fileg & Lakatta, 1988). Thus, apart from peak athletic performance, the adaptations to training can overcome most of the day-to-day functional limitations that might otherwise be imposed by the physiological changes of aging and disuse (Panton et al., 1995).

BIOLOGICAL CHANGES OF AGING INCREASE NUTRITIONAL VULNERABILITY

In addition to the direct effects of aging on exercise capacity noted above, aging may also increase the nutritional vulnerability of the older adult, which will also predispose to disease and dysfunction. As outlined in Table 13.2, these age-related changes impact on energy, protein, and micronutrient requirements; increase the potential for micronutrient toxicity; and may lead to decreased nutrient intake. In the face of increased protein and micronutrient requirements, it is this propensity for both aging and disease to impair energy intake that underlies much of the nutritional deficiencies observed clinically.

In general, all components of energy expenditure are reduced with aging, including basal energy expenditure, expenditure in physical activity, and the thermic effect of feeding. If energy balance is to be achieved, therefore, energy intake must decrease, or adipose

TABLE 13.2 Nutritional Deficiencies which Impair Exercise Tolerance

Deficiency	Physiologic consequence	Primary exercise capacity effected
B12	Central and peripheral nervous system dysfunction	Muscle strength and power
Calcium	Muscle contractile dysfunction, cardiac conduction disturbance	Aerobic capacity, muscle strength, power and endurance
Carbohydrate	Reduced glycogen storage	Aerobic capacity, musculoskeletal endurance
Energy	Sarcopenia, osteopenia	Aerobic capacity, muscle strength, power, and endurance
Iron	Decreased oxygen carrying capacity	Aerobic capacity
Magnesium	Muscle contractile dysfunction, cardiac conduction disturbance	Aerobic capacity, muscle strength, power and endurance
Potassium	Muscle contractile dysfunction, cardiac conduction disturbance	Aerobic capacity, muscle strength, power and endurance
Protein	Sarcopenia, osteopenia	Aerobic capacity, muscle strength, power
Thiamine	Nerve conduction impairment, myopathy, cardiac dysfunction	Aerobic capacity, muscle strength, power and endurance
Vitamin D	Muscle contractile dysfunction and atrophy	Aerobic capacity, muscle strength, power, and endurance

tissue will accumulate. Since most individuals in fact gain fat mass with age (Elmstahl, 1987; Going, Williams, & Lohman, 1994; Shimokata et al., 1988; Vaughan, Zurlo, & Ravussin, 1991), this means that there must be a mismatch, and the fall in energy expenditure is commonly met with a less than equivalent fall in energy intake. This may happen for a variety of reasons, including a change in the neurotransmitter control of satiety and hunger, an uncoupling of needs and intake (Poehlman, Melby, & Badylak, 1991; Roberts, Fuss, Evans, Heyman, & Young, 1993), psychosocial factors dictating food intake patterns, and the ready availability of energy-dense processed foodstuffs in the food supply. Basal energy expenditure is for the most part determined by lean body mass (Ferraro et al., 1992; Poehlman et al., 1993), and thus losses of muscle mass with aging largely predict the fall in basal metabolism with age. Therefore, the changes in muscle mass described earlier, which are so important for musculoskeletal function in old age, are also central to nutritional balance. There are advantages to raising energy requirements in elderly persons, in that protein and micronutrient intake will also increase if a variety of foods are consumed to meet these needs, and more food can be consumed without augmenting adipose tissue stores. Energy requirements can be increased either by increasing muscle mass (thus increasing resting energy expenditure) or by increasing energy expenditure in physical activity. Resistance training is particularly powerful in this regard, as it has the capacity to influence both of these major components of energy expenditure (Treuth et al., 1994), whereas aerobic training does not typically increase muscle mass or protein turnover significantly.

NUTRITIONAL DEFICIENCIES IMPAIR EXERCISE TOLERANCE

If nutritional deficiencies do develop due to age-related vulnerability or disease, they may add to the risk of impaired exercise tolerance already present in the older adult. As shown in Table 13.3, many different nutrients impact on exercise capacity. Most of these nutrients affect exercise capacity broadly, including both cardiovascular and musculoskeletal performance tasks. Although it is important to prevent such deficiency syndromes, there is little scientific evidence that consuming excessive amounts (above the Recommended Dietary Allowances or RDA (National Research Council, 1989)) of protein or micronutrients in supplement form is able to enhance athletic performance, despite billions of dollars invested in industry and advertising to suggest the contrary. In fact, isolated amino acid supplements may impair the uptake and utilization of other essential amino acids from diet, and vitamins and minerals (particularly fat soluble vitamins) may be toxic in high doses, as listed in Table 13.2.

The most common deficiency states in elderly persons related to exercise and functional capacity are energy, protein, potassium,

TABLE 13.3 Physiologic Changes of Aging which Impair Exercise Capacity

Physiologic change	Habitual exercise minimizes change
Altered neural recruitment, electrical characteristics	unknown
Decreased capillary density in skeletal muscle	yes
Decreased glucose transport and glycogen storage capacity in skeletal muscle	yes
Decreased ligament and tendon strength	yes
Decreased maximal aerobic capacity	yes
Decreased maximal heart rate	no
Decreased maximal muscle strength	yes
Decreased muscle endurance	yes
Decreased muscle mass	yes
Decreased muscle power	yes
Decreased nerve conduction velocity	yes
Decreased oxidative and glycolytic enzyme capacity in skeletal muscle	yes
Decreased pulmonary flow rates	no
Decreased stroke volume	yes
Decreased tissue elasticity and joint range of motion	yes
Degeneration of cartilage	yes
Increased fat mass and percent body fat	yes
Increased heart rate and blood pressure response to sub-maximal exercise	yes
Loss of motor neurons and motor units	unknown

magnesium, vitamin B_{12}, and vitamin D (Garry, Goodwin, Hunt, Hooper, & Leonard, 1982). Energy and protein are of particular concern in hospitalized, institutionalized, and acutely ill individuals, as protein-calorie malnutrition is relatively rare in elderly persons in other settings (Casper, 1995; Fischer & Johnson, 1990). Potassium and magnesium deficiencies generally result from chronic use of diuretic therapy or chronic diarrhea, and are vastly underestimated by the simple use of serum levels to monitor nutrient status. Thus, anyone prescribed nonpotassium sparing (and therefore nonmagnesium sparing) diuretics over the long term should be suspected of having low tissue stores of these minerals and advised regarding dietary or pharmacological supplementation. Vitamin D deficiency

is quite prevalent in elderly persons, both institutionalized and community-dwelling (Vir & Love, 1978), as the feasibility and efficacy of
skin production of this vitamin falls significantly with age, despite
ever increasing requirements (see Table 13.2) (Holick, 1986; Morley,
1986). Although the adverse bone effects of osteomalacia and its
contribution to osteoporosis are well-described, the relationship of
vitamin D to muscle atrophy and weakness is less widely appreciated
(Boland, 1986). The greatly exaggerated risk of injurious falls in the
vitamin D-deficient elder is likely a combination of a heightened
risk of falling due to muscle weakness and a more fragile skeleton
with which to absorb the kinetic energy of the fall (Lauritzen,
McNair, & Lund, 1993; Parfitt et al., 1982).

NUTRITIONAL STATUS AND BODY COMPOSITION IS RELATED TO DISEASE ETIOLOGY AND OUTCOMES

The complex interaction of disease, aging, nutrition, and exercise
is evident when one attempts to summarize both the risk factors for
common geriatric diseases and the sequelae of those diseases, as
shown in Table 13.4. Most of the common chronic diseases of elderly
persons are present on this list, emphasizing the central role these
factors play in optimizing health and preventing disease. Excess body
weight and fat (obesity) is a risk factor for cardiovascular disease,
cancer (breast, endometrial, colon, prostate), diabetes, hypertension, osteoarthritis, and stroke. In most individuals, obesity is caused
by an energy imbalance, and is related to either excess dietary intake,
or low levels of physical activity and muscle mass, or both (Roberts
et al., 1994). Thus, effective preventive counselling must address
both aspects of this equation.

On the other hand, low intakes of energy and protein may be
related to immunosenescence as well as osteoporosis, and again
preventing this by increasing macronutrient intake may be possible
only if energy requirements are increased as well, something that
resistance training has been shown to do in both healthy (Campbell,
Crim, Dallal, Young, & Evans, 1994) and frail elderly persons (Fiatarone et al., 1994). More commonly, we see protein and calorie under-
nutrition and low levels of muscle mass (sarcopenia) resulting from
chronic disease, as in cancer, congestive heart failure, cirrhosis,

TABLE 13.4   Diseases Related to Nutritional Status and Body Composition

Disease	Nutritional risk factor	Nutritional sequelae of disease or treatment
CAD	Obesity, low folate, antioxidants, high cholesterol	
Cancer	Obesity, low antioxidants, fiber, phytochemicals	Sarcopenia, protein calorie malnutrition, low folate
Cataracts	Low vitamin C	
CHF	High sodium	Sarcopenia, low potassium, magnesium, calcium
Cirrhosis	High alcohol	Protein calorie malnutrition, low vitamin D
COPD		Sarcopenia, low calcium, vitamin D
CRF	High protein	Sarcopenia, low protein, vitamin D, high potassium, magnesium
Chronic infection	Low protein, energy, zinc, vitamin E, other antioxidants	Sarcopenia
Dementia	Low B1, B3, B6, B12	Protein calorie malnutrition
Depression	Low folate	Hyperphagia, anorexia
Diabetes	Obesity, low chromium, fiber	
Diverticulosis	Low fiber	Low iron
Epilepsy		Low folate, vitamin D
Hypertension	High sodium, low calcium, low magnesium and potassium obesity, low fruits and vegetables	Low potassium, magnesium
Macular degeneration	Low phytochemicals, antioxidants	
Osteoarthritis	Obesity	Low iron
Osteoporosis	Low calcium, vitamin D, energy, high protein, sodium, alcohol	
Parkinson's Disease		Sarcopenia, protein calorie malnutrition
Rheumatoid arthritis		Sarcopenia, low iron, calcium, vitamin D
Stroke	Obesity, high cholesterol	Protein calorie malnutrition
Ulcer disease		Low iron, B12, folate, calcium, zinc, vitamin C

chronic obstructive pulmonary disease, chronic renal failure, chronic infections, dementia, Parkinson's disease, rheumatoid arthritis, and stroke. In these situations, the change in body composition may be due to a combination of primary disease pathophysiology (e.g., cytokines in congestive heart failure and rheumatoid arthritis), anorexia (chronic liver disease), disuse (stroke), or disease treatment (low protein diet for renal failure, corticosteroid treatment for chronic lung disease). Again, optimal prevention and treatment of these diseases require an understanding of the nutritional and physical activity factors underlying such outcomes.

EXERCISE EFFECTS ON BODY COMPOSITION AND RELATED DISEASE

Relation of Body Composition to Disease

There are many reasons to integrate exercise into the conceptual model of successful aging, but clearly one of the most potent pathways from physical activity to health status involves the modulation of body composition by habitual exercise patterns. Body composition is the division of the body mass into its component parts, along the lines of physical, chemical, or other properties of the tissues. Some of the most common methods divide the body into fat and fat-free (or lean) mass, using various techniques such as hydrostatic weighing; isotopic measurements of total body water; dual energy x-ray absorptiometry; computerized tomography; or elemental analysis of total body potassium, carbon, nitrogen, and calcium, for example (Going et al., 1994; Lohman, 1992). Lean body mass includes muscle, bone, and visceral organs. Adipose tissue may be divided into its subcutaneous, truncal, appendicular, and visceral components if regional imaging techniques such as magnetic resonance imaging or computed tomography scanning are utilized (Despres, 1998).

Using this approach, one can then divide chronic diseases and geriatric syndromes into those that are potentially modifiable by exercise if an underlying derangement in body composition is addressed, as shown in Table 13.5. An increase in bone mass is achievable by either resistive or weight-bearing aerobic exercise, and will be useful for both prevention and treatment of osteoporosis and

TABLE 13.5 Clinical Syndromes in which Modulation of Body Composition by Exercise May Be Preventive (P) or Therapeutic (T)

Decreased total or visceral adipose tissue mass	Increased bone mass	Increased muscle mass
Atherosclerosis (P,T)	Osteoporosis (P,T)	Chronic obstructive pul-
Breast cancer (P)	Injurious falls (P,T)	monary disease (T)
Colon cancer (P)	Functional	Chronic renal failure
Degenerative arthritis	dependency	(T)
(P,T)	(P,T)	Congestive heart
Diabetes mellitus, Type		failure
II (P,T)		(T)
Gout (P,T)		Diabetes mellitus, Type
Hyperlipidemia (P,T)		II (P,T)
Hypertension (P,T)		Frailty, functional de-
Low back pain (P,T)		pendency (P,T)
Low self-esteem (P, T)		Gait and balance disor-
Mobility impairment,		ders, falls (P,T)
disability (P,T)		HIV infection (T)
Peripheral vascular dis-		Low back pain (P,T)
ease (P,T)		Neuromuscular disease
Sleep apnea (P,T)		(T)
Stroke (P)		Osteoporosis (P,T)
Vascular impotence (P)		Parkinson's disease (T)
Venous disease (P,T)		Protein-calorie
		malnutri-
		tion, marasmus (T)
		Rheumatoid arthritis
		(T)
		Stroke (T)

related fractures and disability. Decreases in adipose tissue accumulation are achievable by both aerobic and resistive training, usually in conjunction with an energy-restricted diet. This is both preventive and therapeutic for many common chronic diseases and preventive in the case of cancer, stroke, and vascular impotence. An increase in muscle mass, by contrast, is only achievable with progressive resistance training or generalized weight gain (Fiatarone & Evans, 1993), and with the exception of its potential role in prevention for diabetes, functional dependency and falls and fractures, is primarily important in the treatment of chronic diseases and disabilities (Fiatarone & Evans, 1990). It is notable that the treatment of disease-related sarcopenia with exercise is an area that is not addressed at all by the pharmacologic management of conditions such as congestive heart failure and Parkinson's disease, and therefore it is likely that such adjunctive treatment will impact significantly on related morbidity in these patients. For some diseases, like Type II diabetes mellitus, it can be seen that there are advantages to both minimizing fat tissue as well as maximizing muscle tissue, since these compartments have opposite independent effects on insulin resistance in elderly persons (Despres, 1998).

Decreasing Adipose Tissue Mass

Major reviews and meta-analyses provide little evidence for the ability of exercise to significantly modify body weight or total body fat as an isolated intervention in normal elders (Epstein & Wing, 1980; Ballor & Keesey, 1991; King, Haskell, Taylor, Kraemer, & DeBusk, 1991; Thompson, Jarvic, & Lahey, 1982), even after one year of training. As shown in Table 13.6, the most significant losses of weight and body fat occur in studies of men, in which relatively high doses, intensities, and durations of exercise are utilized, and the response appears to be most robust in younger populations who are not morbidly obese.

There are very limited data on the efficacy of exercise as an isolated treatment for reduction of body fat in already obese individuals and no randomized controlled trials using only aerobic exercise in the

TABLE 13.6 Factors Predictive of Greater Adipose Tissue Losses via Exercise

Induction of an overall energy deficit
Greater dose of exercise (intensity and duration)
Male gender
Younger age
Lower body mass index

treatment of obesity in elderly persons. In a study of middle-aged obese women, Despres and colleagues found that aerobic exercise resulted in reductions in abdominal adipose tissue as well as the ratio of subcutaneous abdominal to thigh fat (Despres, Pouliot, & Moorjani, 1991), indicating preferential losses of central adiposity, just as has been seen in nonobese older adults (Kohrt, Obert, & Holloszy, 1992; Schwartz et al., 1991). Other reasons to advocate such exercise in this group include increases in aerobic fitness (Ruoti, Troup, & Berger, 1994) and insulin sensitivity (Hersey et al., 1994; Katzel et al., 1995), which may occur with exercise independently of weight loss in elderly persons.

Like aerobic training, progressive resistive exercise in the absence of dietary energy restriction appears to have only a small impact on total body weight or adipose tissue mass in young or old individuals. However, there is evidence of reduction in intra-abdominal fat stores with resistance training in two studies of normal weight elders (Treuth et al., 1994; Treuth, Hunter, Szabo, Weinsier, Goran, & Berland, 1995), with no overall changes in body weight or composition. Thus, like aerobic training (Schwartz et al., 1991; Kohrt et al., 1992), resistance training appears capable of reducing metabolically undesirable central fat deposits in the absence of significant weight loss or caloric restriction in normal weight elderly persons.

Energy expenditure and intake, and therefore body weight, may both be influenced by aerobic and resistance training in unique ways, as shown in Table 13.7. It is of note that energy expenditure specific to the type of exercise employed may not be the most important factor in choosing an exercise modality for weight loss. Rather, the regularity and dose of exercise, its effects on other components of energy expenditure as well as concomitant changes in dietary intake are likely to be far more important determinants of efficacy in reducing body fat.

Resistance training studies in healthy elderly persons suggest favorable shifts in energy balance even in the absence of weight loss or increases in fat-free mass, which may be mechanistic in the reduction in obesity described above. Campbell has reported that total energy requirements for weight maintenance are increased approximately 15% after 12 weeks of resistance training in older men and women (Campbell, Crim, Young, & Evans, 1994). Treuth has also described increased resting energy expenditure as well as fat oxidation after

TABLE 13.7   Alterations in Energy Balance Potentially Related to Adipose Tissue Reduction with Exercise

Effect	Observed with aerobic training in elderly	Observed with resistance training in elderly
Excess energy expenditure in exercise session	yes	yes
Increased spontaneous physical activity level apart from prescribed exercise	no	yes
Increased resting metabolic rate	variable	yes
Increased fat oxidation	yes	yes
Increased thermic effect of feeding	variable	yes
Increased energy requirements of larger muscle mass	no	yes
Increased protein turnover in skeletal muscle	no	yes
Better adherence to hypocaloric diet	yes	no

resistance training in postmenopausal women (Treuth, Hunter, Weinsier, & Kell, 1995). Over the long term, such adaptations within muscle tissue may significantly affect energy balance and contribute to the maintenance of a healthful body weight while minimizing fat deposition.

The combination of weight lifting and hypocaloric dieting has been of increasing interest in recent years for the treatment of obesity. There is one randomized controlled trial comparing resistance training to endurance training after hypocaloric dieting in obese older women. After 11 weeks of dieting, Ballor et al. randomly allocated 18 older women to moderate intensity resistance or aerobic exercise training for an additional 12 week (Ballor, Harvey-Berino, Ades, Cryan, & Calles-Escandon, 1996). Weight remained stable in the weight lifters, as the decline in fat mass was more than replaced by a gain in fat-free mass, and resting energy expenditure and thermic effect of feeding increased. By contrast, the endurance training group lost fat and fat-free mass, which combined to produce a significant drop in total body weight, but did not show beneficial shifts in energy expenditure. In the long-term control of body weight and adipose tissue deposition, these body composition and energy expenditure adaptations seen with resistance training may be extremely important in minimizing the tendency for weight and fat to be regained after dieting has ceased (weight cycling) (van Dale & Saris, 1989).

Increasing Muscle Mass

There are numerous studies in normal healthy older adults that indicate that high intensity resistance training is associated with increases in lean body mass or muscle area, usually with minimal alteration of total body weight (Cartee, 1994; Charette et al., 1991; Lillegard & Terrio, 1994; McCartney et al., 1995). However, the observed adaptive response of skeletal muscle to resistance training in these studies is quite variable, likely influenced by the intensity and duration of the intervention, subject characteristics, and the precision of the measurement technique itself (Cartee, 1994; Evans, 1996; Nelson et al., 1996).

Unfortunately, most studies to date have included only healthy individuals (Brown, McCartney, & Sale, 1990; Campbell, Crim, Young et al., 1994; Charette et al., 1991; Frontera, Meredeth, O'Reilly, Knuttgen, & Evans, 1988; Larsson, 1982; Lexell, Downham, Larsson, Bruhn, & Morsing, 1995; Pyka et al., 1994). Little clinical information other than age to allow insight into the wide range of muscle tissue responsiveness to weightlifting regimens. It is clear from these studies and our own (Fiatarone et al., 1994; Pu, Johnson, Forman, Piazza, & Fiatarone, 1997; Fiatarone, Singh et al., 1999) including frail elders, that advancing age impairs the hypertrophic response to resistance training, for reasons not yet identified. Taken together, the existing literature suggests that both exercise-related variables as well as individual characteristics contribute to the wide range of lean tissue responsiveness to resistance training. The factors thus far identified as important in this regard are summarized in Table 13.8. Because hypertrophy requires synthesis of new proteins and structural changes, neural adaptation is the primary cause of immediate changes in strength in response to resistance training, and longer periods of training are associated with greater gains in muscle tissue. Exercise that does not involve high loading forces on the muscle is generally ineffective with regard to gains in both strength and muscle mass. Although it is possible to see changes in whole body lean tissue

TABLE 13.8   Factors Associated with More Robust Hypertrophic Response of Skeletal Muscle to Progressive Resistance Training in the Elderly

Training factors	Subject characteristics
Higher intensity of applied load (relative to one repetition maximum)	Younger age
	Relatively healthy clinical status
Eccentric and concentric loading	Previously untrained status
Longer duration of training	Positive energy balance before and during training
	More IGF-1 present in skeletal muscle at baseline

with progressive resistance training even in the face of hypocaloric dieting in healthy middle-aged and older women (Ballor, Katch, Becque, & Marks, 1988; Ballor et al., 1996), in chronically diseased elderly persons, even eucaloric energy intake appears to inhibit muscle growth, and energy supplementation is necessary to induce significant hypertrophy with weight lifting exercise in our experience (Fiatarone SingH et al., 1994). Further research is required to separate the effects of advanced age, nutritional deficiencies, hormonal status, disease attributes, and extreme sedentariness in clinical populations that may impair their ability to augment lean tissue with this mode of exercise relative to healthy peers.

USING EXERCISE TO COUNTERACT TREATMENT SIDE EFFECTS

In addition to its usefulness in optimal aging and the prevention and treatment of disease, exercise may be considered as a specific intervention to offset adverse side effects of standard medical therapies, as summarized in Table 13.9. Multiple medications may be implicated in anorexia and decreased nutritional intake in elderly persons, with resultant weight loss and depletion of lean tissue. Progressive resistance training has been shown to allow augmentation of energy intake in frail elders with a nutritional supplement, whereas sedentary peers had no increase in total energy intake when given the same supplement (Fiatarone et al., 1994). Chronic cortico-

TABLE 13.9   Counteracting Adverse Consequences of Chronic Disease Treatment with Exercise

Disease treatment	Adverse consequence	Effective exercise modalities
Anorexia secondary to drug therapy (digoxin, serotonin re-uptake inhibitors, theophylline, multiple drug regimens)	Weight loss, sarcopenia	Progressive resistance exercise[*]
Corticosteroid treatment for chronic pulmonary disease or inflammatory arthritis	Myopathy Osteopenia, osteoporotic fracture	Progressive resistance exercise Progressive resistance exercise and endurance exercise
Hypocaloric dieting for obesity	Loss of lean body mass (muscle and bone)	Progressive resistance exercise
Low protein diet for chronic renal failure or liver failure	Weight loss, sarcopenia	Progressive resistance exercise
Postural hypotension secondary to drug therapy (diuretics, antihypertensives, parkinsonian drugs, antidepressants)	Postural symptoms, falls, fractures	Endurance exercise
Slowed gastrointestinal motility secondary to anticholinergics, narcotics, calcium channel blockers, iron therapy	Constipation, fecal impaction, reduced food intake	Progressive resistance exercise and endurance training[*]
Thyroid replacement for hypothyroidism	Osteopenia	Progressive resistance exercise and endurance exercise
Treatment with beta-blockers or alpha-methyl dopa for hypertension or heart disease	Depression	Progressive resistance training or endurance training[*]

[*]clinical trial evidence not yet available

steroid therapy causes large losses of muscle and bone mass, as well as a proximal myopathy, which is reversible with progressive resistance training, even in heart transplant recipients (Braith, Mills, Welsch, Keller, & Pollock, 1996; Braith, Welsch, Mills, Keller, & Pollock, 1998). This finding has very significant implications for patients with rheumatoid arthritis, chronic lung disease, and other illnesses where long periods of catabolic immunosuppressive therapy are indicated. Restriction of energy (Ballor et al., 1988; Ballor et al., 1996) intake in obesity and protein (Castaneda et al., 1999) intake in chronic renal failure both result in losses of muscle mass and strength that can be completely offset by the concurrent prescription of progressive resistance training in elderly persons (see Figure 13.1). In fact, the strength gains and muscle mass increases are similar to those seen in normal elders after training, despite the dietary restrictions in these studies.

This work has important implications for the clinical management of chronic renal failure and liver disease in that the necessary protein restriction can be accomplished without negative consequences on health and functioning that would otherwise occur. For some conditions (slowed gastrointestinal transit time, depression, osteopenia related to drug therapy), aerobic training may provide similar benefits to resistance training, and the choice of which modality to use may be made in the context of other clinical features and individual preferences.

THE EXERCISE PRESCRIPTION

The exercise prescription for the older adult involves more than simply giving advice on what type of exercise to do. A stepwise process of assessment and individualized goal setting and monitoring is more likely to result in successful behavioral modification of sedentary adults. The first step is to assess the exercise needs/goals based on history and physical and individual preferences. The presence of particular risk factors, family history of diseases, current health status and functional level, and physical exam findings will produce a picture of potentially remediable factors that may be responsive to aerobic or resistive training or both.

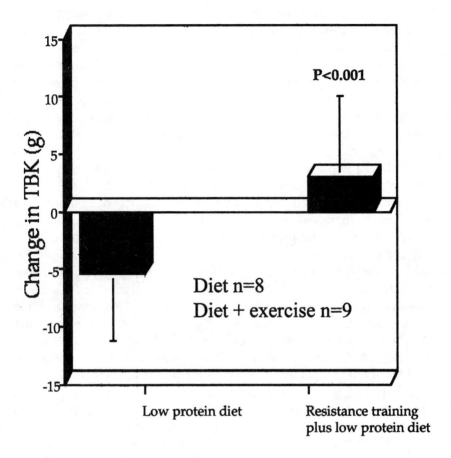

FIGURE 13.1 Effect of resistance training on body composition during dietary treatment of chronic renal failure. Elderly patients with chronic renal failure ($n = 17$) were prescribed and supervised on a low protein diet (0.6 g/kg per day) and then randomized to high intensity progressive resistance training 3 days per week or a control group for 12 weeks. Changes in total body potassium as an index of active cell mass were significantly different between the groups, after adjustment in an ANCOVA model for baseline total body potassium, gender, etiology of chronic renal failure, and level of protein intake ($p<.001$). Exercise completely offset the adverse consequences of the low protein diet on body composition.

Data drawn from: Castaneda et al. (1999). Resistance training prevents muscle wasting in renal disease. *FASEB, 13,* A877.

Prior to initiating recommendations, however, it is necessary to identify behavioral readiness to change lifestyle, and then provide appropriate counselling for the current stage of readiness (King, Taylor, Haskell, & Debusk, 1988). If someone is already contemplating or experimenting with exercise, for example, it may be enough to provide education and access to start a program, whereas for "precontemplators" more work must be done to move them to a stage where they can accept such training, or the prescription will likely fail.

Medical and physical activity history taking will next identify potential risk factors for exercise-related adverse events that can then be avoided by altering the prescription or adding safety elements. For example, a woman with a history of recurrent exacerbations of knee osteoarthritis may be prescribed resistive exercises rather than walking for her arthritis to avoid disease flares that might prevent her adherence to the exercise prescription. An older man with severe visual impairment secondary to macular degeneration and a balance disorder might be advised to use a stationary bike rather than walking for aerobic exercise to minimize his potential for injurious falls. Although more than one exercise need may be identified, these may be then prioritized based on the severity of the deficit to be addressed and the likelihood of adverse events secondary to the exercise itself. It is better to shape a new behavior by advocating change in small doses or steps, so choosing a single feasible and important goal in terms of a new exercise behavior is the best way to begin.

Next, the exercise prescription should be formulated, in the same way that a pharmacologic prescription is given, including the specific exercise modality and dose desired, as outlined in Table 13.10. These recommendations are based on the most recent standards of the American College of Sports Medicine as well as current experts in geriatric exercise physiology and represent dosages of exercise that produce clinically significant changes in physiology, risk profile, or disease status (Fletcher, Balady, Hartley, Haskell, & Pollock, 1995; Mazzeo et al., 1998; Pollock et al. 1998).

Because many older adults will be novices at such exercise regimens, it is usually necessary to provide or refer them to someone for specific training, equipment advice, facility options, safety precautions, and so forth. Some useful resources include physical therapists, fitness centers catering to an older clientele, and personal trainers with special qualifications to work with older adults. It is usually not

TABLE 13.10   Exercise Recommendations for Older Adults

Modality	Resistance training	Cardiovascu-lar endurance training	Flexibility training	Balance training
Dose				
Frequency	2–3 days/wk	3–5 days/wk	2–7 days/wk	1–7 days/wk
Volume	1–3 sets of 8–12 repetitions, 6–10 major muscle groups	20–60 min	4 repetitions, 30 sec/stretch, 6–10 major muscle groups	1–2 sets of 4–10 different exercises including static and dynamic postures
Intensity	15–17 on Borg Scale (80% 1RM), 10 sec/repetition	12–13 on Borg Scale (45–80% maximal heart rate reserve)	Stretch to maximal painfree distance and hold	Progressive difficulty as tolerated
Requirements	Slow speed Good form No breath holding Increase weight progressively	Low impact activity Weight-bearing if possible	Nonballistic movements	Safe environment or monitoring Gradual increase in difficulty

sufficient to provide written or videotaped instructions without any period of hands-on training and supervision, as there is often a significant amount of insecurity present that will otherwise impede adequate progression in the exercise program.

Once the prescription has been agreed on, the health care provider or educator should set up a behavioral program for adoption, adherence, and relapse prevention. Techniques that have been found to be particularly effective include making short-term, achievable goals, record keeping by the individual, providing external rewards for progress, giving timely feedback on attainment of goals, and anticipating common barriers and risks for relapse and planning for them.

Monitoring compliance, benefits, and adverse events over time is essential for the success of the exercise prescription. If patients do not feel that the behavior is important to the caregiver or intrinsically tied to their health and functioning, they will be far less likely to adhere to it in the long term. Such monitoring will allow modification of the exercise prescription over time as health status, goals, and behavioral stage changes.

SPECIFIC EXERCISE RECOMMENDATIONS FOR OLDER ADULTS

In addition to the standard exercise prescription described above, geriatric patients may have specific needs that require specialized recommendations, such as gait and balance disorders, frailty, psychological syndromes, or multiple comorbid diseases. Balance training is still in the process of undergoing rigorous scientific testing to determine the efficacy and feasibility of various regimens, but a rationale approach based on current accepted theory is shown in Table 13.10. Examples of balance enhancing activities include Tai Chi movements, standing yoga postures, tandem standing and walking, standing on one leg, stepping over objects, climbing up and down steps, turning, standing on heels and toes. Many of these movements can be done throughout the day or while waiting in lines or performing other functional and mobility tasks, and are therefore easily incorporated into a daily regimen. The exact doses needed for optimal improvements in balance are not yet known, but it is clear that balance is a highly trainable function, as is aerobic capacity and strength. The intensity of balance training is increased by decreasing the base of support (e.g., progressing from standing on two feet while holding onto the back of a chair to standing on one foot with no hand support); by decreasing other sensory input (e.g., closing eyes or standing on a foam pillow); or by perturbing the center of mass (e.g., holding a heavy object out to one side while maintaining balance, standing on one leg while lifting other leg out behind body, or leaning forward as far as possible without falling or moving feet). As with other modalities of training, progression to higher levels of intensity is critical to the physiologic and clinical benefits achieved.

Common geriatric syndromes that fall outside of the boundaries of single disease entities are often ideally treated with an exercise prescription and are at the same time often not easily treated with standard medical approaches, emphasizing the benefit of this integrated approach to care. Examples of such conditions and their suggested prescriptive elements are given in Table 13.11.

NUTRITIONAL NEEDS OF THE EXERCISING OLDER ADULT

For the most part, nutritional recommendations for the older adult do not change markedly when physical activity levels increase, and in fact exercise may lower nutritional risk by enhancing appetite and food intake and improving nitrogen retention (Campbell, Crim, Dallal, et al., 1994; Shephard, 1989; Wilmore, 1983). However, a few specific suggestions may be made in the circumstances described below:

TABLE 13.11   Choice of Exercise for Common Geriatric Syndromes

Syndrome	Therapeutic exercise recommendation
Anorexia	Endurance or resistance training before meals
Constipation	Endurance or resistance exercise
Depression, anxiety, low self-efficacy	Individual or group exercises including endurance, resistive, and calisthenic activities as preferred
Fatigue	Endurance training in the morning hours, increase duration and intensity as tolerated
Functional dependency	Walking, stair-climbing for endurance Resistance training of upper and lower extremities
Incontinence (stress)	Pelvic muscle strengthening (Kegel exercises); mobility improvement with endurance, balance, and resistance training as needed
Insomnia	Endurance or resistance exercise in mid-late afternoon
Low back pain, spinal stenosis	Resistance training to strengthen the back extensor muscles, rectus abdominus, and hip and knee extensor muscle groups
Recurrent falls, gait and balance disorders	Lower extremity resistance training for hip, knee and ankle Balance training, Tai chi, yoga, ballet Walking in safe or supported environment Training in use of ambulatory device as needed
Weakness	Moderate to high intensity resistance training for all major muscle groups

1. Encourage extra water intake (500–1000 mL) on exercise days, especially in those on diuretics or very low sodium diets, during high ambient temperatures or humid conditions, after recovery from dehydrating illnesses or fevers; sport drink formulations are unnecessary for fluid replacement under normal conditions and in noncompetitive athletes.
2. If a goal is fat/weight loss, combine exercise with a balanced hypocaloric diet and supplement with multivitamin at RDA levels.
3. If the goal is weight maintenance, counsel on increased energy intake (with normal ratios of fat/carbohydrate/protein) as food rather than supplements; encourage dietary diversity to fulfil energy requirements and supply micronutrient needs.
4. If a goal is weight gain, add nutrient and calorically dense food snacks between meals and after exercise sessions.
5. There is no need to supplement protein beyond 1.0 to 1.2 g/kg per day, which can be achieved with diverse dietary sources rather than amino acid or protein supplements.
6. In diabetics, time exercise sessions for the postprandial peaks in blood glucose (1.5–2 hours after a meal); keep high carbohydrate and concentrated sugar snacks available during exercise sessions for brittle or insulin-dependent diabetics; don't exercise after prolonged fasting or skipping meals or during acute illness of any kind.
7. Increase dietary or pharmacological sources of potassium and magnesium if levels are marginal or low, particularly in high risk coronary artery disease or arrhythmia-prone patients on diuretics or digoxin.

SUMMARY

The optimal health and functioning ("successful aging") of the elderly is obviously a multifactorial process, dependent on genetic substrate, environmental factors, social and political forces, and lifestyle choices, among other things. The recognition of the overlapping roles played by physical activity levels and nutritional status assumes increasing importance as we seek to identify modifiable elements in this puzzle that will prevent or delay the onset of many chronic diseases and disabilities. The potential for exercise to lead to improved quality of life on many levels is evidenced by a large body of research over the past several decades. The challenge for gerontologists and health care providers now is to apply and integrate this knowledge into other aspects of planning and care for aged persons.

REFERENCES

Asmussen, E., & Heeboll-Nielsen, M. (1961). Isometric muscle strength of adult men and women. In E. Asmussen, A. Fredsted, & E. Ryge (Eds.), *Community Testing Observation, 11*, (pp. 1–43). Copenhagen, Denmark: Institute of Danish National Association Infantile Paralysis.

Ballor, D., & Keesey, R. (1991). A meta-analysis of the factors affecting exercise-induced changes in body mass, fat mass, and fat-free mass in males and females. *International Journal of Obesity, 15*, 717–726.

Ballor, D. L., Harvey-Berino, J. R., Ades, P. A., Cryan, J., & Calles-Escandon, J. (1996). Contrasting effects of resistance and aerobic training on body composition and metabolism after diet-induced weight loss. *Metabolism: Clinical and Experimental, 45*, 179–183.

Ballor, D. L., Katch, V. L., Becque, M. D., & Marks, C. R. (1988). Resistance weight training during caloric restriction enhances lean body weight maintenance. *American Journal of Clinical Nutrition, 47*, 19–25.

Boland, R. (1986). Role of vitamin D in skeletal muscle function. *Endocrinological Reviews, 7*, 434–448.

Bortz, W. M. (1989). Redefining human aging. *Journal of the American Geriatrics Society, 37*, 1092–1096.

Braith, R., Mills, R., Welsch, M., Keller, J., & Pollock, M. (1996). Resistance exercise training restores bone mineral density in heart transplant recipients. *Journal of the American College Cardiology, 28*, 1471–1477.

Braith, R., Welsch, M., Mills, R., Keller, J., & Pollock, M. (1998). Resistance exercise prevents glucocorticoid-induced myopathy in heart transplant recipients. *Medicine and Science in Sports and Exercise, 30*, 483–489.

Brown, A., McCartney, N., & Sale, D. (1990). Positive adaptations to weight-lifting training in the elderly. *Journal of Applied Physiology, 69*, 1725–1733.

Campbell, W. W., Crim, M. C., Dallal, G., Young, V. R., & Evans, W. J. (1994). Increased protein requirements in the elderly: New data and retrospective reassessments. *American Journal of Clinical Nutrition, 60*, 501–509.

Campbell, W. W., Crim, M. C., Young, V. R., & Evans, W. J. (1994). Increased energy requirements and changes in body composition with resistance training in older adults. *American Journal of Clinical Nutrition, 60,* 167–175.

Cartee, G. D. (1994). Aging skeletal muscle: Response to exercise. *Exercise and Sport Sciences Reviews, 22,* 91–120.

Casper, R. C. (1995). Nutrition and its relationship to aging. *Experimental Gerontology, 30,* 299–314.

Castaneda, C., Gordon, P., Uhlin, K., Kehayias, J., Levey, A., Dwyei, J., Roubenoff, R., & Fiatarone Sengh, M. (1998). Resistance training prevents muscle wasting in renal disease. *FASEB Journal, 3,* A877.

Charette, S., McEvoy, L., Pyka, G., Snow-Harter, C., Guido, D., Wiswell, R. A., & Marcus, R. (1991). Muscle hypertrophy response to resistance training in older women. *Journal of Applied Physiology, 70,* 1912–1916.

Despres, J.-P. (1998). Body fat distribution, exercise and nutrition: Implications for prevention of atherogenic dyslipidemia, coronary heart disease, and non-insulin dependent diabetes mellitus. In D. Lamb & R. Murray (Eds.), *Perspectives in exercise science and sports medicine: Exercise, nutrition and weight control* (Vol. 11) (pp. 107–150). Carmel, IN: Cooper Publishing Group.

Despres, J.-P., Pouliot, M., & Moorjani, S. (1991). Loss of abdominal fat and metabolic response to exercise training in obese women. *American Journal of Physiology, 24,* E159–167.

Elmstahl, S. (1987). Energy expenditure, energy intake and body composition in geriatric long-stay patients. *Comparative Gerontology, A1,* 118–125.

Epstein, L., & Wing, R. (1980). Aerobic exercise and weight. *Addictive Behavior, 5,* 371–388.

Evans, W. J. (1996). Reversing sarcopenia: How weight training can build strength and vitality. *Geriatrics, 51,* 46–47, 51–53, quiz 54.

Ferraro, R., Lillioja, S., Fontvieille, A. M., Rising, R., Bogardus, C., & Ravussin, E. (1992). Lower sedentary metabolic rate in women compared with men. *Journal of Clinical Investigation, 90,* 780–784.

Fiatarone, M. A., & Evans, W. J. (1990). Exercise in the oldest old. *Topics in Geriatric Rehabilitation, 5,* 63–77.

Fiatarone, M. A., & Evans, W. J. (1993). The etiology and reversibility of muscle dysfunction in the elderly. *Journal of Gerontology, 48,* 77–83.

Fiatarone, M. A., O'Neill, E. F., Ryan, N. D., Clements, K. M., Solares, G. R., Nelson, M. E., Roberts, S. B., Kehayias, J. J., Lipsitz, L. A., & Evans, W. J. (1994). Exercise training and nutritional supplementation for physical frailty in very elderly people. *New England Journal of Medicine, 330,* 1769–1775.

Fiatarone Singh, M. A., Ding, W., Manfredi, T. J., Solares, G. S., O'Neill, E. F., Clements, K. M., Ryan, N. D., Kehayias, J. J., Fielding, R. A., & Evans, W. J. (1999). Insulin-like growth factor I in skeletal muscle after weight-lifting exercise in frail elders. *American Journal of Physiology, 277,* E136–E143.

Fischer, J., & Johnson, M. A. (1990). Low body weight and weight loss in the aged. *Journal of the American Dietetic Association, 90,* 1697–1706.

Fleg, J. L., & Lakatta, E. G. (1988). Role of muscle loss in the age-associated reduction in VO_2 max. *Journal of Applied Physiology, 65,* 1147–1151.

Fletcher, G., Balady, G., Hartley, L., Haskell, W., & Pollock, M. (1995). Exercise standards: A statement for healthcare professionals from the American Heart Association. *Circulation, 91,* 580–616.

Frontera, W., Hughes, V., Lutz, K., & Evans, W. J. (1991). A cross-sectional study of muscle strength and mass in 45- to 78-year-old men and women. *Journal of Applied Physiology, 71,* 644–650.

Frontera, W. R., Meredith, C. N., O'Reilly, K. P., Knuttgen, H. G., & Evans, W. J. (1988). Strength conditioning in older men: Skeletal muscle hypertrophy and improved function. *Journal of Applied Physiology, 64,* 1038–1044.

Garry, P. J., Goodwin, J. S., Hunt, W. C., Hooper, E. M., & Leonard, A. G. (1982). Nutritional status in a healthy elderly population. *American Journal of Clinical Nutrition, 36,* 319.

Going, S., Williams, D., & Lohman, T. (1994). Aging and body composition: Biological changes and methodological issues. *Exercise and Sports Science Review, 22,* 411–458.

Heath, G., Hagberg, J., Ehsani, A., & Holloszy, J. (1981). A physiological comparison of young and older endurance athletes. *Journal of Applied Physiology, 51,* 634–640.

Hersey, W. C., Graves, J. E., Pollock, M. L., Gingerich, R., Shireman, R. B., Heath, G. W., Spierto, F., McCole, S. D., & Hagberg, J. M. (1994). Endurance exercise training improves body composition and plasma insulin responses in 70- to 79-year-old men and women. *Metabolism: Clinical and Experimental, 43,* 847–854.

Holick, M. (1986). Vitamin D synthesis by the aging skin. In *Nutrition and aging: Brystol Meyers Symposia 1986* (pp. 45–58). Orlando, FL: Academic.

Katzel, L. I., Bleecker, E. R., Colman, E. G., Rogus, E. M., Sorkin, J. D., & Goldberg, A. P. (1995). Effects of weight loss vs aerobic exercise training on risk factors for coronary disease in healthy, obese, middle-aged and older men: A randomized controlled trial [see comments]. *Journal of the American Medical Association, 274,* 1915–1921.

King, A., Haskell, W., Taylor, C., Kraemer, H., & DeBusk, R. (1991). Group- vs home-based exercise training in healthy older men and women: A community-based clinical trial. *Journal of the American Medical Association, 266,* 1535–1542.

King, A., Taylor, C., Haskell, W., & Debusk, R. (1988). Strategies for increasing early adherence to and long-term maintenance of home-based exercise training in healthy middle-aged men and women. *American Journal of Cardiology, 61*, 628–632.

Klitgaard, H., Mantoni, M., Schiaffino, S., Ausoni, S., Gorza, L., Laurent-Winter, C., Schnohr, P., & Saltin, B. (1990). Function, morphology and protein expression of ageing skeletal muscle: A cross-sectional study of elderly men with different training backgrounds. *Acta Physiology Scand., 140*, 41–54.

Kohrt, W. N., Obert, K. A., & Holloszy, J. O. (1992). Exercise training improves fat distribution patterns in 60- to 70-year-old men and women. *Journal of Gerontology, 47*, M99–105.

Larsson, L. (1982). Physical training effects on muscle morphology in sedentary males as different ages. *Med. Sci. Sports Exercise, 14*, 203–206.

Larsson, L. G., Grimby, G., & Karlsson, J. (1979). Muscle strength and speed of movement in relation to age and muscle morphology. *Journal of Applied Physiology, 46*, 451–456.

Lauritzen, J. B., McNair, P. A., & Lund, B. (1993). Risk factors for hip fractures: A review. *Danish Medical Bulletin, 40*, 479–485.

Lehmann, N., Schmid, P., & Keul, J. (1984). Age- and exercise-related sympathetic activity in untrained volunteers, trained athletes and patients with impaired left-entricular contractility. *European Heart Journal, 5*(Suppl E), 1–7.

Lexell, J., Downham, D., Larsson, Y., Bruhn, E., & Morsing, B. (1995). Heavy-resistance training in older Scandinavian men and women: Short- and long-term effects on arm and leg muscles. *Scandinavian Journal of Medicine and Science in Sports, 5*, 329–341.

Lillegard, W. A., & Terrio, J. D. (1994). Appropriate Strength Training. *Medical Clinics of North America, 78*, 457–477.

Lohman, T. (1992). *Advances in Body Composition Assessment.* Champaign, IL: Human Kinetics Publishers.

Mazzeo, R., Cavanaugh, P., Evans, W. J., Fiatarone, M., Hagberg, J., McAuley, E., & Startzell, J. (1998). Exercise and physical activity for older adults. *Med Sci Sports Exercise, 30*, 992–1008.

Mazzeo, R. S., Brooks, G. A., & Horvath, S. M. (1984). Effects of age on metabolic responses to endurance training in rats. *Journal of Applied Physiology, 57*, 1369–1374.

McCartney, N., Hicks, A., Martin, J., & Webber, C. (1995). Long-term resistance training in the elderly: Effects on dynamic strength, exercise capacity, muscle, and bone. *Journal of Gerontology, 50*, B97–104.

Meredith, C., Frontera, W., Fisher, E., & Hughes, V. (1989). Peripheral effects of endurance training in young and old subjects. *Journal of Applied Physiology, 66*, 2844–2849.

Meredith, C. N., Zackin, M. J., Frontera, W. R., & Evans, W. J. (1987). Body composition and aerobic capacity in young and middle-aged endurance-trained men. *Medicine and Science in Sports and Exercise, 19,* 557–563.

Morley, J. E. (1986). Nutritional Status of the Elderly. *American Journal of Medicine, 81,* 679–695.

National Research Council (1989). *Recommended Dietary Allowances.* Washington, DC: National Academy of Sciences.

Nelson, M., Fiatarone, M. A., Layne, J., Trice, I., Economos, C. D., Fielding, R. A., Ma, R., Pierson, R. N., & Evans, W. J. (1996). Analysis of body-composition techniques and models for detecting change in soft tissue with strength training. *American Journal of Clinical Nutrition, 63,* 678–686.

Panton, L. B., Guillen, G. J., Williams, L., Graves, J. E., Vivas, C., Cedrel, M., Pollock, M. L., Giarzarella, L., Krumerman, J., & Derendorf, H. (1995). The lack of effect of aerobic exercise training on propranolol pharmacokinetics in young and elderly adults. *Journal of Clinical Pharmacology, 35,* 885–894.

Parfitt, A. M., Gallagher J. C., Heaney, R. P., Johnston, C. C., Neer, R., & Whedon, G. D. (1982). Vitamin D and bone health in the elderly. *American Journal of Clinical Nutrition, 36,* 1014–1031.

Poehlman, E. T., Goran, M. I., Gardner, A. W., Ades, P. A., Arciero, P. J., Katzman-Rooks, S. M., Montgomery, S. M., Toth, M. J., & Sutherland, P. T. (1993). Determinants of decline in resting metabolic rate in aging females. *American Journal of Physiology, 264,* E450–455.

Poehlman, E. T., Melby, C. L., & Badylak, S. F. (1991). Relation of age and physical exercise status on metabolic rate in younger and older healthy men. *Journal of Gerontology, 46,* B54–58.

Pollock, M., Gaesser, G., Butcher, J., Despres, J. P., Dishman, R. K., Franklin, B. A., & Garber, C. E. (1998). The recommended quantity and quality of exercise for developing and maintaining cardiorespiratory and muscular fitness, and flexibility in healthy adults. *Medicine and Science in Sports and Exercise, 30,* 975–991.

Pollock, M., Miller, H., Janeway, R., Linnerud, A., Robertson, B.. & Valentino, R. (1971). Effects of walking on body composition and cardiovascular function of middle-aged men. *Journal of Applied Physiology, 30,* 126–130.

Pollock, M. L., Foster, C., Knapp, D., Rod, J. L., & Schmidt, D. H. (1987). Effect of age and training on aerobic capacity and body composition of master athletes. *Journal of Applied Physiology, 62,* 725–731.

Poulin, M. J., Paterson, D. H., Govindasamy, D., & Cunningham, D. A. (1992). Endurance training of older men: Responses to submaximal exercise. *Journal of Applied Physiology, 73,* 452–457.

Pu, C., Johnson, M., Forman, D., Piazza, L., & Fiatarone, M. A. (1997). High-intensity progressive resistance training in older women with chronic heart failure. *Medicine and Science in Sports Exercise, 29,* S148.

Pyka, G., Taaffe, D. R., & Marcus, R. (1994). Effect of a sustained program of resistance training on the acute growth hormone response to resistance exercise in older adults. *Hormone and Metabolic Research, 26,* 330–333.

Rogers, M. A., Hagberg, J. M., Martin, W. H. M., Ehsani, A. A., & Holloszy, J. O. (1990). Decline in V02 max with aging master athletes and sedentary men. *Journal of Applied Physiology, 68,* 2195–2199.

Roberts, S. B., Fuss, P., Evans, W. J., Heyman, M. B., & Young, V. R. (1993). Energy expenditure, aging and body composition. *Journal of Nutrition, 123* (Suppl 2), 474–480.

Roberts, S. B., Fuss, P., Heyman, M. B., Evans, W. J., Tsay, R., Rasmussen, H., Fiatarone, M. A., Cortrella, J., Dallal, G. E., & Young, V. R. (1994). Control of food intake in older men. *Journal of the American Medical Association, 272,* 1601–1606.

Ruoti, R. G., Troup, J. T., & Berger, R. A. (1994). The effects of nonswimming water exercises on older adults. *Journal of Orthopaedic and Sports Physical Therapy, 19,* 140–145.

Schwartz, R. S., Shuman, W. P., Larson, V., Cain, K. C., Fellingham, G. W., Beard, J. C., Kahn, S. E., Stratton, J. R., Cerqueria, M. D., & Abass, I. B. (1991). The effect of intensive endurance exercise training on body fat distribution in young and older men. *Metabolism: Clinical and Experimental, 40,* 545–551.

Seals, D. R., Hagberg, J. M., Hurley, B. F., Ehsani, A. A., & Holloszy, J. O. (1984). Endurance training in older men and women I: Cardiovascular responses to training. *Journal of Applied Physiology, 57,* 1024–1029.

Shephard, R. J. (1989). Nutritional benefits of exercise. *Journal of Sports Medicine and Physical Fitness, 29,* 83–90.

Shimokata, H., Andres, R., Coon, P., Elahi, D., Muller, D., & Tobin, J. (1988). Studies in the distribution of body fat II: Longitudinal effects of changes in weight. *International Journal of Obesity, 13,* 455–464.

Skelton, D. A., Young, A., Greig, C. A., & Malbut, K. E. (1995). Effects of resistance training on strength, power, and selected functional abilities of women aged 75 and older. *Journal of the American Geriatrics Society, 43,* 1081–1087.

Stratton, J. R., Cerqueira, M. D., Schwartz, R. S., Levey, W. C., Verth, R. C., Kahn, S. E., & Abrass, I. B. (1992). Differences in cardiovascular responses to isopreterenol in relation to age and exercise training in healthy men. *Circulation, 86,* 504–512.

Thompson, J., Jarvic, G., & Lahey, R. (1982). Exercise and obesity: Etiology, physiology, and intervention. *Psychological Bulletin, 91,* 55–79.

Treuth, M., Hunter, G., Szabo, T., Weinsier, R., Goran, M., & Berland, L. (1995). Reduction in intra-abdominal adipose tissue after strength training in older women. *Journal of Applied Physiology, 78,* 1425–1431.

Treuth, M., Hunter, G., Weinsier, R., & Kell, S. (1995). Energy expenditure and substrate utilization in older women after strength training: 24-h calorimeter results. *Journal of Applied Physiology, 78,* 2140–2146.

Treuth, M., Ryan, A., Pratley, R., Rubin, M. A., Miller, J. P., Nicklas, B. J., Sorkin, J., Harman, S. M., Goldberg, A. P., & Hurley, B. F. (1994). Effects of strength training on total and regional body composition in older men. *Journal of Applied Physiology, 77,* 614–620.

Van Dale, D., & Saris, W. (1989). Repetitive weight loss and weight regain: Effects on weight reduction, resting metabolic rate, and lipolytic activity before and after exercise and/or diet treatment. *American Journal of Clinical Nutrition, 49,* 409–416.

Vaughan, L., Zurlo, F., & Ravussin, E. (1991). Aging and energy expenditure. *American Journal of Clinical Nutrition, 53,* 821–825.

Vir, S., & Love, A. (1978). Vitamin D status of elderly at home and institutionalized in hospital. *International Journal of Vitamin and Nutrition Research, 48,* 123–130.

Wilmore, J. (1983). Appetite and body composition consequent to physical activity. *Res Quarterly, 54,* 415–425.

CHAPTER 14

Falls Among Elderly Persons

Jonathan Howland, Elizabeth Walker Peterson, and Margie E. Lachman

F alls are a common and serious health problem among elderly persons. Each year about 25% of elders between the ages of 65 to 74 who live independently experience a fall. This increases to about one third among those 75 years and older (Nevitt, 1990).

While only about 10 to 15% of falls among elderly persons result in serious injury, the effects of injurious falls can be devastating. Fall-related mortality is high in older adults (18 per 100,000 vs 2.7 per 100,000 in younger populations), with rates especially high for those 85 and older (131.2 per 100,000). The excessive rates for older people have been specially targeted for reduction in the Department of Health and Human Services' Year 2000 Objectives for the Nation (Department of Health and Human Services, 1990). Overall, falls are the second leading cause of unintentional injury death and are the most common cause of hospital admissions for trauma. They are the source of 87% of all fractures in elderly persons (Baker, O'Neill, Ginsburg, & Li, 1992). Hip fractures alone result in more hospital admissions than any other injury and are the primary cause of about 250,000 hospital admissions each year. People over 65 sustain 85% of all hip fractures (Baker et al., 1992). The likelihood of dying from a fall increases precipitously with age. A third of all fall fatalities occur among people over 85, although this age group comprises only about 1% of the population (Baker et al., 1992). To put this in perspective, there are more deaths from falls among people 85 or older than there are motor vehicle deaths among males between the ages of 18 and 19, the age group at highest risk for traffic fatality (Baker et al., 1992). Falls are also associated with long-term morbidity. Many fall survivors experience accelerated decline in function as a consequence of falling.

Falls are costly. Although the total costs associated with falls are unknown, the yearly costs for acute care associated with fall-related fractures are estimated at $10 billion (Sattin, 1992). It is estimated that falls cost in excess of $6 billion dollars per year. Overall, falls are second only to traffic crashes in total lifetime injury costs, accounting for $37 billion and $49 billion, respectively, in 1985. The higher costs attributed to traffic crashes is a function of differentials in age distribution for these events; younger people are more apt to be involved in traffic crashes while elderly persons are more likely to be injured from falls. The elderly population comprise about 12% of the total population but account for 25% of health care resources expended for trauma. The majority of injuries among elderly persons result from falls.

Fall fatality rates have been decreasing over recent decades. Compared to the period 1977 to 1979, fall death rates for people between the ages of 65 to 85 were more than 20% lower for the period 1984 to 1986. Moreover, there has been a shift in the male to female ratio of fall-related deaths. In 1960, the rate among Whites aged 75 and older was 20% higher for females than males. However, for the period 1980 to 1986, the female rate was 25% lower than the male rate (Baker et al., 1992).

Despite declines in fall fatality rates, it is likely that for the foreseeable future the absolute number of fall-related injuries, and associated costs, will increase as the population ages.

ETIOLOGY OF FALLS

Although falls are common among elderly persons, some individuals are at greater risk than others. Falls are typically multifactorial in nature. In fact, the risk of falling increases with the number of risk factors present (Tinetti, Speechley, & Ginter, 1988). Both intrinsic and extrinsic risk factors contribute to fall risk.

Intrinsic factors include both physiological and behavioral risks. Loss of function associated with aging such as decreased visual acuity, impaired balance and gait, and slowed reaction times have been identified as risks for falling, as have chronic diseases that compromise sensory, cognitive, neurologic, or musculoskeletal functioning (Tinetti, Doucette, Claus, & Marottoli, 1995).

Certain classes of drugs, especially sedatives and hypnotics also increase fall risk (Ray, Griffin, Schaffner, Baugh, & Melton, 1987). Behavioral risk factors include failing to exercise regularly, failing to use prescribed assistive devices (such as walkers) as recommended, climbing on objects to reach items on high shelves, hurrying to answer phones or door bells, and attempting to carry heavy objects or too many objects at one time. Older adults who hesitate to bring concerns about falls (or about their health in general) to the attention of their health care providers or family members place themselves at risk for a fall, as do those who are reluctant to request assistance with activities of daily living (ADLs) or instrumental activities of daily living (IADLs). Therefore, it is important for older adults to learn to use assertive communication skills effectively.

Extrinsic risks are environmental in nature and include household and community hazards. Among community-dwelling older adults, the majority of falls occur in the home; namely in stairways (Lucht, 1971), bedrooms (Wild, Nayak, & Issacs, 1981), and living rooms (Wild et al., 1981). Common environmental hazards include highly polished or wet ground surfaces, poor lighting, lack of handrails on stairs, cluttered spaces (often the result of moving from larger to smaller dwelling spaces), loose or thick pile rugs, irregular ground surfaces, exposed phone cords, poorly planned storage shelves (in kitchens and elsewhere), absence of grab bars near the toilet and in the shower, and improper shoes. Transferring in and out of beds and chairs has been identified as an activity commonly associated with falls (Naylor & Rosin, 1970). Unstable (rolling), low and overly soft beds and chairs are especially problematic. Finally, among institutionalized older adults, the use of physical restraints has been associated with increased falls (Hart & Sliefert, 1983).

FEAR OF FALLING

Fear of falling is a related and important problem that has only recently been the focus of research. Previously, fear of falling was studied as a sequel of experiencing a serious fall. In recent years, however, a number of epidemiological studies have been conducted on fear of falling among the general elderly population.

Howland, Peterson, Levin, Fried, Pordon, and Bak (1993) surveyed community-dwelling elderly residents in two senior-housing projects in metropolitan Boston and found that 47% of respondents were afraid they would fall in coming year. Thirty-five percent said they limited activities they would like to do because they were afraid they would fall. In a similar 1994 study of a sample of community-dwelling elderly residents in St. Louis Arfken, Lach, Birge, and Miller (1994) found that 29% were afraid of falling. In a 1994 study, Auerbach, Bandeen-Roche, Chee, and Fried (1994) queried community-dwelling elderly persons from senior centers in Baltimore. Thirty-one percent said they had been afraid of falling during the past year. In another 1994 study of community-dwelling elderly residents in New Haven, Tinetti, Mendes de Leon, Doucette, and Baker (1994) reported that 43% were afraid of falling, and 19% acknowledged avoiding activities due to this fear. Interestingly, while all of these authors found that a history of falls was associated with fear of falling, they also found that a substantial portion of the population who had not fallen was also afraid of falling. Although each of these studies asked about fear of falling in slightly different ways, there is relative consistency, and it appears as though somewhere between a third and a half of the community-dwelling elderly acknowledge fear of falling.

In addition to being prevalent, fear of falling can be intense. In their 1993 study, Howland et al. (1993) also asked respondents about other fears. In contrast to the 47% who were afraid of falling, 17% were afraid of being robbed in the street; 8% were afraid of forgetting an important appointment; 12% feared financial problems; and, 5% feared losing a cherished item.

While it could be argued that fear of falling is a rational response to the incidence of falls and that caution about falling is an initial and important component of preventing falls, there are several reasons for concern about this fear. First, if the fear of falling is intense enough, it can limit mobility. Tinetti et al. (1988) found that 26% of fallers acknowledged avoiding activities as did 13% of nonfallers. Ten percent of recurrent fallers in a prospective study by Nevitt, Cummings, Kidd, and Black (1989) reported avoiding activity because of fear of falling. In a representative sample of 270 older adults living in senior housing in the Boston area, 17% had fallen to the ground in the past 3 months, whereas 36% reported falls that required medical attention sometime in the past 5 years (Lachman et al., 1998). Activity restriction was found to be a major consequence of fear of falling. Those who had higher fear scores had engaged in fewer activities and reduced their activities more over a 5-year period. More than half of the sample reported that they had cut back on doing a number of activities, such as going out for walks, over the past 5 years. (Lachman et al., 1998). The extent of fear of falling varied across activities. The greatest amount of fear was associated with "going out when it is slippery" and "taking a bath."

By limiting activity, fear of falling can lead to reduced physical conditioning. One consequence of reduced physical conditioning could be increased risk for falls (Nevitt et al., 1989). Thus, while it could be argued that limiting activity due to fear of falling limits opportunities for falling, it might also increase the risk for falling when activity, by necessity, occurs. There is increasing evidence of the role of physical activity in maintaining health status. Fear of falling may therefore have implications for the primary prevention of some chronic conditions. With respect to secondary prevention, fear of falling may reduce compliance with rehabilitation regimens.

Fear of falling impacts negatively on the mental health and overall well-being of older adults in a number of ways. Among older adults, social activity is strongly associated with morale (Graney, 1975; Multran & Reitzes, 1981). Older adults with a fear of falling have the potential to become socially isolated. When persons avoid social roles and activities they increase their vulnerability to poor coping and depression because they lack social supports that serve to buffer against life stressors (Belgrave, 1991; Holahan & Holahan, 1987a, 1987b). Increased use of alcohol, tranquilizers, and hypnotic medications are behavioral manifestations of poor coping, and all are associated with increased fall risk. By avoiding activities, older adults who are fearful of falling also miss opportunities to test their capacities and to maintain a realistic sense of efficacy. Such a pattern may lead to or sustain unrealistic fears of falling. In support of this argument, research has shown that engaging in activities of daily living is related to falls self-efficacy, that is, efficacy beliefs regarding whether one can do the activity without falling (Powell & Meyers, 1995; Tinetti, Richman, & Powell, 1990).

The impact of falls self-efficacy on well-being has been documented by Peterson, Howland, Kielhofner, Lachman, Assmann, Cote, and Jette (1999) in a study that demonstrated the impact of falls self-efficacy on mental health (mood), emotional functioning (extent to which emotional problems interfered with desired activities), social functioning (extent to which health problems interfered with normal social activities), life satisfaction, and leisure activities. Those findings, which show a consistent relationship between falls self-efficacy and well-being independent of risk factors for falls, underscore the importance of falls self-efficacy as a vital characteristic for healthy aging. Evidence of the reciprocal relationship between fear of falling and quality of life was also shown by Lachman et al. (1998). In that study subjects who had greater fear of falling also had lower quality of life, as determined by both health and social indicators.

INTERVENTIONS FOR FALLS AND FEAR OF FALLING

Overview

In recent years, a number of randomized trials have been conducted on interventions designed to prevent falls among elderly persons. The availability of data from randomized trials on the effectiveness of fall prevention programs has important clinical implications. Health care providers working with older adults at risk for falls are now able to provide evidence-based interventions. Because the outcome data yielded by randomized trials is the best available, we surveyed the literature for all large-scale trials that identified falls or fear of falling as the primary outcome of interest. Our review of the literature yielded six studies that met our criteria for discussion in this chapter. Each of the studies enrolled community-dwelling older adults.

Of the six trials presented, all measured impact on falls. One of the studies was conducted on a program specifically addressing fear of falling (Tennstedt et al., 1998). The logic of all interventions presented is to target modifiable risk factors for falls. Recognizing that falls often result from the interaction of several factors, most of the interventions presented take a multifactorial approach, aiming to change several risks simultaneously. Others have focused on a single risk factor, although it is reasonable to assume that intervention for one factor may often have spillover effects for other factors not specifically targeted.

Strategies for reducing falls and fear of falling typically include one or more of the following:

- Modification of behavioral risk factors
- Removal of environmental hazards in the home and in the community
- Lower extremity strength training
- Balance training
- Cognitive restructuring (improving self-efficacy regarding falls prevention)

With respect to exercise regimens, both lack of lower body strength and impaired balance have been identified as risk factors for falls among elderly persons. It has been argued that interventions that focus only on improving strength through static-posture exercises fail to address the need for controlling balance over a dynamically changing base of support. While it is likely that strength training itself may have some beneficial effects for balance, several investigations have tested a falls prevention strategy that focused on balance training alone. Balance training can be accomplished in several ways, ranging from simple exercises to computerized visual display biofeedback devices. Another balance training approach involves Tai Chi, an ancient Chinese exercise related to marital arts training and used to enhance balance and body awareness.

Results of intervention trials have been mixed. A number of trials have achieved significant reductions in falls overall, while some have shown no reductions and several have shown nonsignificant increases in the incidence of falls. Of the randomized trials reviewed here, only one has shown significant reductions in injurious falls. Several have shown reductions in fear of falling.

At this point, it is difficult to conclude whether a single intervention component or combination of components is effective in reducing falls or fear of falling. The multifactorial nature of most intervention trials makes it difficult to disentangle the effects of specific strategies. Nevertheless, interventions do differ in the intensity of focus on a given strategy.

INTERVENTIONS DESIGNED TO REDUCE FALLS

Exercise Strategies

Wolf, Barnhart, Kutner, McNeely, Coogler, Xu, and the Atlanta FIC-SIT Group (1996) conducted a randomized trial comparing the efficacy of two methods of exercise approaches on biomedical, functional, and psychosocial indicators of frailty. Both falls and fear of falling were primary outcome measures of interest. Two hundred community-dwelling, ambulatory participants 70 years and older were randomized to one of three groups: 15 weeks of group Tai Chi training; 15 weeks of computerized balance training; and 15 weeks of discussion groups on health topics of interest to elders lead by a gerontological nurse/researcher (control). The subjects randomized to the Tai Chi group participated in Tai Chi classes that emphasized all components of movement that typically become limited with aging. Specifically, the progression involved a gradual reduction of the base of support until single limb stance was achieved, increased body and trunk rotation, and reciprocal arm movements (Wolf, Coogler, Green, & Xu, 1993). Subjects were encouraged to practice at least 15 minutes twice a day, but home practice was not monitored. Compared to the control group, the Tai Chi participants experienced significant reductions in falls and fear of falling. Surprisingly, these effects were not found for the computerized balance training group. These results suggest that an inexpensive, low intensity routine program that can be practiced by individuals at home can have beneficial outcomes in terms of falls reduction.

Campbell, Robertson, Gardner, Norton, Tilyard, and Buchner (1997) conducted a randomized trial of a falls prevention intervention that combined strength and balance training, as required by individual participants. The program was designed to be administered by a general medical practice. Participants ($N = 233$) were women 80 years or older who lived in the community. The intervention was an individually tailored exercise program delivered in the home by a physical therapist. It consisted of four 1-hour home visits during the first 2 months with follow-up motivational phone calls. Strength training included moderate intensity exercises with cuff weights for a variety of lower extremity muscle and muscle groups; stair climbing; knee squats; and active-range-of-movement exercises. Balance training included standing with one foot in front of the other; walking placing one foot directly in front of the other; walking backwards and walking sideways; and walking on toes and walking on heels. Intervention participants were instructed to perform their assigned exercises independently for 30 minutes at least three times per week. They were also encouraged to walk outside their home at least three times per week. Controls received an equal number of social visits from a research nurse. After 6 months, balance had improved significantly in the treatment group relative to controls. After 1 year there were significantly fewer falls in the treatment group than in the control group (88 vs. 152). Additionally, the treatment group was significantly less likely to experience a first fall with serious injury.

Multifactorial Strategies

The randomized trial conducted by Hornbrook, Stevens, Wingfield, Hollis, Greenlick, and Ory (1994) addressed home safety, exercise, and behavioral risks. Participants ($N = 3182$) were community-dwelling, ambulatory elderly persons aged 65 years who were members of a group model health maintenance organization. All study participants (intervention and control) had their homes inspected for fall hazards by a member of the project staff, were informed of hazards identified, and were given a consumer safety booklet. Control participants were not advised on mitigation. Participants in the intervention group received specific advice on mitigating identified hazards, including fact sheets outlining procedures for obtaining technical and financial assistance in making safety repairs and modifications in the home. In addition, those randomized to the intervention were invited to participate in a series of four weekly, 90-minute group meetings led by a health behaviorist and a physical therapist. These sessions included didactic presentations and discussions on environmental and behavioral risks for falls, as well as opportunities to practice exercises designed to increase strength and balance. Intervention subjects were provided with a manual describing the exercises and were instructed to exercise at home. Further, participants were advised to begin walking at least three times per week and to monitor their exercise using a specially designed calendar. Finally, intervention subjects were offered financial or technical assistance to complete any repairs remaining at the end of the fourth weekly session. After the first four sessions, quarterly maintenance sessions were held. Forty-four percent of the control participants and 39% of intervention participants reported one or more falls over the 23-month study period. Twenty-six percent of control participants and 24% of intervention participants reported injurious falls. Neither difference was statistically significant.

Tinetti, Baker, McAvay, Claus, Garrett, Gottschalk, Koch, Trainor, and Horowitz (1994) conducted a trial of a multifactorial falls prevention intervention that included a comprehensive assessment of intrinsic and extrinsic risk factors for falling. The study population was made up of 301 community-dwelling older adults enrolled in a health maintenance organization who were over 70 years of age. Participants were ambulatory and had at least one of seven identified intrinsic fall risk factors as assessed by a nurse and a physical therapist. All participants received an initial evaluation conducted by a nurse practitioner and a physical therapist. It included a evaluation of postural blood pressure; toilet and tub safety; a room-by-room fall hazard evaluation; gross muscle and range of motion testing; and gait, balance, and transfer assessments. Participants were then randomized (by physician practice) to either a control group (usual care plus social visits) or to an intervention group. The number of visits control and intervention subjects received was based on the baseline assessments. The intervention phase of the program (which involved the first 3 months after the baseline assessment) involved a series of home visits led by a nurse practitioner, a physical therapist, or both depending on the risk factors identified during the initial assessment. Risk factors were prioritized to avoid overburdening subjects. The intervention included education about the risks of medications for falls; a review of medications with the primary care physician;

strength, balance and transfer training; behavioral recommendations to prevent orthostatic hypotension such as elevating the bed and simple exercises (i.e., ankle pumps); and education about ways to improve the safety of the home (e.g., installation of grab bars in the bathroom, removal of hazards). Simple illustrated instructions were provided for each exercise program. Intervention subjects were instructed to perform the exercises twice a day for 15 to 20 minutes per session. Intervention subjects were given the option of carrying out recommended environmental remediations on their own or having them completed by a research staff carpenter (Tinetti, Baker, Garrett, Gottschalk, Koch, & Horwitz, 1993). During the 3-month maintenance phase of the intervention, subjects were expected to continue their previously prescribed abatement program. Intervention subjects received an average of 7.8 home visits. Participants randomized to control received an average of 6.2 home social visits from social work students. There was a significant difference between the intervention and control groups with respect to length of time to first fall and proportion of participants who fell (35% vs. 47%) during the 1-year follow-up period. Fear of falling, as measured by the Falls Self-Efficacy Scale, was significantly mitigated for the intervention group relative to control when adjusted for baseline scores.

Reinsch, MacRae, Lachenbruch, and Tobis (1992) conducted a trial of two primary fall prevention strategies—exercise and cognitive-behavioral—using 230 community-dwelling elders (60-years old and over) randomized by intervention site (senior centers) to one of four study groups: exercise, cognitive-behavioral, exercise-cognitive, and discussion control (group discussions of health issues not necessarily concerning falls prevention). The exercise and exercise-cognitive intervention groups met for 1 hour, three days per week, for 1 year; the cognitive-behavioral and discussion control groups met for 1 hour per day, 1 day a week, for 1 year. The core exercise program involved a specific number of "stand-ups" from a sitting position and "step-ups" to a 6-inch step. The cognitive-behavioral intervention used a curriculum on fall risk reduction (including home environmental hazards), relaxation training, and videogames to improve reaction time. The exercise-cognition intervention included one class per week focusing on the cognitive-behavioral component and two classes per week on exercise but also included relaxation training.

No significant differences were found between the four groups during the intervention year for time to first fall or incidence of serious falls (requiring medical attention). Fear of falling was not lowered after 1 year and did not differ between the treatment and control group.

INTERVENTION DESIGNED TO REDUCE FEAR OF FALLING

Tennstedt et al. (in press) developed and evaluated an intervention specifically aimed at reducing fear of falling. The study population consisted of 434 residents of senior housing aged 60 or older who had restricted activities because they were concerned they might fall. Because fear of falling is experienced by both fallers and nonfallers, fall experience was not a prerequisite for inclusion in the study. Randomization occurred by housing site. The purpose of the intervention (titled "A Matter of Balance") was to reduce fear of falling and consequently increase social and physical functioning. The intervention consisted of eight 2-hour group sessions that met twice a week for a month. To increase participants' sense of control and perceived ability to make change, the intervention featured a strong cognitive restructuring component. Throughout the intervention, cognitive restructuring activities were used to help the participants recognize and evaluate their beliefs about fall risk, fall prevention, and aging and to dispel myths about falling. Videotapes were used to expose intervention subjects to positive role models. To enhance participants confidence in their own abilities to make adaptive changes in their lives, many opportunities to build fall prevention skills were provided. The intervention addressed physical, environmental, and cognitive risk factors for falls through a variety of techniques including group discussion, mutual problem solving, exercises designed to improve range of motion and strength, assertiveness training, and home assignments. Individualized risk reduction strategies were created by participants through the use of behavioral goal setting and contracts. These contracts, known as "personal action planners," focused on identifying and mitigating home hazards, engaging in physical exercise, finding safer approaches to ADL and IADL, and resuming former activities. All cognitive restructuring and skill-building activities were reinforced by didactic material (presented by a trained group facilitator) on the incidence of falls, risk factors for falls, and strategies to reduce fall risk. Intervention subjects participated in balance assessments at the beginning and end of the program to provide them with objective feedback on their balance capabilities. Participants randomized (by housing development) to control received a single attention session. In that session, information on fall prevention (including a video produced by the American Association of Retired Persons) which focused on changing the environment to reduce hazards was presented. At 1-year follow-up, intervention participants, relative to controls, were significantly less afraid of falling (as measured by the Falls Self-Efficacy Scale), had a greater sense of control over falls, had better overall scores on the Sickness Impact Profile (SIP), the SIP Physical score, the SIP Mobility Range score, and the SIP Social Behavior score. Falls were monitored in the intervention and control groups to insure that the program did not increase falls as a consequence of increasing activity. There were no significant differences between groups in either the number of participants who fell or in the number of falls during the follow-up period.

SUMMARY OF KEY INTERVENTION COMPONENTS

Environmental Modification and Fall Prevention

Falls often occur during routine activities, therefore it is important to create an environment that supports an older adult in completing ADLs and IADLs independently. The list of potential hazards in the home and community is infinite, however, a careful assessment of common typical activities and the environments in which they routinely occur is possible and a frequently recommended component of a fall risk assessment. Falls often occur as a result of the interaction of risk factors; therefore, by reducing environmental hazards, fall risk should be lowered.

While none of the studies described in this chapter involved trials of environmental strategies alone, most included a component on household hazards. The interventions of Hornbrook et al. (1994) and Tinetti et al. (1994) both identified hazards and facilitated remediation; the intervention of Reinsch et al. (1992) provided information about home hazards but did not facilitate changes. During the fear of falling intervention, participants conducted their own assessments after learning about common hazards and then used personal action planners to identify environmental hazards and plan solutions. While the project staff did not help to mitigate problems of individual participants, the study groups shared expertise and may have helped each other correct hazards in the home. It is interesting to note that the intervention with the most emphasis on environment (Hornbrook et al., 1994) did not show significant effects for falls. Because many falls occur outside the home (Hornbrook et al., 1991), safety improvements may have little impact. While the outcomes of study conducted by Tinetti et al. (1994) contrast favorably with the studies led by Hornbrook and Reinsch (both of which included an environmental component), it is not possible to tell the extent to which the environmental components contributed to the reduction in falls among the intervention group in that study. The results of this comparison suggest that environmental modifications are an important component of fall prevention strategies, however, by themselves such modifications are not sufficient to prevent falls.

Exercise and Fall Prevention

The studies conducted by Wolf et al. (1996), Hornbrook et al. (1994), and Tinetti et al. (1994) were part of a multicentered program funded jointly by the National Institute on Aging and the National Institute for Nursing Research—the Frailty and Injuries: Cooperative Studies of Intervention Techniques (FICSIT). The FICSIT studies were designed as a cooperative effort to gather a common set of data about functional, physiological, psychosocial, and environmental variables affecting older people while serving as an exploration of novel interventions to improve frailty or reduce the effects of falls (Buchner et al., 1993). Tinetti et al. (1994) and Hornbrook et al. (1994) identified fall prevention among community-dwelling older adults as the primary outcome of interest. Balance and falls, respectively, were the primary and secondary outcomes addressed by Wolf et al. (1996). Only two of the studies, the aforementioned multifactorial intervention study by Tinetti et al. and the Tai Chi intervention study by Wolf et al. (1996) showed significant reductions in falls. Because research methods were coordinated, meta-analysis of different exercise strategies could be performed across individual studies. Pooled estimates were developed for the effects on falling of exercise, resistance training, balance training, endurance training, and flexibility training. Of these, only balance training showed significant results for falls reduction (Province et al., 1995).

In summary, among the studies discussed, the study conducted by Wolf et al. (1996) involving only Tai Chi balance training significantly reduced falls, but the companion study using computerized biofeedback balance training did not. Two studies combining strengthening and balance training (Tinetti et al., 1994; Campbell et al., 1997) showed significant reductions in falls. The two studies including strength training, but not balance training (Hornbrook et al., 1994; Reinsch et al., 1992) did not show significant reductions in falls. Taken together, these studies suggest the value of balance training for reducing falls. It is, however, unclear why the computerized biofeedback balance training intervention failed to yield significant outcomes. One possible explanation is that participants in the Tai Chi trial were able to practice their exercise at home, in addition to their group sessions, whereas the participants in the computerized biofeedback intervention trial were unable to replicate these exercises when not at the study site. Tai Chi participants were encouraged to practice at least 15 minutes per day at home, but compliance was not monitored. The possibility that the effectiveness of balance training is a function of the extent to which the method allows for discretionary increases in dosage by home practice is consistent with the significant findings of the Tinetti et al. (1994) and the Campbell et al. (1997) studies, both of which used "low-tech" balance training exercises that participants were able to practice in their homes.

Falls Self-Efficacy, Cognitive Restructuring, and Fall Prevention

As can be seen by the review of interventions designed to reduce falls and fear of falling, many of the approaches taken to reduce falls involve changing the behaviors of older adults. Adaptive behaviors associated with fall prevention include (but are not limited to) exercising regularly, communicating assertively, and finding alternative approaches to potentially risky activities (such as using unstable step stools to reach overhead objects). Research shows that optimal performance requires not only the necessary skills but also adaptive self-conceptions (Bandura, 1989). With respect to fear of falling, if older adults believe they have poor balance and limited strength and there is nothing they can do to improve it, they are unlikely to use effort to learn or implement new strategies. Moreover, they are likely to curtail activities and complicate their problems through disuse and deconditioning. If, however, control beliefs are enhanced along with teaching skills, this combination is likely to increase effort and persistence, thereby maximizing the effectiveness of skill learning (e.g., using a walker or doing appropriate exercises), as well as to reduce depression and anxiety (Lachman, Jette, Tennstedt, Howland, Harris, & Peterson, 1997).

Lachman et al. (1997) presented a conceptual framework outlining the importance of multifaceted interventions in the context of promoting exercise among sedentary older adults. This strategy entails the combination of teaching compensatory strategies to combat age-related losses, offering incentives or rewards and social support to increase motivation, and instructing participants in techniques for enhancing beliefs about control and self-efficacy over the aging process. The belief that one does not have control over mobility and other physical aspects of the aging process is likely to result in anxieties such as fear of falling (Lachman et al., 1997). This suggests that interventions designed to address fear of falling should also focus on beliefs about control as well as associated fears. This integrated approach was used in the previously described "Matter of Balance" intervention (Tennstedt et al., 1998), which was specifically designed to improve falls' self-efficacy. Several of the other studies discussed in this chapter also described falls self-efficacy or fear of falling as outcomes of interest.

Falls self-efficacy refers to efficacy beliefs regarding whether one can engage in an activity with out falling. (Tinetti et al., 1990). Self-efficacy is behavior specific and future oriented. That is, it pertains to an individual's perceived ability to use particular cognitive or behavioral skills in a specific situation at some point in the future. As we have seen by the review of tested interventions designed to prevent falls and fear of falling, many different skills are associated with fall prevention. It is appropriate, therefore, that the studies measuring falls self-efficacy employed a variety of methods to achieve this outcome. Gonzalez, Goeppinger, and Lorig (1990) identified four empirically verified ways to enhance self-efficacy: skills mastery, modeling, reinterpretation of signs and symptoms, and persuasion. Examples of how these strategies were used in the interventions discussed in this chapter are presented below.

Skills Mastery

By engaging study participants in exercise training, all of the interventions described in this chapter provided opportunities for skill mastery associated with fall prevention. Further studies are needed to understand the dose-response relationship between time spent practicing fall prevention skills and success in fall prevention.

Modeling

Peer networks are valuable sources of adaptive role models because peers are often realistic figures for self-comparison. Indeed, creation of such patient networks has been shown to improve the likelihood that a target group or individual will adopt a new behavior. Among the studies examined, results of the group intervention were mixed compared to the strong results for the individualized interventions. Further research is needed to determine the contribution that peer networks (facilitated through group interventions) make in establishing long-term intervention effects.

Reinterpretation of Signs and Symptoms

What people believe about their condition or how they interpret symptoms can affect their ability to deal with it (Bandura, 1982). In the study described by Tennstedt et al. (1998), a number of activities were provided to foster participants' awareness of maladaptive attitudes toward fall prevention and aging. Further, participants were taught to recognize the connection between thoughts ("My balance is so bad I can't do things on my own."), feelings (anxiety), and behaviors (restricted activity). Reflecting on thinking patterns was novel for many of the participants in the fear of falling intervention, however, the facilitators of that program describe this aspect of self-efficacy training as essential to the success of that program (Peterson, 1998).

Persuasion

Whether interventions are conducted one on one or in group settings, persuasion can be found in feedback from peers or an "expert" (such as a health care provider with experience in fall prevention). Realistic goals, once achieved, also provide older adults with persuasive, objective proof that progress in fall prevention is possible. Goal setting and evaluation does not have to be a complicated process. For example, in the study conducted by Tinetti et al. (1994), simply advancing to a new color of Theraband or Theraputty indicated to intervention subjects that their strength was improving.

In summary, research findings suggest that falls self-efficacy can be enhanced through targeted interventions. Behavioral theory and the results of the trials conducted indicate that building falls self-efficacy is a useful component of fall prevention programs.

CAN FALLS AND FEAR OF FALLING AMONG ELDERLY PERSONS BE PREVENTED?

On balance, the current literature on falls-prevention trials suggests cautious optimism, with several caveats. First, the studies considered have focused on older adults who are well enough to live in the community. Therefore the results of the studies discussed may not be applicable to the approximately 5% of the senior population living in institutions. As suggested by Hornbrook et al. (1994) it is likely that health problems (as opposed to environmental or behavioral factors) play a larger role in more serious falls. Thus, it may be that strategies that are effective for the well elderly population would not be effective for frail elderly persons who are at highest risk for serious falls. Intensive programs targeted at frail elderly persons may be necessary to prevent the most injurious (and costly) falls; this logic also applies to noninstitutionalized elderly persons who are home bound, either due to dementia, frailty, or fear of falling. Again, these higher risk individuals may be unable or unwilling to comply with the intervention programs of demonstrated efficacy for more active elderly populations. Finally, as is always the case with rigorous intervention studies, the quality of the successful programs may not be replicable when programs are implemented within the context of the existing health care delivery system. Nevertheless, it appears as though falls risk-reduction is possible for large numbers elderly persons living independently. Longitudinal studies are necessary to determine whether moderate intensity falls prevention programs are useful in preventing serious falls in the long run.

Exercise, and specifically balance training, are the common components to the effective interventions. The Tai Chi intervention study would suggest that balance training is sufficient to yield significant falls reduction. From the published reports, it is difficult to compare the doses of strength and balance training delivered in the two studies that combined both in effective interventions. Further research is needed to determine the relative merits of strength and balance training and whether the two types of exercise work synergistically.

In looking for further clues to success, based on our review of the trials presented, we suspect that the most effective interventions are those that: (a) allow participants to tailor interventions to meet their own needs (with respect to both pace and content); (b) provide opportunities to experience success; and (c) focus on internal (inherent) abilities. Comparison of the studies suggests that interventions conducted in the home may lend themselves to such characteristics. Alternatively, providing training that can be replicated independently by participants in the home is a useful strategy. If a group format is used, participants can be encouraged to practice skills learned in the group sessions at home. Such a strategy was used by Wolf et al. (1996). Interventions fully or partially based in the home have a number of advantages. Home-based programs allow for individualized interventions derived from assessments. In other words, compliance and effectiveness may be increased when individuals are asked to do only what is specifically required based on their status. Home-based programs also allow individuals to work on new skills on their own schedule, when their motivation is highest. Finally, interventions based fully or partially in the home may empower older adults by allowing them to experience success in their own living environment, instead of in a clinic or simulated home environment. Whether utilizing one on one or group education, future fall prevention interventions should include elements of customization and skill development exercises that participants can practice at home on their own schedules.

The intervention studied by Tennstedt et al. (1998) is an example of a group intervention that allowed for customization. By working on individually created behavioral contracts, participants developed skills by independently identifying needs and devising solutions that met their needs given the context of their lives. To be effective, fall prevention programs must expand beyond the life of the program. Abilities and needs change as we age, therefore older adults need to be taught how to recognize and respond to changes associated with aging. The fear of falling intervention provided additional benefits to participants, including opportunities for peer support and sharing of resources, peer modeling, social reinforcement, and the development of peer group norms regarding the appropriateness of falls prevention behaviors.

It appears that remediation of environmental hazards alone is not sufficient for falls reduction, although perhaps useful as an adjunct to other strategies. Mitigation of environmental hazards might yield psychological benefits if assessment and alteration is done by the individual as part of enhancing self-efficacy about falls prevention. It is equally evident that instruction on behavioral changes alone will not suffice to reduce falls risk, although again this strategy could be a component to increase the individual's sense of control over the likelihood of falling. In other words, it appears that the most successful strategies require older adults to become active participants in the intervention. In the study led by Tinetti, for example, risk factors were prioritized, however, participants were ultimately responsible for selecting the intervention strategy.

Finally, it is noteworthy that all of the interventions described delivered a program in conjunction with or with consent from participants' physicians. Many of the programs were interdisciplinary in nature. Fall prevention programs with the most potential for success are most likely those that facilitate communication across disciplines.

Involvement of primary health care providers may increase compliance and effectiveness because participants' view the interventions within the context of their overall health care.

Two related issues, intensity and cost, should be considered. The most intensive interventions, in terms of time, were those tested by Reinsch et al. (1992). Participants were asked to meet for 1 hour per week, 3 days a week, for 1 year—a total of 156 hours. These interventions were not effective. In the intervention developed by Hornbrook et al. (1994), which strongly facilitated mitigation of environmental home hazards, the average cost per household for safety alterations was $78, a substantial amount for many community-dwelling elderly persons living on limited fixed incomes. This intervention also involved 10.5 hours of group sessions. It did not significantly reduce falls. The intervention developed by Tinetti et al. (1994) involved an average of 7.8 home visits and cost $891 per intervention participant. Although we do not have cost data for the home-based exercise intervention developed by Campbell et al. (1997), presumably it was less expensive, compared to the Tinetti et al. (1994) intervention because it involved only four home visits. Both of these programs were effective. The Tai Chi intervention involved approximately 45 minutes of instructor contact time per week for 15 weeks, for a total of 11.25 hours. Thus, it appears as though interventions need not be costly in terms of resources or participant out-of-home time commitment to be effective.

In summary, the research to date suggests that relatively low-cost, low intensity, "low-tech" interventions can be effective in reducing falls for a large segment of the community-dwelling population. Fear of falling, as well, seems subject to modification. The trial of the fear of falling intervention developed by Tennstedt et al. (1998) demonstrates that fear of falling and some associated physical and psychosocial outcomes can be modified. The Tai Chi falls prevention program developed by Wolf et al. (1996) and the multifactorial intervention developed by Tinetti et al. (1994) also showed significant reductions in fear of falling. This is encouraging news for a society with an expanding elderly population.

It is likely that research on interventions to prevent falls and fear of falling will continue in response to an increasing demand for effective programs. This demand is rooted in a concern for the injury and in the meaning society ascribes to falls. Falls are important sentinel events in nursing home admissions. Indeed, it is estimated that 40% of these admissions are precipitated by falling (Tinetti et al., 1988). Thus, concern about falls reflects, in part, concern with loss of independence (Peterson & Howland, 1992). For this reason, many elders feel constrained from sharing their fear and experience of falling with family members and health care providers. In this regard, falls can be isolating, cutting one off from important social support. A demand for fall prevention programs will reflect a broader demand for interventions that enhance and maintain functioning in general in later years.

REFERENCES

Arfken, C. L., Lach, H. W., Birge, S. J., & Miller, J. P. (1994). The prevalence and correlates of fear of falling in elderly persons living in the community. *American Journal of Public Health, 84,* 565–570.

Auerbach, H. P., Bandeen-Roche, K., Chee, E., & Fried, L. P. (1994). *Fear of falling: Characteristics of fallers and non-fallers.* Paper presented at the Annual Scientific Meetings of Gerontology Society of America. Atlanta, GA.

Baker, S. P., O'Neill, B., Ginsburg, M. J., & Li, G. (1992). *The Injury Fact Book* (2nd ed.). New York: Oxford University Press.

Bandura, A. (1982). Self-efficacy mechanism in human agency. *American Psychologist, 37,* 122–147.

Bandura, A. (1989). Regulation of cognitive processes through perceived self-efficacy. *Developmental Psychology, 25,* 729–735.

Belgrave, F. Z. (1991). Psychosocial predictors of adjustment to disability in African Americans. *Journal of Rehabilitation, 57,* 37–40.

Buchner, D. M., Hornbrook, M. C., Kutner, N. G., Tinetti, M. E., Ory, M. G., Mulrow, C. D., Schechtman, K. B., Gerety, M. B., Fiatarone, M. A., & Wolf, S. L. (1993). Development of the common data base for the FICSIT trials. *Journal of the American Geriatrics Society, 41,* 297–308.

Campbell, J. A., Robertson, M. C., Gardner, M. M., Norton, R. N., Tilyard, M. W., & Buchner, D. M. (1997). Randomised controlled trial of a general practice program for home based exercise to prevent falls in elderly women. *The British Medical Journal, 315,* 1065–1069.

Department of Health and Human Services. (1990). *Healthy People 2000: National health promotion and disease prevention objectives.* Washington, DC: U.S. Government Printing Office.

Gonzalez, V. M., Goeppinger, J., & Lorig, K. (1990). Four psychosocial theories and their application. *Arthritis Care and Research, 3,* 132–143.

Graney, M. J. (1975). Happiness and social participation in aging. *Journal of Gerontology, 30,* 701.

Hart, M. A., & Sliefert, M. K. (1983). Monitoring patient incidents in a long-term care facility. *Quality Review Bullentin, 9,* 356–365.

Holahan, C. K., & Holahan, C. J. (1987a). Life stress, hassels, and self-efficacy in aging: A replication and extension. *Journal of Applied Social Psychology, 17,* 574–592.

Holahan, C. K., & Holahan, C. J. (1987b). Self-efficacy, social support, and depression in aging: A longitudinal analysis. *Journal of Gerontology, 42,* 65–68.

Hornbrook, M. C., Stevens, V. J., Wingfield, D. J., Hollis, J. F., Greenlick, M. R., & Ory, M. G. (1994). Preventing falls among community-dwelling older persons: Results from a randomized trial. *The Gerontologist, 34,* 16–23.

Hornbrook, M. C., Wingfield, D. J., Stevens, V. J., Hollis, J. F., & Greenlick, M. R. (1991). Falls among older persons: Antecedents and consequences. In R. Weindruch, E. C. Hadley, & M. G. Ory (Eds.), *Reducing frailty and falls in older persons* (pp. 106–125). Springfield, IL: Charles C. Thomas.

Howland, J., Peterson, E. W., Levin, W., Fried, L., Pordon, D., & Bak, S. (1993). Fear of falling among the community-dwelling elderly. *Journal of Aging and Health, 5,* 229–243.

Lachman, M. E., Howland, J., Tennstedt, S., Jette, A., Assmann, S., & Peterson, E. W. (1998). Fear of falling and activity restriction: The Survey of Activities and Fear of Falling. *Journal of Gerontology, 53,* 43–50.

Lachman, M. E., Jette, A., Tennstedt, S., Howland, J., Harris, B. A., & Peterson, E. (1997). A cognitive-behavioral model for promoting regular physical activity in older adults. *Psychology, Health, and Medicine, 2,* 251–261.

Lucht, U. (1971). Prospective study of accidental falls and resulting injuries in the homes of elderly people. *Acta Sociomedica Scand, 2,* 105–120.

Multran, E., & Reitzes, D. (1981). Retirement, identity and well-being: Realignment of role relationships. *Journal of Gerontology, 36,* 733.

Naylor, R., & Rosin, A. J. (1970). Falling as a cause of admission to a geriatric unit. *Practitioner, 205,* 327–330.

Nevitt, M. C. (1990). Falls in older persons: Risk factors and prevention. In Institute of Medicine (Ed.), *The second fifty years: Promoting health and preventing disability.* Washington, DC: National Academy Press.

Nevitt, M. C., Cummings, S. R., Kidd, S., & Black, D. (1989). Risk factors for recurrent nonsyncopal falls: A prospective study. *Journal of the American Medical Association, 261,* 2663–2668.

Peterson, E. W. (1998). *The fear of falling program: A matter of balance.* Paper presented at the meeting of the Boston University Roybal Center for Research on applied Gerontology, Boston, MA.

Peterson, E. W., & Howland, J. (1992). Gerontology special interest section newsletter. *American Occupational Therapy Association, 15,* 1–3.

Peterson, E. W., Howland, J., Kielhofner, G., Lachman, M. E., Assmann, S., Cote, J., & Jette, A. (1999). Falls self-efficacy and occupational adaptation among elders. *Physical and Occupational Therapy in Geriatrics, 16,* 1–16.

Powell, E., & Meyers, A. M. (1995). The activities-specific balance confidence scale. *Journal of Gerontology, 50,* 128–134.

Province, M. A., Hadley, E. C., Hornbrook, M. A., Lipsitz, L. A., Miller, J. P., Mulrow, C. D., Ory, M. G., Sattin, R. W., Tinetti, M. E., & Wolf, S. L. (1995). The effects of exercise on falls in elderly patients: A preplanned meta-analysis of the FICSIT trials. *Journal of the American Medical Association, 273,* 1341–1347.

Ray, W. A., Griffin, M. R., Schaffner, W., Baugh, D. K., & Melton, L. J., III. (1987). Psychotropic drug use and risk of hip fracture. *New England Journal of Medicine, 316,* 363–369.

Reinsch, S., MacRae, P., Lachenbruch, P. A., & Tobis, J. S. (1992). Attempts to prevent falls and injury: A prospective community study. *The Gerontologist, 32,* 450–456.

Sattin, R. W. (1992). Falls among older persons: A public health perspective. *Annual Review of Public Health, 13,* 489–508.

Tennstedt, S., Howland, J., Lachman, M., Peterson, E., Kasten, L., & Jette, A. (1998). A randomized controlled trial of a group intervention to reduce fear of falling and associated activity restriction in older adults. *Journal of Gerontology, 53,* 384–392.

Tinetti, M. E., Baker, D. I., Garrett, P. A., Gottschalk, M., Kosch, M. L., & Horowitz, R. I. (1993). Yale FICSIT: Risk factor abatement strategy for fall prevention. *Journal of the American Geriatrics Society, 41,* 315–320.

Tinetti, M. E., Baker, D. L., McAvay, G., Claus, E. B., Garrett, P., Gottschalk, M., Koch, M. L., Trainor, K., & Horowitz, R. I. (1994). A multifactorial intervention to reduce the risk of falling among elderly people living in the community. *New England Journal of Medicine, 331,* 821–827.

Tinetti, M. E., Doucette, J., Claus, E., & Marottoli, R. (1995). Risk factors for serious injury during falls by older persons in the community. *Journal of the American Geriatrics Society, 43,* 1214–1221.

Tinetti, M. E., Mendes de Leon, C. F., Doucette, J. T., & Baker, D. I. (1994). Fear of falling and falls-related efficacy in relationship to functioning among community-living elders. *Journal of Gerontology, 49,* 140–147.

Tinetti, M. E., Richman, D., & Powell, L. (1990). Falls efficacy as a measure of fear of falling. *Journal of Gerontology, 45,* 239–243.

Tinetti, M. E., Speechley, M., & Ginter, S. F. (1988). Risk factors for falls among elderly persons living in the community. *New England Journal of Medicine, 319,* 1701–1707.

Wild, D., Nayak, U. S. L., & Issacs, B. (1981). Prognosis of falls in old people at home. *Journal of Epidemiology and Community Health, 35,* 200–204.

Wolf, S. I., Barnhart, H. X., Kutner, N. G., McNeely, E., Coogler, C., Xu, T., & the Atlanta FICSIT Group. (1996). Reducing frailty and falls in older persons: An investigation of Tai Chi and computerized balance training. *Journal of the American Geriatrics Society, 44,* 489–497.

Wolf, S. L., Coogler, C. E., Green, R. C., & Xu, T. (1993). Novel interventions to prevent falls in the elderly. In H. M. Perry III, J. E. Morely, & R. M. Coe (Eds.), *Aging and musculoskeletal disorders* (pp. 178–196). New York: Springer.

CHAPTER 15

Geriatric Rehabilitation

Linda Thalheimer

G eriatric rehabilitation is complex and challenging. The complexity manifests itself in the numerous areas of natural decline in the aging population: muscle strength, aerobic capacity, vasomotor stability, selective attention and complex problem solving, and all five senses. Moreover, additional declines in muscle strength and function are evident with hospitalization stays as short as 2 days (Creditor, 1993; Hirsch, Sommers, Olsen, Mullen, & Winograd, 1990). The challenge of geriatric rehabilitation is in the need to assess and treat multiple diagnoses in both medical and functional terms while accommodating ingrained lifestyle patterns. It is complicated by diagnoses that may not be founded in straightforward symptoms (Jenkyn & Reeves, 1981), and by new cost containment measures that support the expedient discharge of patients. Patients are, therefore, being forced into rehabilitative settings with increasing levels of ambiguous, unresolved diagnoses.

THE DOMAINS OF FUNCTION

Understanding the domains of function as defined in the Trifocus Geriatric Evaluation Form (TRI-VAL) (Thalheimer, 1991) can simplify functional assessment and the development of rehabilitation goals. As shown in Figure 15.1, the TRI-VAL is designed for independent assessment of the three domains of function: physical; cognitive; and motivational skills. Based on this assessment, the rehabilitation team can set practical and realistic goals more easily by addressing them interdependently in the plan of care.

ASSESSMENT OF THE DOMAINS OF FUNCTION

Physical Functioning

Physical skills are defined in terms of muscle strength, joint range, coordination, balance, and endurance. Functionally these can be assessed by direct observation of the effort exerted and the balance displayed when the patient rises from a chair, ambulates across the room, dons/doffs shoes and socks, toilets, and combs hair. More objective tests for physical skill level can include the evaluation of muscle strength with manual muscle testing, range of motion with goniometric measurements, coordination with demonstration of heel to shin, hand to nose, and fine motor skill tests. The Get Up and Go Test and timed single leg standing are good indicators of balance and fall risk (Tinetti, 1986). Mobility trials with monitoring of heart rate, blood pressure, respiration, and oxygen saturation are important when assessing endurance.

Cognitive Functioning

Cognitive skills include attention, memory, organization, problem solving, and judgment. A short digit span may be indicative of poor attention. Poor attention is usually associated with poor memory. Memory can be defined functionally in terms of learning: long-term memory (the ability to retrieve "old learning") and short-term memory (the ability to retain "new learning"). Validation of long-term memory with a family member or friend will help to assess the quality of long-term memory, as a patient may be able to give a detailed taped recording of special past events, which may or may not be accurate. Short-term memory can be assessed functionally

PHYSICAL FUNCTIONING (P) *Physical Assistance*	COGNITIVE FUNCTIONING (C) *Cueing, Supervision*	MOTIVATION (M) *Coaxing, Encouragement*
1. INDEPENDENT-No physical assistance required. Does not use adaptive devices.	1. INDEPENDENT-No cueing or supervision required. Insight into own abilities, understanding of purpose, safety and organization of task.	1. INDEPENDENT-Highly motivated. No coaxing or encouragement needed. Strong desire for independently performing task.
2. INDEPENDENT with limitations- Use of adaptive devices, limited energy, and /or time.	2. INDEPENDENT with limitations- Limited insight into disability, safety and/or quality of task.	2. INDEPENDENT with limitations- Generally motivated to perform task, but easily accepts assistance.
3. MINIMAL-Minimal physical assistance required to INITIATE task and/or set-up.	3. MINIMAL-Cueing and /or supervision required to INITIATE task.	3. MINIMAL-Encouragement and/or coaxing required to INITIATE task.
4. MODERATE-Physical assistance required OCCASIONALLY during task.	4. MODERATE- Cueing and /or supervision required OCCASIONALLY during task.	4. MODERATE-Encouragement and/or coaxing required OCCASIONALLY during task.
5. MAXIMAL-Physical assistance required THROUGHOUT task.	5. MAXIMAL- Cueing and /or supervision required THROUGHOUT task.	5. MAXIMAL-Encouragement and/or coaxing required THROUGHOUT task.
6. DEPENDENT-Requires heavy physical assistance.	6. DEPENDENT-Cueing ineffective.	6. DEPENDENT-Refusal to perform activity.

ADL Activities of Daily Living	Date____			Source of Report____
	P	C	M	Comments:
Feeding				Diet_____
Hygiene				
Dressing				
Showering/Bathing				
Toileting				
Bed Mobility				
Transfers				
Household Mobility				☐ ambulation_____ ☐ wheelchair

Score NA if not performed 2° to role delineation ≥10 yrs

IADL Instrumental Activities of Daily Living	Date____			Source of Report____
	P	C	M	Comments:
Telephone Skills				
Managing Medication				
Managing Money				
Food Preparation				
Shopping				
Laundry/Cleaning				
Community Mobility				☐ ambulation_____ ☐ wheelchair
Transportation				

SENSORY/AIDS ☐ Visual Impairment ☐ Glasses
☐ Hearing Impairment ☐ (R) ☐ (L) Hearing Aid

FIGURE 15.1 TRI-VAL Geriatric Functional Evaluation.

Developed by Linda Thalheimer, 1991

during the interview based on the patients' knowledge of their medical condition, their length of stay, and the type of setting in which they are residing. Additional memory testing is important to identify a patient's potential to learn with multiple repetition, association cues, and recall with the use of visual reminders. The learning patterns and skills identified during the assessment process enable the rehabilitation team to tailor its rehabilitation programs based on learning style as well as to enhance realistic goal setting. Organization, problem solving, and judgment are higher level cognitive skills that can be assessed functionally: observing safety, set-up and management of morning activities, as well as interpersonal communication strategies. These higher level skills can also be assessed with more formalized tests of clock drawing, coin switch, leather craft activities (Allen, 1990), and linguistic tests.

Motivational Functioning

Motivation includes the patient's perception of priorities, quality, and effort. Motivation toward rehabilitation is created when the potential outcome is weighed greater than the exertion of effort. The demands of rehabilitative therapy often require a substantial daily commitment of time and energy, exertion, and the potential of pain. The goal of therapy is, most frequently, increased independence in a population that may no longer perceive its value. The value of independence may be magnified by the influence of lifelong behavior patterns. Research has shown that the outcomes of repetitive life experiences, such as daily obligations and demands, relate more strongly to psychological well-being than do major life events (Kanner, Coyne, Schaefer, & Lazarus, 1981).

GOAL SETTING WITH THE DOMAINS OF FUNCTION

Once assessment of functional skills has been completed, the focus on individual domains of function within each skill area must be determined in terms of the potential for improvement and then identified as a rehabilitation goal. For each skill area, motivation, cognition, and physical skills should be assessed as to why the deficit is present and whether it is remediable. For each deficit that is remediable, the modality to improve the skill should be identified and defined as skilled or unskilled for rehabilitation therapists. Skilled therapy requires that the complexity and sophistication of the intervention is such that it can only be performed safely and effectively by or under the supervision of a skilled therapist. Program development and training for skill acquisition will often require skilled intervention, while the execution of certain programs will be considered repetitive or unskilled. Unskilled services should be more appropriately delegated to nursing, the activities department, or social service. Goals for each discipline can then be effectively and efficiently established.

LIMITATIONS AND THERAPEUTIC INTERVENTIONS FOR THE DOMAINS OF FUNCTION

Physical Functioning

The most common limitations to physical functioning in the geriatric population are pain, generalized weakness, and impaired balance as well as the more debilitating effects of Parkinson's disease, hip fracture, and stroke. Rehabilitation therapists can be very effective in treating each of these areas following a full medical work-up to establish diagnosis. Chronic pain, especially debilitating back pain, may be reduced by abdominal and postural strengthening exercises, heat modalities, and facial/tendon release techniques to reduce spasms. Patients with chronic back pain have also shown benefit from cognitive-behavior modification programs with improved functional outcomes, as well as moderate decreases in pain (Basler, 1997).

Generalized weakness is common after bed rest during hospitalization or self-imposed immobility in the home. The deconditioning effects on muscle strength and balance are functionally significant following even short periods of bed rest or immobility that may prevent a discharge to a previous home setting. Rehabilitation therapies using monitored exercise and balance programs provide modalities for restoring strength and mobility to these patients. Skilled therapy services are often required when secondary diagnosis of cardiac and respiratory conditions are present to insure safe and effective muscle reconditioning. Vital signs should be monitored to appropriately modify and develop reconditioning exercise programs. Strengthening of the patient with Parkinson's should include exercises that have repetitive continuous movements like that of the arm and leg erganometers or arm wheels.

Balance is another area of physical function that is a common problem addressed by rehabilitation therapists. Although the reason is not clear, many elderly patients will lose their ability to assess accurately their center of gravity. Several studies have linked peripheral nerve dysfunction in elderly persons with postural instability and falls. One such study showed that peripheral nerve dysfunction subjects who fell demonstrated significantly worse vibratory sense at the ankle and finger and had significantly decreased unipedal stance time (3.1 seconds vs. 9.1 seconds) (Richardson & Hurvitz, 1995). Ability to take a balance challenge standing needs to be assessed in all directions. While most older patients do lose their balance backward, there are those who will also lose their balance forward or to either side. Cognitively intact patients do exceptionally well with formal balance exercises, and patients with dementia can often show significant progress with accommodated balance programs. Footwear should be addressed when optimizing balance. Studies by Robbins and colleagues from Concordia University in Montreal Canada concluded that common athletic shoes impair equilibrium in both young and older men and are associated with more than twice the number of balance failures compared with thin soled shoes (Skol Corporation, 1995). Impaired balance due to stroke may be successfully accommodated with Bobath exercises, which are based on neurodevelopmental techniques for regaining motor control (Borgman & Passarella, 1991) and a variety of positioning and mobility aids.

The loss of continence is also a significant physical impairment that can impact independence and self-esteem. Following elimination of remedial causes such as a urinary tract infection, diagnosis of stress, urge, overflow, or functional incontinence should be assessed. Kegal exercise training, with or without biofeedback techniques, in conjunction with scheduled toileting programs, are often effective in reducing incontinence (Resnick, 1995).

Swallowing disorders are common among patients with Parkinson's and following a stroke. Since aspiration is often silent with the Parkinson's patient and difficult to assess in the stroke patient, swallowing disorders are best diagnosed with a modified barium swallow (MBS). The MBS provides valuable information regarding motility patterns during swallow so that effective treatment interventions regarding diet and liquid consistency, intake technique, and postural programs can be appropriately determined.

Physical limitations to hip fracture are dependent on the type of fracture and the type of repair. Typically, hemiarthroplasty or total hip arthroplasty require precautions that include limiting hip flexion to 90 degrees and internal rotation and adduction to prevent dislocation. If there are no extenuating circumstances, such as impaired bone density, there is usually no need for weight bearing precautions. Fractures that require pins and plates often require strict weight bearing precautions to prevent movement of the hardware, although there are usually no limitations on movement. The freedom to return to ambulating without concern of weight bearing is a significant advantage for cognitively impaired patients. Surgeons may opt for a hip replacement even when the fracture can be repaired to optimize recovery and minimize the potential need for restraints in this population.

Cognitive Functioning

The most common limitations to cognitive skills are attention, memory, and judgment impairments. Cognitive limitations impact physical learning and safety in returning to independence. Attention impairments are frequently related to medication effects, an infarct, or depression. Diagnosis, therefore, is significant. Poor attention impacts the ability to learn. When a patient demonstrates poor attention, rehabilitation strategies based on learning are likely to be ineffective. Functional maintenance programs established to assess and develop environmental accommodation and provide staff training are appropriate for optimizing functional performance. Rehabilitation therapy, in conjunction with family or nursing care, can play an important role in designing or accommodating settings that may include structuring the daily routine, setting and the interaction method while performing the daily routine, utilization of visual cues, verbal cues, and limiting distraction. Patients with memory deficits who show some evidence of learning may benefit from sequencing signs, reminder notebooks, and task simplification programs in conjunction with behavior modification.

Motivational Functioning

Limitations to motivation include fear, hopelessness, despair, and learned helplessness. Patients who have been hospitalized because of a fall may be fearful that they will fall again. Some are so fearful that they decline in function in all aspects of functional mobility and are hesitant to participate in therapy. It is necessary for the therapist to gain the confidence of the patient to enable a successful outcome. The demands of rehabilitation therapy often require substantial daily commitment of time, energy exertion, and potential of pain. Patients who feel hopeless or depressed may be unable to envision a good outcome, and therefore may be less motivated toward therapy. Depressed and anxious patients are less likely to do well in rehabilitation, meet rehabilitation goals, and regain the ability to live independently after leaving the hospital. Brief interventions of behavioral therapy for depressed and anxious patients during the rehabilitation period can enhance rehabilitation effort and outcome (Lopez & Mermelstein, 1995). Still other patients may already have developed a sense of learned helplessness or enjoy the secondary effects of the social interaction of assistance. These residents will also have impaired motivation toward therapy.

A study of geriatric nursing home residents utilized verbal cues vs. physical assistance for the performance of a psycho-motor task verified the concept of learned helplessness. The group that was provided with verbal cues showed an improvement in self-confidence and physical performance. The group that was physically assisted was associated with a loss of functional capacity (Avorn & Langer, 1982). This study was equally important in identifying the effectiveness of training on performance and self-confidence. It is important for the therapist to assess motivation and enable patients to be objective both with the therapist and themselves. Ongoing communication with the patients as to their goals and priorities cannot be overemphasized. Goals that the patient identifies as important must be addressed first, and hopefully, with the attainment of short-term goals, more aggressive long-term goals may be set and obtained. If the patient does not concur with the plan of care, goals should be revised.

Effective coping skills can reduce the likelihood that a disability will result in a decline in functional performance. Acquisition and use of adaptive strategies can potentially improve health and well being through enhancing perception of personal control. And outcomes of everyday life events, which can be influenced by the use of adaptive strategies, may be more strongly linked to older adults' health and well-being than are major life events (Clark et al., 1996).

Initial goals are based on premorbid function, medical indications, and the patient's motivation toward treatment intervention. Goals need to be frequently revalidated as cognitive skills, physical ability, and behavior are continually assessed during treatment and nursing interventions. "Rating scales can be helpful but must be interpreted judiciously. Some disabled people may vary in their performance within the day, from day to day, from person to person, and between home and hospital" (Mulley, 1994, p. S29). Rehabilitation goals do not have to be grandiose to guarantee the return to independent living. Goals can be as basic as including the optimizing of body alignment in wheelchairs, training for functional bedroom mobility, pain control, and enhancing participation in daily living skills.

A team approach is most effective. The rehabilitation team varies from facility to facility depending on staffing; however, typically the team consists of the physician or psychiatrist, nurse, social worker, occupational therapist, physical therapist, speech therapist, respiratory therapist, dietitian, activity director, pharmacist, and, most importantly, the patient. Successful rehabilitation teams revolve around the patient, accommodating, as much as possible, the patient's goals, style, and values. Communication is essential among all disciplines to achieve optimal rehabilitation benefits. Common communication techniques include blackboards; nursing Kardex; regular inservicing by rehabilitation staff, equipment, and positioning lists; and routine family and interdisciplinary meetings. Goal setting is a team process based on interdisciplinary communication. Like a puzzle, each discipline provides a piece in the total development of realistic goals.

The potential of therapeutic interventions with elderly persons is maximized when the therapist acknowledges and accommodates the declines in all five senses and the decline in reaction and learning time. Therapy will be more effective when it ensures adaptive hearing and vision devices are being utilized. The therapy room should have adequate lighting and be free from distracting noises. Communication should be provided with slow, clear speech, instructions provided both verbally and then written for a reference. Repetition is essential during training, and then review of the information is needed to insure that the patient is retaining the correct information. Recall is enhanced with list making with or without the intent to refer back to it (Burack & Lachman, 1996).

REHABILITATION SETTINGS

Rehabilitation should begin in the acute setting for geriatric patients to prevent the potential physiological side effects of orthostasis, impaired balance, and muscle wasting. Therapy may continue in a tertiary care unit, a rehabilitation hospital, a skilled nursing facility, or at home with outpatient or home therapy services. The location of therapy intervention is dependent on the complexity of the diagnoses, the potential for return to a community setting in a "reasonable" time period, finances (health insurance), location, and personal preference. Patients with good potential outcomes who can tolerate several hours of therapy intervention a day and who can benefit from on-site physicians are good candidates for a rehabilitation facility. Skilled nursing facilities provide more cost effective therapy intervention but have significantly less physician involvement.

MOBILITY AIDS AND ADAPTIVE DEVICES

Each year there is an increasing selection and availability of assistive devices and mobility aids to increase the potential for independence in all areas of daily living: mobility, feeding, dressing, and homemaking. Most adaptive devices, including mobility aids, again require the assessment of physical functioning, cognitive ability, and motivation. Once an aide is determined appropriate for a patient, it must be fitted to the patient, and the patient must be trained in its proper use.

Canes

The foremost recommendation when evaluating a patient for mobility devices will often start with proper footwear. Mobility devices include canes and walkers. Canes are designed to provide a source of added stability. Aluminum adjustable height canes are most frequently prescribed because of the ease of sizing. Wood may be used out of personal preference but must be cut to size. Canes are held in the hand opposite the disability, and the elbow should be just slightly flexed at 20 to 30 degrees. Tripod and quad canes, most frequently used with stroke patients, provide even greater stability with the widened base of support, but tend to slow the ambulating process. There are distinct right and left sides to the quad canes, and a moderate level of cognition is required to assure use in the correct hand; otherwise, the base of the cane becomes a tripping hazard.

Walkers

Walkers provide greater stability than the cane. Walkers come in folding and nonfolding versions, an option important to know for those who will be frequently transported in cars. Standard walkers have four legs, while rolling walkers may have two wheels in front or wheels on each leg. Standard walkers are especially useful for those people with weight-bearing precautions as well as those who need maximal stability with slowed ambulation. The hemiwalker is designed for maximal stability with the hemiplegic patient who does not have two functional upper extremities to maneuver a standard walker.

Rolling walkers are very useful for patients with many types of limitations: Parkinson's, compression fracture, severe kyphosis, limited upper extremity range or strength, and impaired cognition. The rolling walker may also be chosen by those who feel a standard walker "slows them down." The patient with Parkinson's benefits because there is no need to initiate the repetitive lifting and replacing of the walker. These patients will often carry their standard walkers. Those with back pain benefit from the ability to use the rolling walker as a support to their spine as well as a relief from having to lift against gravity with the standard walker. Patients who lack the cognition to learn walker placement may also benefit from the rolling walker. A slight variation in the rolling walker is swivel front wheels that ease maneuvering the walker around turns. The easier a walker or mobility aid is to maneuver, the more successfully it can be used. A walker is a two-handed operation, preventing functional manipulation of objects. A walker bag or basket is imperative for the safety of a person using a walker functionally, for without one the person must abandon the walker to manipulate the items.

Wheelchairs

Wheelchairs should be user-specific. The method of wheelchair propulsion, either with hands, feet or a combination of the two must be identified. The width, depth, and seat-to-floor height of the patient should be measured. Seat-to-floor height is a critical measurement for patients who will be propelling the chair with their feet. Standard wheelchairs are designed to be pushed by the arms or by another person, so it is not surprising that its seat-to-floor height is inappropriately high (19 to 20"), for the majority of geriatric patients. Special low-height wheelchairs are necessary not only for independent and safe mobility but for proper posturing within the wheelchair. When a wheelchair does not fit, a sliding recline is the most typical result. Hemiplegic patients benefit from one arm drive wheelchairs that enable control of both wheels on one side of the wheelchair. Extensions or rubber grips on wheels are adaptations for those with impaired hand coordination. Swing away/removable footrests enhance wheelchair mobility and improve transfer safety. Brake extensions are useful to provide torque to enhance brake operation and, therefore, safety.

Proper positioning within a wheelchair always starts at the base and progresses up the torso to the head, as necessary. Cushions vary from maximal support to maximal pressure reduction. The decision to choose more support or pressure reduction is related to sitting balance and the potential for pressure areas. Often, choosing an appropriate cushion is a compromise of the two.

Recliner backs, lumbar supports, lateral supports, arm troughs, and lap trays are all means to improve body alignment. There are many customized wheelchair backs that can be attached to standard wheelchairs that provide independently or in combination recline, lateral, and lumbar support. Modification of the back and base of the wheelchair to create a tilt-in-space provides for optimal body alignment while accommodating disabilities of severe trunk weakness, severe kyphosis, or extensor patterns, minimizing the need for positioning belts while enhancing feeding and functional socialization.

Other Adaptive Equipment

Almost any physical limitation can be accommodated with some form of adaptive equipment. Patients must be involved in the choice of adaptive equipment to maximize motivation. It is important to assess the cognitive skill level of the patient in terms of learning to use the equipment and being able to remember to use it when alone. Hemiplegic patients benefit from devices that will allow them to perform one-handed activities. These devices include reachers, dressing sticks, rocker knives, and elastic shoelaces. With a combination of techniques and adaptive devices, a patient can learn to remaster basic activities of daily living tasks. A flaccid upper extremity must be provided with long-term pain management by the use of slings during transfers and arm troughs or trays when sitting in a wheelchair. Patients with multiple disabilities including hip replacements will benefit from the dressing stick or reacher for maneuvering items out of reach and getting pants over the feet, a long handled shoe horn, a sock aid and elastic shoelaces to don shoes and socks, and a raised toilet seat and toilet rail frame. Shower aids include a tub bench, shower hose extension, and long handled sponge for the back as well as the lower extremities. A simple "soap on a rope" can reduce risk of falls by preventing attempts to retrieve a dropped bar of soap. Feeding aids may include a high friction mat, plate guard, and rocker knife. There are multiple variations for utensils and cups. Aids for those with decreased hand function include built-up handles on items ranging from writing utensils to tooth brushes. Patients with Parkinson's may benefit from weighted utensils to decrease their tremors. The variety of adaptive devices is extensive, but most will require skilled intervention in assessment, trial, and training.

SUMMARY

The World Health Organization defines rehabilitation as "an active process by which those people who are disabled by injury or disease achieve a full recovery, or, if full recovery is not possible, realize their optimal physical, mental and social potential and are integrated into their most appropriate environment" (World Health Organization, 1980). Geriatric rehabilitation is specialized. To effectively reach goals, it requires attention to detail and the obscure; assessment of the domains of function, physical, cognitive, and motivational; assessment of family and community resources; understanding of the roles of the interdisciplinary team members and the motivation to communicate; awareness of the abundance of adaptive devices available, including wheelchairs and postural supports; knowledge of the options of rehabilitation settings; and the ability to appropriately set goals with all of these factors combined. As life expectancy continues to be extended, geriatric rehabilitation must be viewed as a key component in maximizing the quality of life of our aging population.

REFERENCES

Allen, C. (1990). *Allen Cognitive Level (ACL) Test Manual.* Colchester, CT: S & S/Worldwide.

Avorn, J., & Langer, E. (1982). Induced disability in nursing Home patients: A controlled trial. *Journal of the American Geriatric Society, 30,* 397–400.

Basler, H. D. (1997). Incorporation of cognitive-behavioral treatment into the medical care of chronic low back patients: A controlled randomized study in German pain treatment center. *Patient Education and Counseling, 31,* 113–124.

Borgman, M. F., & Passarella, P. M. (1991). Nursing care of the stroke patient using Bobath principles: An approach to altered movement. *Nursing Clinics North America, 26,* 1019–1035.

Burack, O., & Lachman, M. (1996). The effects of list-making on recall in young and elderly adults. *Journal of Gerontology, 51,* 226–228.

Clark, F., Carlson, M., Zemke, G., Patteson, B., Ennevor, B., Rankin-Martinez, A., Hobson, L., Carndall, L., Mandel, D., Lipson, L. (1996). Life domains and adaptive strategies of group of low-income, well older Adults. *American Journal of Occupational Therapy, 50,* 99–108.

Creditor, M. (1993). Hazards of hospitalization of the elderly. *Annals of Internal Medicine, 118,* 219–223.

Hirsch, C. H., Sommers, L., Olsen, A., Mullen, L., & Winograd, C. H. (1990). The natural history of functional morbidity in hospitalized older patients. *Journal of the American Geriatrics Society, 38,* 1296–1303.

Jenkyn, L. R., & Reeves, A. G. (1981). Neurologic signs in uncomplicated aging. *Seminal Neurology, 1,* 21.

Kanner, A. C., Coyne, J. C., Schaefer, C., & Lazarus, R. S. (1981). Comparisons of two modes of stress management: Daily hassles and uplift versus major life events. *Journal of Behavioral Medicine, 4,* 1–39.

Lopez, M. A., & Mermelstein, R. J. (1995). A cognitive-behavioral program to improve geriatric rehabilitation outcome. *The Gerontologist, 35,* 696–700.

Mulley, G. P. (1994). Principles of rehabilitation. *The Revue of Clinical Gerontology, 4,* 61–69.

Resnick, N. M. (1995). Urinary incontinence. *Lancet, 346,* 94–99.

Richardson, J. K., & Hurvitz, E. A. (1995). Peripheral neuropathy: A true risk factor for fall. *Journal of Gerontology, 50,* 211–215.

Skol Corporation (1995). Do athletic shoes pose an injury risk For frail back patients? [The Back Letter]. *Sports and the Spine, 10,* 513.

Thalheimer, L. (1991). Tri-val geriatric functional evaluation. Paper presented at the Geriatric Medicine Course, Division on Aging, Harvard Medical School, Boston, MA.

Tinetti, M. E. (1986). Performance-oriented assessment of Mobility problems in elderly patients. *Journal of American Geriatrics Society, 34,* 119–126.

World Health Organization (1980). *World health Organization International classification of impairment, disability and handicap: A manual of classification related to the consequences of disease.* Geneva, Switzerland: Author.

CHAPTER 16

The Invisible Epidemic: Alcohol Abuse and Dependence in Older Adults

Yeon Kyung Chee and Sue E. Levkoff

S ubstance abuse, particularly alcohol abuse and dependence, is one of the fastest growing health problems facing the country. Many older individuals experience chemical dependency, which affects their ability to function independently and the quality of their lives. Although prevalence rates vary in epidemiologic studies among elderly persons due to differences in case detection methods and populations studied, it is clear that elderly individuals experience alcohol-abuse and dependence. In addition, substantial numbers of elders are at risk for alcohol-related problems, without experiencing either alcohol abuse or dependence.

In community-based studies, this "invisible epidemic" affects from 2 to 17% of adults aged 60 and over (Adams, Barry, & Fleming, 1996; Bucholz, Sheline, & Helzer, 1995; D'Archangelo, 1993; Gomberg, 1995; Minnis, 1988). Higher rates, from 15 to 44%, have been found among samples of geriatric inpatients and outpatients (Marcus, 1993; Solomon, Manepalli, Ireland, & Mahon, 1993). Despite the magnitude of the problems and their associated costs, families, physicians, and other health care professionals often fail to recognize and adequately treat this problem. One of key reasons that alcohol problems are not identified is due to the stigma associated with labeling older persons as "alcoholics." With census figures documenting that there will be over 32 million older Americans in 2000 (U.S. Bureau of Census, 1996), if the alcoholism rate remains the same, there are 50% more elderly persons with drinking problems than 20 years earlier (Gurnack & Hoffman, 1992).

Alcoholism is the third most prevalent behavioral health disorder among elderly men, surpassed only by dementia and anxiety disorders (Myers et al., 1984). Men are disproportionately more likely to be alcoholic than women (Bucholz et al., 1995), but women live longer and therefore represent greater numbers of abusers in old age. In 1994, among adults 65 to 69, there were 82 men for every 100 women. Among those 85 to 89, there were 44 men for every 100 women, and the disparity is even greater for those 90 and older (U.S. Bureau of the Census, 1996). Moreover, men are more likely to be diagnosed, possibly due to the fact that women often drink alone and are thus less likely to reveal an alcohol problem to others, and due to the fact that there is a tendency among physicians to attribute early signs of alcohol abuse in women to depression (The National Center for Addictions and Substance Abuse at Columbia University [CASA], 1998). This suggests that the available prevalence rates of alcohol misuse among older women may be lower than the actual scope of the problem to the extent that physicians fail to recognize many cases of alcohol abuse (Coleman & Veach, 1990; Dawson, 1994; Moore et al., 1989; Saitz, Mulvey, Plough, & Samet, 1997). One serious consequence of this lack of recognition is that older women are less likely to be referred to alcohol abuse counseling or treatment (CASA, 1998).

There is mounting concern in both the clinical and policy communities of the importance of providing adequate health care services in response to this problem. In this chapter, we discuss elements that are essential to understanding this burgeoning epidemic.

DEFINITIONS AND CRITERIA

It is well known that variations exist in the definitions of problem drinking. Screening for alcohol dependence relies on a variety of instruments and different operational definitions. Self-reported alcohol consumption often underestimates prevalence of the problem. Two among the most frequently used criteria are those contained in the American Psychiatric Association's *Diagnostic and Statistical Manual of Mental Disorders, 4th Edition (DSM-IV)* and the definition issued jointly by the National Council on Alcoholism and Drug Dependence [NCADD] and the American Society of Addiction Medicine [ASAM].

The *DSM-IV* (1994) uses the terms "substance abuse" to describe maladaptive patterns of substance use, including alcohol, within a 12-month period with the presence of one or more of the following symptoms resulting in: (a) failure in fulfilling role obligations at work, school, or home; (b) physical hazard; (c) legal problems; and (d) social or interpersonal problems.

According to the NCADD-ASAM (Morse & Flavin, 1992), alcoholism is defined as "a primary, chronic disease with genetic, psychosocial, and environmental factors influencing its development and manifestation. The disease is often progressive and fatal. It is characterized by impaired control over drinking, preoccupation with the drug alcohol, use of alcohol despite adverse consequences, and distortions in thinking, most notably denial."

There has been a call for more age-specific definitions and patterns of alcohol misuse among older adults (Gomberg, 1990). Many experts regard the *DSM-IV* criteria as too stringent for older adults (Adams, 1998; Blow, 1999a; The Center for Substance Abuse Treatment [CSAT], 1998). They rely instead on other definitions, such as binge drinking, at-risk, heavy, and problem drinking in place of the *DSM-IV* model of substance abuse. These other definitions allow for more flexibility in characterizing the diverse drinking patterns found among older adults (CSAT, 1998).

In the classification scheme for alcohol misuse in older persons developed by Blow (1999b), an at-risk drinker is one whose patterns of alcohol use, although not yet causing problems, may bring about adverse consequences, either to the drinker or to others. In this classification system, heavy and problem drinking signify more hazardous levels of consumption (Blow, 1999b; CSAT, 1998). Binge drinking is defined as alternating periods of abstinence with relatively short periods of loss of control over drinking (CSAT, 1998). For older adults, CSAT (1998) defines a binge as any drinking occasion in which an individual consumes four or more standard drinks.

Regular moderate use of alcohol is probably less dangerous than binge drinking on occasion (Blow, 1999a). Binge drinking may cause serious adverse medical consequences because older people retain higher blood alcohol levels per drink and tolerance falls with age (Adams, 1998; Stoddard & Thompson, 1996). Binge drinking in older adults is the most risky form and pattern of drinking, so much recent work has focused on this group.

It is important to note that the definitions of problem drinking may have a major impact on the results of alcoholism treatment and research. These different conceptualizations have significant implications in ascertaining treatment goals: whether the goals are to prevent relapse or to reduce at-risk drinking or hazardous drinking (See below Abstinence Model and Hazard Reduction Model under Treatment).

EPIDEMIOLOGY

It is estimated that 2.5 million older adults in the United States have problems related to alcohol (CASA, 1998). The projected aging of the population has serious implications for both the numbers of alcohol-related problems likely to occur among older adults and the subsequent costs involved in responding to them. Currently, rates for alcohol-related hospitalizations among older patients are similar to those for myocardial infarctions, indicating a significant problem for older individuals (Adams, Yuan, Barboriak, & Rimm, 1993).

These figures, however, probably represent an underestimation of the actual magnitude of the problem (Rains & Ditzler, 1993). It is believed that the reported rates of alcoholism among elderly persons are relatively lower than actual rates. Studies consistently find that older adults are less likely to receive a primary diagnosis of alcoholism than are younger adults (Beresford, Blow, Brower, Adams, & Hall, 1988; Blazer, Crowell, & George, 1987; Booth, Blow,

Cook, Bunn, & Fortney, 1992; Geller et al., 1989; Meyers, Goldman, Hingson, Scotch, & Mangione, 1981–1982; Molgaard, Nakamura, Stanford, Peddecord, & Morton, 1990; Stinson, Dufour, & Bertolucci, 1989). Problems with identification or case finding for older problem drinkers include: (a) ageism and lack of visibility (i.e., typical manifestations of alcohol problems, such as getting into fights and driving under the influence of alcohol, are often not relevant for older adults); (b) symptoms of alcohol problems are less apparent in older adults such as unmanageable hypertension, gait disturbances, difficulty with diabetes control; and (c) the volume of absolute consumption of alcohol is lower in older adults (Adams, 1998; Blow, 1999a).

Community-based prevalence studies have found that lower-income elderly persons consume less alcohol than higher-income elderly persons (Liberto, Oslin, & Ruskin, 1992) and that the relationship between ethnic origin and alcohol consumption is inconsistent (Gomberg & Nelson, 1995). However, an interaction seems to exist between socioeconomic status, ethnicity, and alcohol consumption. Among low-income men, African-Americans have more drinking problems, while, among higher income men, the difference in drinking problems between African-Americans and Whites is not significant (Gomberg & Zuker, 1998). In a recent study comparing drinking patterns among African-American and White older men in their mid-sixties, Gomberg and Nelson (1995) reported that African-American alcoholic men drink larger quantities, prefer high-alcohol-content beverages, are more likely to drink in public areas, and manifest more health problems. Determinants of alcohol-related problems appear to be a history of alcohol use or abuse, social isolation, being male, and being single, as well as being relatively well-educated (Barry & Ackerman, 1999).

Occurrence of Late Onset Alcoholism

While a number of cross-sectional studies demonstrate a decline in alcohol use and misuse in old age, this decline may be partially due to mortality for long-term drinkers (Barnes, 1979; McKim & Quinlin, 1991; Meyers et al., 1981–1982). Several studies describe the phenomenon of "late onset alcoholism," where an older person begins problem drinking in old age (Atkinson, Tolson, & Turner, 1990;

Finlayson, Hurt, Davis, & Morse, 1988; Liberto & Oslin, 1996; Schonfeld & Dupree, 1991), or an increase in the incidence of alcohol abuse and alcoholism after age 60 (Glynn, Bouchard, Lo Castro, & Laird, 1985). One third of older alcoholics are estimated to have begun their alcohol abuse after the age of 65 (Beresford et al., 1988).

Compared to early onset drinkers, these late onset drinkers are more likely to be triggered by stress from negative life events such as widowhood, loss of friends or family, or loss of familiar living arrangements, particularly in women (Brennan & Moos, 1990; Finlayson et al., 1988). When there is a question of late onset, a drinking history should be taken into account. There are also people with intermittent histories of heavy drinking. Their history may suggest that they have been on and off the use of alcohol at particular times in their lives. Because late onset problem drinkers have a shorter history of problem drinking and therefore fewer health problems than early onset drinkers do, health care providers tend to overlook their drinking (CSAT, 1998).

Similarly, late onset drinkers include higher proportions of women, higher socioeconomic status, less family history of alcoholism, and less alcohol-related chronic illnesses than early onset drinkers (CSAT, 1998). Although there is controversy regarding the issue of whether there are differences in treatment outcomes (Atkinson, 1994), some studies suggest that late onset alcoholics may respond better than early onset alcoholics to brief intervention techniques (See below under Treatment) because late onset problems tend to be milder and are more sensitive to informal social pressure (Atkinson, 1994; Moos, Brennan, & Moos, 1991).

Older Women and Alcohol Abuse

Although women constitute the majority of older adults, knowledge of alcohol problems among older women is limited because most research on substance abuse has largely studied male subjects. Also, there are more older women living alone, and thus, there are fewer significant others to identify the use of alcohol as a problem (Moore et al., 1989). Clinical research consistently reports late onset of problem drinking among older women (Gomberg, 1995; Hurt, 1988; Moos et al., 1991). In one study by Gomberg (1995), women reported a mean age at onset of 46.2 years, whereas men reported 27.0 years. Furthermore, 38% of older female patients but 4% of older male patients reported onset within the last 10 years.

It is estimated that alcoholism affects up to 10% of older women, contributing to functional disability (Byyny & Speroff, 1996). However, the excess use or misuse of alcohol is often overlooked and misdiagnosed (Byyny & Speroff, 1996). Women drink less in public places and are therefore less likely to drive while intoxicated or engage in other behaviors that might reveal problems related to alcohol (Gomberg, 1995).

Women also metabolize alcohol differently than men. Compared to men, lower levels of intake produce higher blood alcohol concentration. This is attributed to lower dilution because of the lower body water content in women. In addition, an older woman is at high risk for alcohol abuse if there is a family history of alcoholism and if there has been personal habitual alcohol use (Byyny & Speroff, 1996).

Gender differences in the patterns and identification of alcohol abuse have implications for intervention. Women of all ages are less likely than men to appear at treatment facilities. Outreach and educational efforts should be targeted especially to older women who are socially isolated. Moreover, compared to men, the current cohort of women have less insurance coverage and supplemental income, such as a pension, and they are less likely to have worked and more likely to live in poverty. Thus, they would be less likely to seek treatment for a lack of financial resources. Families, physicians, senior centers, and retirement community staff could play important roles in helping women who have drinking problems (CSAT, 1998).

RISK FACTORS

Losses

As individuals age, they experience a number of losses, including the loss of spouse, other family members, and friends, to death or separation. The highest rate of completed suicide among all population groups is in older White men who become excessively depressed and drink heavily following the death of their spouses

(Brennan & Moos, 1990; Fulop et al., 1993; National Institute on Alcohol Abuse and Alcoholism [NIAAA], 1995). Retirement may mean loss of income as well as work-related network and self-esteem (Bossé, 1993; Thériault, 1994). Losses related to retirement are seen as the psychological issues to be considered for older alcoholics by behavioral health care providers (Stoddard & Thompson, 1996).

Substance Abuse Earlier in Life

A strong relationship exists between developing substance abuse earlier in life and experiencing a recurrence in later life (CSAT, 1998). Some recovering alcoholics with long periods of sobriety may undergo a recurrence of alcoholic drinking due to major losses or an excess of discretionary time (Atkinson & Ganzini, 1994). Among the 10% of older men who reported a history of heavy drinking at some point of their lives, widespread physical and social problems occurred in later life (Colsher & Wallace, 1990). Drinking problems early in life confer a greater than fivefold risk of late life behavioral health problems, despite cessation of heavy drinking. Research suggests that a previous drinking problem is the strongest indicator of a drinking problem in later life (Welte & Mirand, 1992).

Comorbid Psychiatric Disorders

Estimates of comorbid psychiatric disorders occurring in older alcohol abusers vary from 12 to 30% or more (Finlayson et al., 1988; Koenig & Blazer, 1996). Although research does not support the notion that mood disorders precede alcoholism in older adults, there is evidence that they may be either precipitating or maintenance factors in late onset drinking. Depression, for example, appears to precipitate drinking, particularly among women. Some problem drinkers of both sexes who do not meet the clinical criteria for depression often report feeling depressed prior to the first drink on a drinking day (Dupree, Broskowski, & Schonfeld, 1984; Schonfeld & Dupree, 1991).

Patients with severe cognitive impairment generally drink less than nonimpaired alcohol users. However, among individuals who are only mildly impaired, alcohol use may increase as a reaction to lower self-esteem and perceived loss of memory. Late onset alcohol abuse is less associated with psychiatric problems and more likely linked to losses in old age (CSAT, 1998; Moos et al., 1991).

Family History

There is a substantial amount of research implicating genetic factors as significant determinants of alcohol-related behaviors throughout the life span (Carminelli, Heath, & Robinette, 1993; Heller & McClearn, 1995; Swan, Carminelli, Rosenman, Fabsitz, & Christian, 1990). Researchers who studied the genetic tendency of a group of male alcohol abusers suggested that there may be a greater genetic etiology of the problem in early onset than in late onset (Atkinson, Tolson, & Turner, 1990).

SCREENING

As has been noted, elderly alcoholics represent an "invisible epidemic." The screening and detection of alcoholism in elderly persons is often missed because of a low awareness of suspicion, denial and concealment by patients and families, and attribution of symptoms to aging (Council on Scientific Affairs, American Medical Association, 1996; Blow, 1999a). Additionally, physicians often fail to ask questions regarding drinking behavior because of fears of insulting or embarrassing their older patients. Detailed information should be obtained from the patient with respect to drinking behavior, and this information should be supplemented by family members. Historic information may be limited for those who have no family or relatives. Along with screening, further diagnostic work-up should include physical examination; laboratory tests; psychiatric evaluation; and a history of use of medications, particularly psychoactive drugs such as sedatives and hypnotics, and illegal drugs. Clinical symptoms may also indicate the diagnosis of problem drinking. Liver disease, trauma, fractures, and irregular sleeping pattern may be associated with alcohol abuse.

The CAGE questions have been widely used for screening in the general population (Bush, Shaw, Cleary, Delbanco, & Aronson, 1987). The questionnaire consists of four items usually with a cut-off point of 1 as positive (Table 16.1). However, Adams and her colleagues screened 5000 older adults in primary care using the CAGE questionnaire, and it performed poorly in detecting heavy and binge drinkers among older adults (Adams et al., 1996).

Identifying older binge drinkers can be as difficult as identifying older individuals with other kinds of drinking problems due to a lack of clues that exhibit signs of excessive drinking, such as drunk driving (CSAT, 1998), and a misconception that older persons are less likely to have social occasions in which they engage in binge drinking. It may also be more difficult to detect binge drinking in older persons who have less access to health care services and thus may present to the health care system long after the binge episode. Oslin and Blow developed a screening instrument to detect binge drinking and alcohol dependence among older adults for a multisite study funded by the Substance Abuse and Mental Health Service Administration [SAMHSA], the Veterans Administrations, and the Health Resource and Service Administration [HRSA] (Barry, Oslin, & Blow, in press) (Table 16.2).

The World Health Organization developed the Alcohol Use Disorder Identification Test (AUDIT), a 10-item questionnaire that includes items about quantity, frequency, and binge drinking behavior, along with questions about alcohol-related problems in the previous 12 months (Saunders, Aasland, Babor, De La Fuente, & Grant, 1993). The AUDIT tends to exclude alcohol consumed in small amounts (Roberts, 1999).

TABLE 16.1 The CAGE Questionnaire

Directions: Answer yes or no to the following:

- Have you ever felt you ought to **C**ut down?
- Have you ever been **A**nnoyed by criticism of your drinking?
- Have you ever felt **G**uilty about your drinking?
- Have you ever felt the need for an **E**ye opener?

Source: Ewing, J. A. (1984). Detecting alcoholism: The CAGE questionnaire. *Journal of the American Medical Association, 252,* 1905. Reprinted with permission of the American Medical Association.

TABLE 16.2   Binge Drinking Questions

- Have you had any alcoholic beverages in the last year (e.g., beer, wine, wine coolers, or hard liquor like vodka, gin, or whiskey)? Yes/No
- In the last three months, on average, how many days per week did you drink? _____ days
- During the last 3 months, on average how many drinks will you consume on a day that you drink? _____ drinks
- During the last 3 months, on days that you drank any alcohol, how many times did you drinks in one day? _____ times

Source: Barry, K. L., Oslin, D. W., & Blow, F. C. (in press). Prevention and management of alcohol problems in older adults. A brief intervention.

Note: A single mixed drink = 1 drink
A 12 oz. beer = 1 drink
A shot of hard liquor = 1 drink
A pint of hard liquor = 11 drinks
A fifth of hard liquor = 18 drinks
A 4 oz. glass of wine = 1 drink
A pint of wine = 5 drinks
A bottle of wine (40 oz.) = 8 drinks

The Michigan Alcoholism Screening Test-Geriatric Version (MAST-G) is a 24 item yes/no screening test, including several age-appropriate questions with a score of 5 or more yes answers being indicative of a problem. The MAST-G was tested on more than 900 older adults in a variety of settings including nursing homes, primary care settings, congregate meal sites, and housing sites (Table 16.3) (Blow et al., 1992). This is one of the only screens developed specifically for an older population and has high psychometric properties. The MAST-G has a sensitivity of 93.9%, specificity of 78.1%, positive predictive value of 87.2%, and negative predictive value of 88.9% (Blow et al., 1992).

The CAGE questionnaire and the MAST-G have both been validated for use with older adults (Barry & Ackerman, 1999; CSAT, 1998). The MAST-G also has a shorter version consisting of 10 items. Its psychometric properties are similar to those of the MAST-G (Blow et al., 1992; Blow, personal communication, 1999). Validation studies for the AUDIT with older adults are underway (McGann & Spangler, 1997). However, it has been validated cross-culturally at primary care

TABLE 16.3   The Michigan Alcoholism Screening Test-Geriatric Version (MAST-G)

1. After drinking have you ever noticed an increase in your heart rate or beating in your chest?
2. When talking with others, do you ever underestimate how much you actually drink?
3. Does alcohol make you sleep so that you often fall asleep in your chair?
4. After a few drinks have you sometimes not eaten or been able to skip a meal because you didn't feel hungry?
5. Does having a few drinks help decrease your shakiness or tremors?
6. Does alcohol sometimes make it hard for you to remember parts of the day or night?
7. Do you have rules for yourself that you won't drink before a certain time of the day?
8. Have you lost interest in hobbies or activities you used to enjoy?
9. When you wake up in the morning do you ever have trouble remembering part of the night before?
10. Does having a drink help you sleep?
11. Do you hide your alcohol bottles from family members?
12. After a social gathering have you ever felt embarrassed because you drank too much?
13. Have you ever been concerned that drinking might be harmful to your health?
14. Do you like to end an evening with a night cap?
15. Did you find your drinking increased after someone close to you died?
16. In general, would you prefer to have a few drinks at home rather than go out to social events?
17. Are you drinking more now than in the past?
18. Do you usually take a drink to relax or calm your nerves?
19. Do you drink to take your mind off your problems?
20. Have you ever increased your drinking after experiencing a loss in your life?
21. Do you sometimes drive when you have had too much to drink?
22. Has a doctor or nurse ever said they were worried or concerned about your drinking?
23. Have you ever made rules to manage your drinking?
24. When you feel lonely does having a drink help?

Source: Blow, F. C., Brower, J., Schulenberg, J. E., Demo-danenberg, L. M., Young, J. S., & Beresford, T. P. (1992). The Michigan Alcoholism Screening Test—Geriatric version (MAST-G): A new elderly specific screening instrument. *Alcoholism: Clinical and Experimental Research, 16*, 372. Reprinted by permission of Lippincott, Williams, & Wilkins.

settings in Australia, Bulgaria, Kenya, Mexico, and Norway (Saunders et al., 1993).

CONSEQUENCES

Health Services Utilization

Alcohol use is associated with increased use of emergency rooms and hospitals. Estimates of alcohol-related emergency room evaluations and hospital admissions range from 10 to 50% (Barry & Ackerman, 1999). Cost estimates place the treatment of alcohol-related disease at 10 to 15% of total health care costs (McCrady, 1996). Despite the decline in the amount of absolute consumption in alcohol with age, alcohol-related illnesses and use of hospitals persists in elderly persons at rates comparable to the younger population because of the aging process and hence more probable adverse effects of drinking (Barry & Ackerman, 1999).

Physiological Consequences

Among other diseases, cirrhosis; cancers of mouth, larynx, and esophagus; ulcers; respiratory disease; stroke; myocardial infarction; and fractures are positively associated with chronic heavy drinking (Bikle, Stesin, Halloran, Steinbach, & Recker, 1993; Colsher & Wallace, 1990). While the benefit of light drinking on coronary artery disease appears positive, these data need to be interpreted with caution (Barrett, Anda, Croft, Serdula, & Lane, 1995) and recommendations for use of alcohol should be on an individual basis (CSAT, 1998).

Because the aging body is more susceptible to adverse interactions, the potential for interactions between alcohol and medications is likely to be higher in elderly persons, who on average consume large numbers of medications (Council on Scientific Affairs, American Medical Association, 1996). Drug interactions are likely to be more harmful in elderly persons because of slowed metabolic and clearance mechanisms, resulting in a delay in the resolution of the unfavorable reaction.

Chemical dependence may also contribute to difficulties in management of other medical conditions by affecting the patient's ability to seek appropriate care, comply with medications and other treatment, and maintain social networks that are important for community-dwelling elders (Barry & Ackerman, 1999). Elderly alcoholics, compared with nonalcoholics, have been found to have higher morbidity and mortality. Deaths are often caused by accidents and medical complications (McCrady, 1996).

Psychiatric and Psychosocial Consequences

Psychiatric and psychosocial effects of alcohol abuse can be as serious as physiological effects. A history of heavy drinking is positively associated not only with dementia but also with other psychiatric disorders, most notably depression in later life (as discussed earlier) (Saunders et al., 1991). Alcoholism and depression frequently are both implicated in suicides and suicide attempts by elderly persons (CSAT, 1998). Isolation and hopelessness may be even more problematic (Osgood, 1987). Liberto et al. (1992) argued that older persons who became alcoholic early in life tend to be less stable psychologically than those with late onset alcoholism.

TREATMENT

Treatment encompasses detoxification and brief intervention through inpatient/outpatient services, Alcoholics Anonymous (AA), and other support as aftercare. Withdrawal is often the first step in treatment for younger adults but can be potentially life threatening in older patients (Brower, Mudd, Blow, Young, & Hill, 1994). Detoxification of older drinkers results best in a hospital setting in which benzodiazepines and other medication, including psychotropic drugs can be carefully monitored (Barry & Ackerman, 1999; Council on Scientific Affairs, American Medical Association, 1996). Because inpatient programs are expensive, they may serve only limited number of clients. After detoxification, a proper treatment plan needs to be applied to the patient. Treatment approaches include cognitive-behavioral, medical-psychiatric, group-based, family therapy, brief intervention, and 12-step AA. These methods all employ the variations of the mechanisms of motivational and behavioral change.

Cognitive-behavioral techniques teach clients to identify and eventually alter drinking patterns and behaviors. The cognitive-behavioral model enables providers and patients to draw a "drinking behavior chain," which consists of the antecedent situations, thoughts, feelings, and drinking urges that cause alcohol abuse and consequences (CSAT, 1998). This information can lead a given individual to practice a self-management strategy (Dupree et al., 1984).

Medical-psychiatric approaches to modifying drinking behavior in older persons include medications that are used in substance abuse treatment. A medical evaluation of older individuals with chronic mental illness is especially critical due to increased vulnerability to toxic drug side-effects and possible adverse interactions with other prescribed medications.

Group-based approaches seem particularly beneficial to older adults. The most effective aspect of supportive groups is the opportunity to alleviate loneliness and guilt, accept others, and, in return, be accepted by them and create a sense of morale (Gomberg & Zuker, 1998).

Little is available about the effectiveness of family therapy with alcoholics. However, based on the individual's drinking antecedent behaviors, providers can identify the dynamics of marriage and the family, which influence his or her drinking behavior (e.g., Tabisz, Jacyk, Fuchs, & Grymonpre, 1993). Family members can play a critical role in treatment. In fact, married older alcoholics are more likely to comply with treatment regimen when their spouses are involved in the process (Atkinson, Tolson, & Turner, 1993).

Primarily, treatment of alcohol abuse in the elderly should begin with reducing risk factors that can contribute to problem drinking, education about coping strategies for stress that may result from late life changes, and education about the adverse effects of alcohol. This approach, known as brief intervention, ranges from relatively unstructured counseling to more formal therapy, relying on concepts and techniques from motivational and behavioral psychology (Miller & Rollnick, 1991; Samet, Rollnick, & Barnes, 1996). The goal is to motivate the problem drinkers to change their behavior, not to blame. The index of success can be flexible, allowing drinking in moderation, which is called the Hazard Reduction Model, while the Abstinence Model desires total abstinence (Barry et al., in press). Brief intervention usually consists of three sessions over a 12-week period. In the first session, future goals are set to reduce excessive drinking, and the assessment of health habits, reasons for drinking, coping with risky situations, and strategies for cutting down or ultimately quitting are discussed. In the following sessions, current drinking patterns, treatment goals, and intensity of intervention are reviewed. After these initial treatment sessions, pharmacotherapy or increasing the frequency of visits can be considered.

Brief intervention has been shown to be effective in reducing alcohol use in health care settings with other age groups (Barbor & Grant, 1992; Bien, Miller, & Tonigan, 1993; Kahan, Wilson, & Becker, 1995; Wallace, Cutler, & Haines, 1988). There are several studies in progress using this approach for older adults, and the results have been promising (e.g., Chermack, Blow, Hill, & Mudd, 1996). An ongoing study funded by the Substance Abuse and Mental Health Service Administration [SAMHSA], the Veterans Administration, and the Health Resource and Service Administration [HRSA] is applying a brief intervention in a multisite geriatric sample that has screened positive for alcohol abuse and dependence.

In the community, self-help groups are beneficial for long-term support (Campbell, 1997). AA offers a free opportunity for care after institutional treatment. The goal of AA is to defy the isolation of the alcoholic and provide support using a group therapy technique.

Transportation can be an important barrier to treatment, even among motivated individuals. Transportation is especially problematic in rural communities, where there is often a lack of public transportation. In poor urban areas, accessing transportation can be dangerous. A person may be able to go to a hospital for treatment but not to AA or aftercare (Fortney, Booth, Blow, & Bunn, 1995). A shrinking social support network may be a factor causing older adults to withdraw from continuing care because they tend to have fewer friends to support them or participate in the treatment process (CSAT, 1998).

PREVENTION

A wide range of unique issues affect older adults and should enter into discussions about prevention of substance abuse: losses, isolation, loneliness, financial problems, complex medical conditions, multiple medications, reduced mobility, sensory deficits, impaired self-care activities, and demoralization (Blow, 1999a).

Prevention strategies effective with younger populations may translate for use with older adults, although little research has been done in this area. Studies of health promotion and disease prevention suggest that individual-based health education can be a major area of prevention about alcohol and other substance abuse (Gomberg & Zucker, 1998). Families and peers potentially provide important care and support for the persons with alcohol problems. Broad-based membership organizations, such as health care organizations and the American Association of Retired Persons provide access to health information through various modalities (e.g., written materials, the Internet).

Problem drinking among older adults is an area that needs much additional research. Future interventions and research on alcohol abuse must be accompanied by more age-appropriate classification and assessment.

REFERENCES

Adams, W. L. (1998). Alcohol and substance abuse. In E. H. Duthie & P. R. Katz (Eds.), *Practice of geriatrics* (3rd ed.) (pp. 307–316). Philadelphia: W. B. Saunders.

Adams, W. L., Barry, K. L., & Fleming, M. F. (1996). Screening for problem drinking in older primary care patients. *Journal of the American Medical Association, 276,* 1964–1967.

Adams, W. L., Yuan, Z., Barboriak, J. J., & Rimm, A. A. (1993). Alcohol-related hospitalizations of elderly people: Prevalence and geographic location in the United States. *Journal of the American Medical Association, 270,* 1222–1225.

American Psychiatric Association. (1994). *Diagnostic and Statistical Manual of Mental Disorders* (4th ed.). Washington, DC: Author.

Atkinson, R. M. (1994). Late onset problem in older adults. *International Journal of Geriatric Psychiatry, 9,* 321–326.

Atkinson, R. M., & Ganzini, L. (1994). Substance abuse. In C. E. Coffey & J. L. Cummings (Eds.), *Textbook of geriatric neuropsychiatry* (pp. 297–321). Washington, DC: American Psychiatric Press.

Atkinson, R. M., Tolson, R. L., & Turner, J. A. (1990). Late versus early onset problem drinking in older men. *Alcoholism: Clinical and Experimental Research, 14,* 574–579.

Atkinson, R. M., Tolson, R. L., & Turner, J. A. (1993). Factors affecting outpatient treatment compliance of older male problem drinkers. *Journal of Studies on Alcohol, 54,* 102–106.

Babor, T. F., & Grant, M. (1992). Report on Phase II: A randomized clinical trial on brief interventions in primary health care. In *Project on identification and management of alcohol-related problems.* Geneva, Switzerland: World Health Organization.

Barnes, G. M. (1979). Alcohol use among older persons: Findings from a Western New York State general population survey. *Journal of the American Geriatrics Society, 27,* 244–250.

Barrett, D. H., Anda, R. F., Croft, J. B., Serdula, M. K., & Lane, M. J. (1995). The association between alcohol use and health behaviors related to the risk of cardiovascular disease. *Journal of Studies on Alcohol, 56,* 9–15.

Barry, P., & Ackerman, K. (1999). Chemical dependency in the elderly. In W. R. Hazzard, J. P. Blass, W. H. Ettinger, J. B. Halter, & J. G. Ouslander (Eds.), *Principles of geriatric medicine and gerontology* (4th ed.) (pp. 1357–1363). New York: McGraw-Hill.

Barry, K. L., Oslin, D. W., & Blow, F. C. (in press). Prevention and management of alcohol problems in older adults. A brief intervention. New York: Springer.

Beresford, T. P., Blow, F. C., Brower, K. J., Adams, K. M., & Hall, R. C. W. (1988). Alcoholism and aging in the general hospital. *Psychosomatics, 29,* 61–72.

Bien, T. H., Miller, W. R., & Tonigan, J. S. (1993). Brief interventions for alcohol problems: A review. *Addiction, 88,* 315–335.

Bikle, D. D., Stesin, A., Hollaran, B., Steinbach, L., & Recker, R. (1993). Alcohol-induced bone disease. *Alcoholism: Clinical and Experimental Research, 17,* 690–695.

Blazer, D., Crowell, B. A., & George, L. K. (1987). Alcohol abuse and dependence in the rural South. *Archives of General Psychiatry, 44,* 736–740.

Blow, F. C. (1999a). *Overview of substance abuse prevention in aging and critical issues in prevention.* Paper presented at Aging and Substance Abuse Educational In-Service, Rockville, MD.

Blow, F. C. (1999b). The spectrum of alcohol interventions for older adults. In E. S. L. Gomberg, A. M. Hegedus, & R. A. Zucker (Eds.), *Alcohol problems and aging.* Rockville, MD: National Institute on Alcohol Abuse and Alcoholism.

Blow, F. C., Brower, J., Schulenberg, J. E., Demo-Danenberg, L. M., Young, J. S., & Beresford, T. P. (1992). The Michigan Alcoholism Screening Test—Geriatric version (MAST-G): A new elderly specific screening instrument. *Alcoholism: Clinical and experimental Research, 16,* 372.

Booth, B. M., Blow, F. C., Cook, C. A., Bunn, J. Y., & Fortney, J. C. (1992). Age and ethnicity among hospitalized alcoholics: A nationwide study. *Alcoholism: Clinical and Experimental Research, 16,* 1029–1034.

Bossé, R. (1993). Change in social support after retirement: Longitudinal findings from the Normative Aging Study. *Journal of Gerontology, 48,* 210–217.

Brennan, P. L., & Moos, R. H. (1990). Life stressors, social resources, and late-life problem drinking. *Psychology and Aging, 5,* 491–501.

Brower, K. J., Mudd, S., Blow, F. C., Young, J. P., & Hill, E. M. (1994). Severity and treatment of alcohol withdrawal in elderly versus younger patients. *Alcoholism: Clinical and Experimental Research, 18,* 196–201.

Bucholz, K. K., Sheline, Y., & Helzer, J. E. (1995). The epidemiology of alcohol use, problems, and dependence in elders: A review. In T. P. Beresford & E. S. L. Gomberg (Eds.), *Alcohol and Aging* (pp. 19–41). New York: Oxford University Press.

Bush, B., Shaw, S., Cleary, P., Delbanco, T. L., & Aronson, M. D. (1987). Screening for alcohol abuse using the CAGE questionnaire. *The American Journal of Medicine, 82,* 231–235.

Byyny, R. L., & Speroff, L. (1996). *A clinical guide for the care of older women: Primary and preventive care,* 2nd ed. Baltimore, MD: Williams & Wilkins.

Campbell, J. W. (1997). Alcoholism. In R. J. Ham & P. D. Sloane (Eds.), *Primary care geriatrics: A case-based approach* (pp. 365–371). St. Louis, MO: Mosby.

Carminelli, D., Heath, A. C., & Robinette, D. (1993). Genetic analysis of drinking behavior in World War II veteran twins. *Genetic Epidemiology, 10,* 201–213.

The Center for Substance Abuse Treatment [CSAT] (1998). *Substance abuse among older adults:* Treatment Improvement Protocol (TIP) series. Washington, DC: Substance Abuse and Mental Health Services Administration, U.S. Department of Health and Human Services Publication No. (SMA) 98-3179.

Chermack, S. T., Blow, F. C., Hill, E. M., & Mudd, S. A. (1996). The relationship between alcohol symptoms and consumption among older drinkers. *Alcoholism: Clinical and Experimental Research, 20,* 1153–1158.

Coleman, P. R., & Veach, T. L. (1990). Substance abuse and the family physician: A survey of attitudes. *Substance Abuse, 11,* 84–93.

Colsher, P. L., & Wallace, R. B. (1990). Elderly men with histories of heavy drinking: Correlated and consequences. *Journal of Studies on Alcohol, 51,* 528–535.

Council on Scientific Affairs, American Medical Association (1996). Alcoholism in the elderly. *Journal of the American Medical Association, 275,* 797–801.

D'Archngelo, E. (1993). Substance abuse in later life. *Canadian Family Physician, 39,* 1986–1993.

Dawson, D. A. (1994). Are men or women more likely to stop drinking because of alcohol problems? *Drug and Alcohol Dependence, 36,* 57–64.

Dupree, L. W., Broskowski, H., & Schonfeld, L. (1984). The Gerontology Alcohol Project: A behavioral treatment program for elderly alcohol abusers. *The Gerontologist, 24,* 510–516.

Finlayson, R., Hurt, R., Davis, L., & Morse, R. (1988). Alcoholism in elderly persons: A study of the psychiatric and psychosocial features of 216 inpatients. *Mayo Clinic Proceedings, 63,* 761–768.

Fortney, J. C., Booth, B. M., Blow, F. C., & Bunn, J. Y. (1995). The effects of travel barriers and age on the utilization of alcoholism treatment aftercare. *American Journal of Drug and Alcohol Abuse, 21,* 391–406.

Fulop, G., Reinhardt, J., Strain, J. J., Paris, B., Miller, M., & Fillit, H. (1993). Identification of alcoholism and depression in a geriatric medicine outpatient clinic. *Journal of the American Geriatrics Society, 41,* 737–741.

Geller, G., Levine, D. M., Mamon, J. A., Moore, R. D., Bone, L. R., & Stokes, E. J. (1989). Knowledge, attitudes, and reported practices of medical students and house staff regarding the diagnosis and treatment of alcoholism. *Journal of the American Medical Association, 261,* 3115–3120.

Glynn, R. L., Bouchard, G. R., Lo Castro, J. S., & Laird, N. M. (1985). Aging and generational effects on drinking behaviors in men: Results from the Normative Aging Study. *American Journal of Public Health, 75,* 1413–1419.

Gomberg, E. S. L. (1990). Drugs, alcohol, and aging. In L. T. Kozlowski, H. M. Annis, & F. B. Cappell (Eds.), *Research advances in alcohol and drug problems* (Vol. 10). New York: Plenum.

Gomberg, E. S. L. (1995). Older women and alcohol use and abuse. In M. Galanter (Ed.), *Recent developments in alcoholism: Alcoholism and women* (pp. 61–79). New York: Plenum.

Gomberg, E. S. L., & Nelson, B. W. (1995). Black and White older men: Alcohol use and abuse. In T. P. Beresford & E. S. L. Gomberg (Eds.), *Alcohol and aging* (pp. 307–323). New York: Oxford University Press.

Gomberg, E. S. L., & Zucker, R. A. (1998). Substance use and abuse in old age. In I. H. Nordhus, G. R. Vandenbos, S. Berg, & P. Fromholt (Eds.), *Clinical geropsychology* (pp. 189–204). Washington, DC: American Psychological Association.

Gurnack, A. M., & Hoffman, N. G. (1992). Elderly alcohol misuse. *International Journal of Addiction, 27,* 869–878.

Heller, D. A., & McClearn, G. E. (1995). Alcohol, aging, and genetics. In T. P. Beresford & E. S. L. Gomberg (Eds.), *Alcohol and aging* (pp. 99–114). New York: Oxford University Press.

Hurt, R. D., Finlayson, R. E., Morse, R. M., & Davis, L. J. (1988). Alcoholism in elderly persons: Medical aspects and prognosis of 216 patients. *Mayo Clinic Proceedings, 63,* 753–760.

Kahan, M., Wilson, L., & Becker, L. (1995). Effectiveness of physician-based interventions with problem drinkers: A review. *Canadian Medical Journal, 152,* 851–856.

Koenig, H. G., & Blazer, D. G. (1996). Depression. In J. E. Birren (Ed.), *Encyclopedia of gerontology: Age, aging, and the aged* (pp. 415–428). San Diego: Academic Press.

Liberto, J. G., & Oslin, D. W. (1996). Early versus late onset alcoholism in the elderly. In A. M. Gurnack (Ed.), *Drugs and the elderly: Use and abuse of drugs, medicines, alcohol, and tobacco* (pp. 94–112). New York: Springer.

Liberto, J. G., Oslin, D. W., & Ruskin, P. E. (1992). Alcoholism in older persons: A review of the literature. *Hospital and Community Psychiatry, 43,* 975–983.

Marcus, M. T. (1993). Alcohol and other drug abuse in elders. *Journal of ET Nursing, 20,* 106–110.

McCrady, B. S., & Langenbucher, J. W. (1996). Alcoholism treatment and health care system reform. *Archives of General Psychiatry, 53,* 737–746.

McGann, K. P., & Spangler, J. G. (1997). Alcohol, tobacco, and illicit drug use among women. *Primary Care, 24,* 113–122.

McKim, W. A., & Quinlan, L. T. (1991). Changes in alcohol consumption with age. *Canadian Journal of Public Health, 82,* 231–234.

Meyers, A. R., Goldman, E., Hingson, R., Scotch, N., & Mangione, T. (1981–1982). Evidence for cohort or generational differences in the drinking behavior of older adults. *International Journal of Aging and Human Development, 14,* 31–44.

Miller, W. R., & Rollnick, S. (1991). *Motivational interviewing.* New York: Guilford.

Minnis, J. (1988). Toward an understanding of alcohol abuse among the elderly: A sociological perspective. *Journal of Alcohol and Drug Education, 33,* 32–40.

Molgaard, C. A., Nakamura, C. M., Stanford, E. P., Peddecord, K. M., & Morton, D. J. (1990). Prevalence of alcohol consumption among older persons. *Journal of Community Health, 15,* 239–251.

Moore, R. D., Bone, L. R., Geller, G., Marmon, J. A., Stokes, E. J., & Levine, D. M. (1989). Prevention, detection, and treatment of alcoholism in hospitalized patients. *Journal of the American Medical Association, 261,* 403–407.

Moos, R. H., Brennan, P. L., & Moos, B. S. (1991). Short-term processes of remission and nonremission among late-life problem drinkers. *Alcoholism: Clinical and Experimental Research, 15,* 948–955.

Morse, R. M., & Flavin, D. K. (1992). The definition of alcoholism. *Journal of the American Medical Association, 268,* 1012–1014.

Myers, J., Weismann, M., Tishler, G., Holzer, C. E., Leaf, P. J., Orvaschel, H., Anthony, J. C., Boyd, J. H., Burke, J. D., & Kramer, M. (1984). Six month prevalence of psychiatric disorders in three communities: 1980 to 1982. *Archives of General Psychiatry, 41,* 959–967.

The National Center on Addiction and Substance Abuse at Columbia University. (1998). *Under the rug: Substance abuse and the mature women.* Washington, DC: The National Council on Patient Information and Education (NCPIE).

National Institute on Alcohol Abuse and Alcoholism (1995). *The physician's guide to helping patients with alcohol problems.* NIH Publication No. 95-3769. Rockville, MD: Author.

Osgood, N. J. (1987). The alcohol-suicide connection in late life. *Postgraduate Medicine, 81,* 379–394.

Rains, V. S., & Ditzler, T. F. (1993). Alcohol use disorders in cognitively impaired patients referred for geriatric assessment. *Journal of Addiction Disorders, 12,* 55–64.

Roberts, G. D. (1999). Substance abuse. In R. E. Feinstein & A. A. Brewer (Eds.), *Primary care psychiatry and behavioral medicine* (pp. 83–112). New York: Springer.

Saitz, R., Mulvey, K. P., Plough, A., & Samet, J. H. (1997). Physician unawareness of serious substance abuse. *American Journal of Drug and Alcohol Abuse, 23,* 343–354.

Samet, J. H., Rollnick, S., & Barnes, H. (1996). Beyond CAGE: A brief approach after detection of substance abuse. *Archives of Internal Medicine, 156,* 2287–2293.

Saunders, J. B., Aasland, O. G., Babor, T. F., De La Fuente, J. R., & Grant, M. (1993). Development of the Alcohol Use Disorders Identification Test (AUDIT): WHO collaborative projects on early detection of persons with harmful alcohol consumption—II. *Addiction, 88,* 791–804.

Schonfeld, L., & Dupree, L. W. (1991). Antecedents of drinking for early and late onset elderly alcohol abusers. *Journal of Studies on Alcohol, 52,* 587–592.

Solomon, K., Manepalli, J., Ireland, G. A., & Mahon, G. M. (1993). Alcoholism and prescription drug abuse in the elderly: St. Louis University grounds. *Journal of the American Geriatrics Society, 41,* 57–69.

Stinson, F. S., Dufour, M. C., & Bertolucci, D. (1989). Alcohol-related morbidity in the aging population. *Alcohol Health and Research World, 13,* 80–87.

Stoddard, C. E., & Thompson, D. L. (1996). Alcohol and the Elderly: Special concerns for counseling professionals. *Alcoholism Treatment Quarterly, 14,* 59–69.

Swan, G. E., Carminelli, D., Rosenman, R. H., Fabsitz, R. R., & Christian, J. C. (1990). Smoking and alcohol consumption in adult male twins: Genetic heritability and shared environmental influences. *Journal of Substance Abuse, 2,* 39–50.

Tabisz, E. M., Jacyk, W. R., Fuchs, D., & Grymonpre, R. (1993). Chemical dependency in the elderly: The enabling factors. *Canadian Journal of Aging, 17,* 78–88.

Thériault, J. (1994). Retirement as a psychosocial transition: Process of adaptation to change. *International Journal of Aging and Human Development, 38,* 153–170.

Wallace, P., Cutler, S., & Haines, A. (1988). Randomized controlled trial of general practitioner intervention in patients with excessive alcohol consumption. *British Medical Journal, 290,* 1949–1953.

Welte, J. W., & Mirand, A. L. (October, 1992). *Alcohol use by the elderly: Patterns and correlates: A report on the Erie county elder drinking survey.* Buffalo, NY: Research Institute on Addictions.

U.S. Bureau of the Census (1996). *65+ in the United States.* Current population reports, Special Studies, Number P23-190. Washington, DC: U.S. Government Printing Office.

PART IV

Service Provision for the Elderly

CHAPTER 17

Patient-Provider Communication

Margaret Bergmann and Ruth Kandel

I t is a busy day in your office. Your next patient, Mr. G, age 75, is accompanied by his concerned daughter who explains that he has been having a difficult time managing things at home since the death of his wife, such as paying bills and wearing clean clothes. Mr. G denies everything and appears to be defensive when you question him, stating that he "is not crazy." After an exam you direct much of your discussion to the patient's daughter who is anxious, concerned, and seeking your advice. You explain the uncertainty of what these changes signify and suggest that Mr. G will have to be followed over time to see how he progresses. There is just so much you can tell from one brief office encounter. You go on to your next patient but feel unsatisfied about the interaction. Perhaps you will have more of an opportunity next time you see Mr. G to develop a relationship with him, but how?

This chapter will focus on patient-provider communication. We will outline characteristics of a successful encounter, review sensitive issues that need to be considered when interviewing an older individual, and list strategies for clinicians and staff to optimize patient visits. While our focus is on communication in the primary care office setting, much of the information can be generalized to other situations. We use the term *clinicians* to include not only physicians but other providers of health care such as nurse practitioners and physician assistants.

The health care system today is complicated and there is a growing need for clinicians to coordinate medical care and help individuals negotiate the system. Essential features for such providers include an interest and experience in geriatrics as well as compassion and respect for older people. Appreciating that many older individuals have chronic medical problems, there is a subtle but significant shift in the philosophy of geriatric medicine when compared to the traditional curative focus of adult internal medicine. In geriatrics the emphasis is on maximizing autonomy, enabling individuals to develop their maximal functional abilities and maintaining a good quality of life despite chronic medical problems.

In geriatric care there is also an emphasis on the multidisciplinary approach. Geriatric medicine utilizes a team of professionals in dealing with problems, including doctors; nurses; social workers; nursing assistants; occupational, physical and recreational therapists; and nutritionists. Sometimes enabling someone to remain at home requires the assistance of others, such as home health aides, companions, and visiting nurses to complement family efforts. Among doctors and nurses, geriatricians and gerontological nurse practitioners are clinicians who have advanced training and expertise in geriatrics. Their role as primary providers or consultants can be invaluable in the care of older patients.

The practice of geriatrics goes beyond the traditional medical framework that focuses on treatments for a particular disease, and recognizes the complex interplay between medical, social, ethical, and psychological issues. This not only allows but often demands us to provide creative answers that take into account a person's quality of life. For example, a patient, Mrs. A, comes to you with an essential tremor. She initially denies being bothered by this but on examination you notice that she has lost weight and appears sad. When questioning her, Mrs. A comments that she has stopped going to the group dining room in her senior housing facility because she is embarrassed by her shaking. This is an unfortunate loss for her because dining with friends had been an important daily social event.

With this information you realize that the tremor, though benign, is having a significant negative impact on Mrs. A's quality of life. You refer Mrs. A to an occupational therapist who provides weighted utensils and cups to steady her hands while dining. This simple intervention, without any medications, allows the patient the pleasure of dining with others again.

CHARACTERISTICS OF A SUCCESSFUL ENCOUNTER

We view the geriatric provider to be in partnership with the patient and, at times, the family. Within this partnership, the clinician needs to recognize the importance of the following.

An Atmosphere of Mutual Respect

People are unique, having their own personal histories, cultural backgrounds, and religious beliefs that influence how they view themselves and others. This holds true both for patients and clinicians. It is very important for the provider to establish a respectful relationship with older persons and their families. To accomplish this providers need to confront their own attitudes toward aging. There is a tendency, especially if problems with communication exist, for the clinician to direct the conversation to the family member. This might further be supported by the older person who may be deferential to the provider as the main authority figure. It is important for the provider and family not to "gang up" on the patient. Ultimately this leads to isolation of the patient and interferes with the patient-provider relationship.

Good Communication Skills

Providers must encourage honest, open communication. Both the patient and family should feel comfortable talking with the clinician. From the onset of the interview, patient-centered questions could be introduced such as "What would you like me to do for you?" or "What were you hoping would happen today?" (Sledge & Feinstein,

1997). Sometimes, despite best intentions, there are barriers that impair communication between provider and patient. The following have been identified as helpful in overcoming these difficulties: recognition and acknowledgment of the problem; open exploration with the patient; expression of empathy by the provider; and brainstorming alternatives (Quill, 1989).

Sufficient Time

The practice of geriatric care requires time, a much sought after commodity in this hectic and fast-paced health care world. Older individuals often require more time due to multiple medical problems and complicated treatment regimens. Even changing into an exam gown may take considerable time. Creative ways to adjust for this include scheduling more than one appointment to go over concerns in order of importance; dividing an encounter among several clinicians, such as a social worker, physician, and nurse, each of whom can go over health matters in their respective disciplines; and, for newer patients, requesting prior medical evaluations.

Comprehensive Knowledge Base

Providers of care to older persons need to have an understanding of the process of normal aging; the different ways that health problems may present in the aged; and the importance of changes in functional abilities. In addition, clinicians need to appreciate conditions that primarily affect an older population such as cardiovascular problems, neurodegenerative diseases, and loss of mobility. There are a variety of specifically designed geriatric tests that can aid providers in their evaluations (Gallo, Reichel, & Anderson, 1995). Older individuals often experience the same common medical problems that are seen in younger adults, however, the presentation of such problems may be atypical and not system specific. For example, confusion may be the presenting symptom for a number of medical illnesses, including infections or cardiovascular disease. Diagnosing a problem is especially challenging in individuals with dementia, who may have a difficult time articulating their symptoms. Thus, again, the clinician needs to go beyond the obvious clues and look at the individual in his or her entirety to identify the underlying problem.

SENSITIVE TOPICS

The provider of geriatric care needs to be able to address certain sensitive issues that older people may confront over time. Given their sensitive nature, these problems are often not mentioned by provider and patient. The clinician should acknowledge that though some personal problems may be uncomfortable or embarrassing, it is important to discuss them. One helpful way to introduce a difficult topic is to say, "Some people with this condition . . . " (Gastel, 1994). Providers of care to elderly persons should have a substantial knowledge base in each of the following areas.

Neglect and Abuse

Each year many older Americans are victims of physical, psychological, or other forms of abuse and neglect. Embarrassment and fear of reprisal are some reasons why patients may not report this problem. Routine practice protocols should include both subjective and objective assessments of common indicators of mistreatment (Fulmer & Birkenhauer, 1992). Clinicians can provide treatment, support, and referrals when needed. In many states providers are mandated reporters of suspected neglect and abuse.

Depression

Depressive symptoms and illnesses are seen in elderly persons and need to be assessed during routine evaluation. The incidence of suicide rate among older people is higher than in the general population (Greene & Adelman, 1996). Depression in elderly persons may be caused by medical problems or life stressors (Blazer & Cassel, 1994). Diagnosis, however, remains challenging for several reasons. Symptoms of depression are sometimes confused with those of medical illness. Expression of these symptoms may be limited due to resistance to talk about these issues by the current cohort of older persons who may have negative associations with mental illness and psychiatric treatment (Martin, Fleming, & Evans, 1995). People with depression often lack hope and may feel it futile to comment on their feelings of sadness. The situation is further complicated in those individuals with cognitive impairment who may have a difficult time expressing their feelings. The recognition and treatment of depression can have a significant positive impact on a person's life.

Cognitive Impairment

For clinicians involved in the care of older people, questions about cognition are frequently asked. Often a family will come to the clinic with concerns about a loved one's failing memory or functional decline. There are many causes, some reversible, for cognitive impairment, and a medical evaluation is essential in determining proper diagnosis and treatment (Small et al., 1997). For those individuals with dementia, the provider can review treatment options with patients and families. Just as important as medications in the management of dementia are strategies, education, and support. Some general interventions that may be helpful for patients include orientation boards at home, reminder calls on the phone to take medications, and using memory notebooks. Strategies can be developed for patients based on the stage of dementia and cognitive profile. Teaching families different ways to communicate, often as simple as breaking down complicated sentences or tasks, can be invaluable. It is useful to explain to families that some of the cognitive and behavioral changes seen in dementia are due to the disease and may not be within a patient's control. Providing routine activities can be of benefit in terms of overall care. It is often helpful for families to identify what problems with the patient are most distressing. Dementia is truly a family affair often resulting in significant stress for the caregiver, who can be viewed as a hidden patient. There are many services in the community that can provide assistance for the patient and family such as home companions, home health aides, and adult day care.

Caregiving and Caregiver Stress

Working with older individuals may bring clinicians in contact with their families and friends. The provider must at all times respect the older person's right to privacy and independence. Providers should ask the patient's permission before revealing any medically related information to a third party. It is helpful to know whom, within the patient's social network, is willing and able to provide help and support when needed. Clarifying what assistance is needed is equally important because often family members want to help but do not know how.

Special consideration must also be given to the patient as caregiver. Often older patients are in the role of caregiver to a spouse or dependent minors of the family. This can have great impact on whether the patient can "afford to be sick." This can also affect willingness to report health problems. In supporting caregivers it is important to assess their need for assistance and to encourage them not to do the impossible alone. The provider can encourage caregivers to plan ahead and can be a source of referrals for respite services, support groups, reading materials, and counseling as necessary.

Sexuality

Clinicians should be aware that many older persons participate in and continue to enjoy sexual activities. Discussion of sexuality should be routinely included in the care of all patients with a focus on whether aging and health problems affect one's sexual function (Butler & Lewis, 1993). It should not be assumed that older persons are necessarily heterosexual. Providers can evaluate problems and provide information, treatment, and referrals as appropriate.

Urinary Incontinence

Urinary incontinence often goes untreated because patients are embarrassed to mention this problem or mistakenly assume it is a part of normal aging. In noninstitutionalized persons over 60 years of age, the prevalence of incontinence ranges from 15 to 35% and is associated with both substantial physical and psychosocial morbidity (Fantl et al., 1996). It is important to recognize that incontinence can result from multiple predisposing factors not just limited to the lower urinary tract. The mnemonic DIAPPERS (which represents delirium, infection, atrophic urethritis and vaginitis, pharmaceuticals, psychologic conditions, excessive urinary output, restricted mobility, and stool impaction) is helpful in addressing transient causes of incontinence (Resnick, 1984). Independent of etiology, urinary incontinence can be cured or substantially alleviated through a variety of behavioral, medical, and surgical treatments.

End-of-Life Decisions

Especially in geriatric medicine, concerns about death and dying are paramount, and it is the practitioner's responsibility to raise this topic. People have repeatedly stressed that they want to talk about end-of-life decisions but are hesitant to do so (Reilly et al., 1994). Most older patients would welcome the opportunity to discuss their feelings about death and dying as well as the aging process. In addition, by establishing advanced directives, older persons can share with their families their views on such topics as whether to perform cardiopulmonary resuscitation, the use of feeding tubes, and long-term care services. Older individuals should be asked to name a person who is their designated health care proxy with whom they could communicate these directives. Preplanning helps to lessen the burden of critical decision making by relatives during difficult and emotional times. Raising these issues can result in an on-going dialogue that may be revisited over time and strengthens the patient-provider relationship.

TIPS FOR FACILITATING AN EFFECTIVE MEDICAL ENCOUNTER

Because older persons often have lengthy and complex medical histories and take a variety of medications, preplanning of many aspects of the encounter are not only recommended but are essential for providing effective and efficient medical care. This is especially true today in the context of time and cost restraints in managed care. Many strategies can be employed to facilitate the communication process and create a more effective encounter before, during, and after the visit. The goals or objectives of an encounter have been defined as: data gathering to establish diagnoses; communicating information and recommending treatments; and developing and maintaining the relationship between patient and provider (Lazare, Putnam, & Lipkin, 1995).

Before the Visit

Staff should be familiar with the nature of the provider practice and be able to properly describe it to prospective patients. At the time of appointment scheduling, staff should inquire about the reason for the visit and triage appropriately. They can assist patients in identifying the best time of day for travel (i.e., cab availability, traffic volume low) and give or mail directions as necessary. Preprinted instructions can save staff time. A confirmation of appointment policy should be in place, such as having a receptionist call patients 1 day ahead or mailing reminder postcards.

Every effort should be made to create an accessible office. Because older persons can have impairments in mobility, accessibility for walkers and wheelchairs can greatly facilitate and ease visits. The environment should be welcoming and seek to alleviate discomforts. Background noise should be minimized and interruptions avoided.

Staff should remind patients or significant others to bring along basic, though often essential, information such as insurance cards, and request additional medical information from other providers and specialists before the appointment. Older persons often have multiple, diverse health providers, including dentists, podiatrists, therapists, and a variety of medical specialists.

Encouraging patients to write down questions and concerns can save much time in identifying and targeting problems during the encounter. Mailing diaries or logs addressing pertinent information can assist patients in describing and defining health problems. Asking patients to complete questionnaires either at home or in the office can expedite history gathering.

As previously stated, older persons often take numerous medications. Reminding patients to bring a list of all current drugs, including prescription and over the counter medications, as well as commonly forgotten items such as ophthalmic and optic preparations, can save time and prevent misunderstandings. An alternative to this list, which can be difficult and time consuming for some, is to ask patients to "brown bag" medications, which involves placing all drugs in a bag to be brought to the visit.

Lastly, staff should encourage patients, particularly frail individuals or those with dementia, to bring a family member or friend to the visit. Often this person can help provide additional information, remember questions, and review later what has transpired.

During the Visit

Verbal and nonverbal communication serve as the basis of any health encounter and therefore, before initiating any interaction, the clinician must first focus on enhancing communication while eliminating any potential barriers. Visits should be "close encounters" of a meaningful, productive kind and not scary, frustrating, or otherwise difficult. Rapid-fire questioning and fast delivery of information need to be avoided, as does the use of medical terminology or words that are unfamiliar to older patients. Older persons should be addressed by their proper name unless they indicate otherwise. They should not be referred to by their first name without the patient's permission or be called "dear" or "honey." All staff should introduce themselves and explain their roles.

Many older individuals have hearing or visual impairment. Speaking in low tones is important with older persons because hearing loss with age primarily affects high tones. Be sure a patient who has a hearing aid is wearing it and that it is turned on and working. Inquire about what helps (i.e., speaking slowly or facing the patient to facilitate lip reading). Use of simple diagrams and written materials can often enhance communication with the hearing impaired. There are many excellent assistive hearing devices that can be used during a medical encounter to augment and facilitate communication. For those with visual deficits, remind or assist patients to clean and put on eyeglasses. Provide adequate lighting without glare.

Again, use of written materials with large enough type can enhance communication. Alternatively, large pictures or diagrams and tape-recorded instructions can be used.

While taking a history, the provider should help the patient sort out what is most important to the patient and what is medically important. Often an individual can have one problem that prevents focusing on another that may be more medically significant (i.e., skin-tag vs hypercholesterolemia). An area of special concern for miscommunication is when the patient does not speak English. Translation must be available, when necessary, by staff or families. A careful review of medications and compliance is essential. Because side effects, interactions, and misuse can create rather than treat medical problems, it is crucial to ascertain what drugs patients are taking. Benefits and side effects should be discussed. Particularly important questions include whether medications are being taken as directed and if there are any problems interfering with the instructions (i.e., high costs, lack of insurance, or pharmacy availability). The provider can help or enlist help with problems as appropriate.

Eliciting a social and life history, which includes assessment of cultural or ethnic norms and influences, is equally important with older persons. Such information is essential in planning interventions that are realistic and appropriate for the patient's living arrangements and life style. Some areas to discuss include eating habits, tobacco and alcohol use, safety issues, and financial concerns. It is important to clarify what supports are available from family members. Encouraging patients to convey experiences, perceptions, and attitudes regarding health, disease, and death can aid in health care planning and decision making. Such information helps the provider better understand patients and families, respect and support their goals, and make appropriate resource referrals.

Functional status is uniquely important in the assessment of an older person's health. Providers should know a patient's level of everyday functioning on activities of daily living (ADLs), such as bathing, grooming, and toileting, and instrumental activities of daily living (IADLs), such as cooking, banking, and shopping. Ability to perform ADLs and IADLs both reflects and affects a patient's health. Sudden changes in ADLs or IADLs are valuable diagnostic clues in the older person who may not show typical signs of illness. Home visits can be particularly insightful, allowing the provider to see how a patient functions. If assessment in the home environment is not possible, asking the patient to describe a typical day can provide some understanding of the home situation and an individual's level of functioning.

Because education of the patient and family is an integral part of the health care visit, some special strategies are highlighted to enhance this process. Providers tend to underestimate how much patients want to know and may overestimate how long they spend giving information to them. Patient dissatisfaction with care has been tied to insufficient, contradictory, or confusing information (Waitzkin & Stoeckle, 1972). Education is an important part of enabling patients and families to be active and equal partners in their care. General suggestions include encouraging the patient to ask questions; seeking clarification as necessary; and providing additional information through drawings, videos, and pamphlets. The provider may ask patients to repeat their understanding of the conversation, allowing one to correct misconceptions. The patient should be informed about and encouraged to see other team members who can provide additional education and information.

An important area of educational focus is explaining diagnoses and discussing treatments. Older patients should be encouraged to express their beliefs about what is wrong and express the feasibility or acceptability of proposed treatment measures. The provider can refer the patient to the vast network of health information resources available today. One helpful guide *Talking With Your Doctor: A Guide for Older People* is available from the National Institute of Aging (Karp, 1994). There are specific disease and syndrome foundations and support groups such as the Parkinson's Disease Foundation and the Alzheimer's Association. There are also resources with a particular emphasis on aging concerns, including the American Association of Retired Persons and local senior centers and agencies.

In terminating a visit it is important to save time at the end to ask patients if there is anything else they would like to discuss. Patients may not be comfortable until the end of an encounter to express a concern. One should make decisions together and agree on the plan of care. Patients should be encouraged to take notes and be provided with written materials or instructions as appropriate. A summary of the visit highlighting the issues that were addressed can help build a trusting relationship.

After the Visit

Strategies can also be employed to insure continuity and enhance patient-provider communication after an individual encounter. A plan should be developed for ongoing communication with permission and encouragement given to the patient to call about any points of confusion that might arise after the visit. Provider and staff should always convey an open door policy. A specific plan for follow-up appointments or phone contact as necessary should be made clear to patients and documented in the medical record. The primary provider can often be the source and coordinator of referrals for second opinions and specialty consultations. Encouraging patients to maintain a notebook of who, what, when, and where of referrals can enhance and inform the communication process.

SUMMARY

Mr. G, the patient who we introduced at the beginning of the chapter, returns with his daughter for a follow-up exam. In preparation for this visit you have him meet with the social worker who performs a functional evaluation and reviews safety issues. During your medical encounter you ask Mr. G what his main concerns are to which he answers how lonely and isolated he has felt since the death of his wife. You note that Mr. G has lost weight, suffers from insomnia, and has trouble concentrating. Your assessment includes a follow-up neurological exam with emphasis on the mental status exam and signs and symptoms of depression. At the meeting's conclusion you direct your comments to both Mr. G and his daughter and discuss your diagnosis of depression and develop a plan, which includes the social worker's input on what support services are needed at home; a list of senior centers and agencies in the community for Mr. G and his daughter to visit and seek information from; a prescription for an antidepressant medication, reviewing benefits and side effects; and scheduled follow-up appointments. For Mr. G, future encounters will be important in assessing effectiveness of intervention, monitoring symptom progression, and further developing the patient-provider partnership.

Communication is a major tool that providers can employ in dealing with the complexities and challenges of the health care system in general and of geriatric care specifically. Though it is beyond the scope of this chapter to address the vast literature on patient-provider relationship models and communication styles, we encourage the reader to review medical, nursing, and allied health literature for further study. In addressing the unique issues in patient-provider communication when working with older populations, it is our hope that patient care will be enhanced and that this would result in greater satisfaction for both the patient and provider.

REFERENCES

Blazer, D. G., & Cassel, C. K. (1994). Depression in the elderly. *Hospital Practice, 29*, 37–44.

Butler, R. N., & Lewis, M. I. (1993). *Love and sex after 60*. New York: Ballantine Books.

Fantl, J. A., Newman, D. K., Colling, J., DeLancey, J., Keeys, C., Loughery, R., McDowell, B. J., Norton, P., Ouslander, J., Schnelle, J., Staskin, D., Tries, J., Urich, V., Vitousek, S. H., Weiss, D., & Whitmore, K. (1996). *Urinary incontinence in adults: Acute and chronic management: Clinical practice guideline, No. 2 Update.* (AHCPR Publication No. 96-0682). Rockville, MD: U.S. Department of Health and Human Services.

Fulmer, T., & Birkenhauer, D. (1992). Elder mistreatment assessment as a part of everyday practice. *Journal of Gerontological Nursing, 18*, 42–45.

Gallo, J. J., Reichel, W., & Anderson, L. M. (1995). *Handbook of geriatric assessment.* Gaithersburg, MD: Aspen Publishers, Inc.

Gastel, B. (1994). *Working with your older patient: A clinician's handbook.* Bethesda, MD: National Institutes of Health.

Greene, M. G., & Adelman, R. D. (1996). Psychosocial factors in older patients' medical encounters. *Research on Aging, 18*, 84–102.

Karp, F. (Ed.). (1994). *Talking with your doctor: A guide for older people.* Bethesda, MD: National Institutes of Health.

Lazare, A., Putnam, S. M., & Lipkin, M. (1995). Three functions of the medical interview. In M. Lipkin, S. M. Putnam, & A. Lazare (Eds.), *The medical interview: Clinical care, education and research* (pp. 3–19). New York: Springer-Verlag.

Martin, L. M., Fleming, K. C., & Evans, J. M. (1995). Recognition and management of anxiety and depression in elderly patients. *Mayo Clinic Proceedings, 70*, 999–1006.

Quill, T. E. (1989). Recognizing and adjusting to barriers in doctor-patient communication. *Annals of Internal Medicine, 111,* 51–57.

Reilly, B. M., Magnussen, C. R., Ross, J., Ash, J., Papa, L., & Wagner, M. (1994). Can we talk?: Inpatient discussions about advanced directives in a community hospital. *Archives of Internal Medicine, 154,* 2299–2308.

Resnick, N. M. (1984). Urinary incontinence in the elderly. *Medical Grand Rounds, 3,* 281–290.

Sledge, W. H., & Feinstein, A. R. (1997). A clinimetric approach to the components of the patient-physician relationship. *Journal of the American Medical Association, 278,* 2043–2048.

Small, G. W., Rabins, P. V., Barry, P. P., Buckholtz, N. S., DeKorsky, S. T., Ferris, S. H., Finkel, S. I., Gwyther, L. P., Khachaturian, Z. S., Lebowitz, B. D., McRae, T. D., Morris, J. C., Oakley, F., Schneider, L. S., Streim, J. E., Sunderland, T., Teri, L. A., & Tune, L. E. (1997). Diagnosis and treatment of Alzheimer disease and related disorders: Consensus statement of the American Association for Geriatric Psychiatry, the Alzheimer's Association, and the American Geriatric Society. *Journal of the American Medical Association, 278,* 1363–1371.

Waitzkin, H., & Stoeckle, J. (1972). The communication of information about illness: Clinical, sociological, and methodological considerations. *Advances in Psychosomatic Medicine, 8,* 180–215.

CHAPTER 18

Ethical Issues in the Geriatric Patient

Muriel R. Gillick

E thical issues arise near the end of life because of conflict regarding the type and amount of medical care that is appropriate (Gillick, 1994a). Older individuals who have a limited life expectancy and who, in some instances, already suffer from multiple chronic illnesses and extensive disability, are at risk of iatrogenic complications from medical treatment (Gillick, Serrell, & Gillick, 1982). They have less to gain from treatment than their younger counterparts with the same disease because their life expectancy is shorter. In addition, they may be at risk of further functional decline from conventional medical treatment (Fried, Gillick, & Lipsitz, 1997). Usual treatment is thus not necessarily the desired treatment for older people who are frail, have dementia, or are terminally ill. Determining the approach to care that makes most sense is often a major ethical challenge.

WHO DECIDES?

Contemporary Western biomedical ethics—a tradition that is only 30 years old—regards the patient as the central figure in medical decision making. Grounded in the principle of autonomy, or the right to make choices about one's own life, the accepted model of decision-making begins with the physician telling the patient his diagnosis, prognosis, and options for treatment (President's Commission, 1982). Based on an understanding of the pros and cons of the various possible approaches and on the patient's values and preferences, the patient and physician are expected to arrive at a decision about treatment (Emanuel & Emanuel, 1992b). Unfortunately, dementia is a highly prevalent condition in elderly persons, which often prevents their participating in such discussions. Moreover, many cognitively intact older people develop delirium in the setting of acute illness and are also incapable of complex decision making at the time of need. Before proceeding with decision-making, the physician needs to assess whether a patient can make decisions for himself.

ASSESSING DECISION-MAKING CAPACITY

Physicians should not conclude that patients are unable to engage in decision-making process merely because they are ill or have some degree of underlying dementia. A mildly demented individual, for instance, may understand the issues involved in amputation of a gangrenous foot well enough to be able to accept or refuse surgery.

Determinations of *competence* are judicial decisions that involve ruling on the patient's global decision-making ability. Determination of *decision-capacity* is always with reference to a specific medical intervention and can be undertaken by a physician. Psychiatrists are often asked to make this assessment, but all geriatric physicians should be trained to serve this role as well. There is no quantitative test of decision-capacity: neither the Folstein Mini-Mental State nor other tests of cognitive function predict the ability to make medical decisions (Marson, Hawkins, McInturff, & Harrell, 1997). The clinician must be satisfied that the patient meets four criteria: (1) the ability to communicate. It is important to use a translator for a foreign patient, a communications board for an aphasic patient, or to write out questions for a deaf patient; (2) The ability to understand the proposed treatment. Typically, physicians ask that the patient repeat in his or her own words what is being discussed; (3) The ability to grasp the consequences of proceeding with treatment or of declining treatment; and (4) The ability to manipulate information rationally. Patients may start with different assumptions from their physicians— for example, the Jehovah's witness who believes he will forgo everlasting salvation if he receives a blood transfusion—the question is not whether the physician shares their premises but whether the patient's conclusions follow logically from his assumptions (Appelbaum & Grisso, 1988).

DEPRESSION

In general, patients who are decision-capable should be involved in discussions regarding their care. One mitigating circumstance is depression. Patients who are severely depressed may have the cognitive ability to make decisions, but their preferences are affected by their mood disorder. Overriding the wishes of a seemingly decision-capable patient should not be undertaken lightly. If a patient's depression is thought to lead to his or her making choices that are different from those that would be made in other circumstances, psychiatric consultation is warranted. Ideally, decisions about medical care should be delayed until depression has been adequately treated. Sometimes this is not possible, and surrogate decision making is required.

CULTURAL FACTORS

In some cultures, patients do not routinely participate in medical decision making. In those cases, it is usually the family that serves as the surrogate decision maker, even if the patient is capable of discussing his or her wishes. A study of the effect of ethnicity on attitudes toward decision making, conducted in elderly outpatients, found that only 28% of Korean Americans, compared with 65% of White Americans felt patients should make decisions about life-supporting technology (Blackhall, Murphy, Frank, Michel, & Azen, 1995). The conflict between these cultural norms and the American bioethical paradigm creates a challenge for physicians. One possible solution is for physicians to ask patients, particularly those from ethnic groups that tend to favor family decision-making, whether they wish to be involved in discussions about their care.

SURROGATE DECISION MAKING

If a patient is found incapable of participating in health care decisions, or if he or she cedes the right to make decisions to others, a surrogate decision maker must be identified. While next of kin are the presumed surrogate decision makers, it is preferable for patients, while lucid, to explicitly designate a surrogate to speak on their behalf if they are not able to (Annas, 1991). Formal appointment of a substitute decision maker (known as either a health care proxy or a durable power of attorney for health care) is recognized in all 50 states. In addition, some states have passed legislation determining which family member is authorized to make health care decisions if the patient has not selected a proxy (Menikoff, Sachs, & Siegler, 1992).

Whether the surrogate is the next of kin or a formally designated proxy, the usual expectation is that he or she will make health care decisions using *substituted judgment*. This involves making a decision either based on the previously stated wishes of the patient or by inference from their attitudes toward physicians, medical procedures, and health as well as their religious and other values. When the surrogate is unable to determine how best to proceed based on substituted judgment, he or she is typically expected to assess the *best interests* of the patient and decide based on what most people in that condition would choose (Emanuel & Emanuel, 1992a).

If an acutely ill patient is incapable of making health care decisions and has neither a formal nor an informal surrogate, then the physician may need to go to court to seek appointment of a temporary guardian (*guardian ad litem*). The legal route is necessary if the patient is a candidate for any procedure requiring informed consent (e.g., a surgical operation, dialysis, or other invasive treatment or diagnostic test). Rarely, the courts will need to be involved if the patient has not selected a health care proxy and the next of kin cannot agree on an approach to medical care. In such situations, mediation by the physician, the health care team, an external facilitator such as a social worker or psychiatrist, or the institutional ethics committee should precede legal involvement. Even more rarely, the physician or hospital will challenge the legitimacy of the surrogate appointed by the patient. Only if the proxy is clearly acting in his own self-interest rather than that of the patient or is actively mentally ill is a court likely to invalidate a properly executed health care proxy (Lynn, 1988).

ADVANCE MEDICAL PLANNING

In addition to appointing a health care proxy, most ethicists advise that patients in general and geriatric patients in particular engage in some form of advance medical planning. Thinking about and prioritizing general goals for care—prolongation of life, maintaining function, and maximizing comfort, for example—in advance of any particular acute illness can help patients think about specific health care decisions when they arise (Gillick, 1995). Writing down their preferences for care can help guide their health care proxy and is very useful for the primary care physician.

The most widely used written advance directive is the *living will.* Living wills are general statements of the form that patients would not wish heroic measures undertaken in the event that they are terminally ill with no chance of recovery. Some living wills list specific interventions such as cardiopulmonary resuscitation or feeding tubes that the patient might want or not want at the end of life, but most are quite vague and apply only to the dying patient (Bok, 1976).

The *medical directive* is an example of an instructional directive, a document that specifies in far greater detail which interventions the patient would accept in particular circumstances (Emanuel & Emanuel, 1989). The medical directive asks patients to consider four possible clinical situations: irreversible coma, possibly reversible coma but with a very low probability of full recovery, severe cognitive impairment, and severe cognitive impairment plus terminal illness. For each of these predicaments, the patient is asked to consider the following interventions that might be medically indicated: cardiopulmonary resuscitation, a respirator, dialysis, chemotherapy, major surgery, artificial nutrition, minor surgery, intravenous fluids, antibiotics, simple tests, and medication for pain control even if it shortened life. In each case, the potential patients check off whether they would want the intervention, would not want the intervention, would want a limited trial of the intervention, or is uncertain. Despite the seeming comprehensiveness of the medical directive, it does not address many of the kinds of decisions frail elderly patients have to make, such as whether to be treated at home or in the hospital, in the intensive care unit or in a conventional hospital unit. This kind of directive may also give the illusion of precision because of the number of scenarios it presents, whereas in fact patients cannot make such choices without clarifying what goals the interventions aim to achieve (Brett, 1991).

Another type of advance medical planning is the *values history* (Lambert, Gibson, & Nathanson, 1990). This involves patients completing a questionnaire intended to elucidate which aspects of life are most important to them. For example, the future patient is asked which is preferable, dying at home or in the hospital, as well as questions about religious preferences and attitudes toward pain and suffering. Answering the questions may be a useful way for individuals to be encouraged to think about difficult and important issues regarding care at the end of life. The utility of the values history in guiding clinical care has not been established.

DECISIONS TO LIMIT CARE

Advance planning medical planning is designed to facilitate decision making in the acute situation if the patient is unable to participate in such discussions, either because of underlying dementia or temporary incapacity. If the patient has indicated preferences about care prior to the development of a medical problem, those preferences should be respected. If there is a surrogate, the surrogate should be told about the prior statements. A surrogate may, of course, make a different decision from the one agreed on in the past, just as a patient is entitled to change his or her own mind. However, surrogates should take very seriously the preferences the patient expressed when lucid.

When advance planning has not taken place, or previous discussions are not applicable to the acute situation facing a decision-incapable patient, surrogates are often asked to participate in decisions to authorize or to limit treatment. In deciding to accept or reject a proposed medical treatment, the surrogate needs to consider the *benefits* and *burdens* of the treatment. This formulation is the basis of secular biomedical thinking (President's Commission, 1983). It is also consistent with much of religious medical ethical thinking, as exemplified by the Catholic Church, which has argued that a person has a moral obligation to use ordinary or proportionate means of preserving his or her life. Proportionate means are those that in the judgment of the patient offer a reasonable hope of benefit and do not entail an excessive burden or impose excessive expense on the family or the community (National Conference of Catholic Bishops, 1995). Burdens should be understood to include short-term pain and suffering from the treatment as well as long-term impairment of function that may arise from the treatment. Benefits should be taken to include both the prolongation of life and salutary effects on function or generalized well being.

Patients, and by extension, their surrogates, have a right to refuse medical treatments. This principle has been tested in numerous court cases involving the refusal of cardiopulmonary resuscitation, ventilators, antibiotics, amputation, dialysis, chemotherapy, and artificial nutrition (Weir & Gostin, 1990). Some states limit the kinds of treatment over which a surrogate has jurisdiction (in California, for example, surrogates cannot authorize electric shock treatments) and some states only allow certain treatments to be limited if the patient left explicit directives to do so (in New York and Missouri, for example, artificial nutrition and hydration may not be withheld unless there is clear and convincing evidence of the patient's wishes). In the Cruzan case, one of the few right to die cases to come before the United States Supreme Court, however, the court held that all types of medical treatment are ethically and legally equivalent (Weir & Gostin, 1990).

Sometimes health care personnel are reluctant to withdraw treatment once it has been initiated, though they would have considered failing to institute the treatment in the first place. Most philosophers do not distinguish between withdrawing and withholding treatment (Brock, 1989). In both cases, the goal is to avoid a burdensome or ineffective treatment. The basis of a limited trial of therapy, for example, is to attempt treatment, but with the understanding that the treatment can be discontinued if it proves ineffective. If withdrawing treatment were not permissible, then more patients might opt to withhold treatment initially so as to avoid being faced with enduring unwanted therapy indefinitely.

FUTILITY

Physicians sometimes argue that there are instances in which medical care is simply futile, and no discussion with the patient or surrogate is necessary. Physicians are under no obligation to provide ineffective treatment, such as laetrile for cancer or antibiotics for a viral upper respiratory infection. However, they must be careful that they are not calling treatment futile that merely has a low likelihood of success or that can prolong life but cannot restore a patient to normal function. Ventilator support for an irreversibly comatose patient or artificial nutrition and hydration for a patient in a persistent vegetative state cannot be expected to restore those individuals to health, but are perfectly consistent with the goal of prolongation of life. Ethicists continue to struggle to define *futility*, with some believing that a treatment is futile if it is physiologically incapable of achieving the state goal (Truog, Brett, & Frader, 1992), and others arguing that treatment is futile if it is statistically unlikely to achieve the desired goal (Schneiderman, Jecker, & Jonsen, 1990). Physicians need to clarify with their patients the goals of treatment to determine whether a treatment is consistent with those goals, rather than to refuse treatment based on an ill-defined criterion of futility.

PHYSICIAN-ASSISTED SUICIDE

A small number of patients near the end of their lives find their existence so unbearable that they wish to go beyond withholding or withdrawing treatment and request assistance in dying. Public opinion surveys have found that many more people wish to have the option of physician-assisted suicide than would actually use such an option if it existed (Blendon, Szalay, & Knox, 1992). The major argument in favor of physician-assisted suicide is that it would enable patients to have greater control over their last days of life, assuaging their fear that death will be undignified and painful (Cassel & Meier, 1990).

Legalization of physician-assisted suicide (PAS) rai
cerns (Foley, 1997). One concern is that since more t
Americans have no health insurance, physician-assiste
be used as a substitute for prohibitively expensive
unable to pay for their medical care. A second fear is
assisted suicide would quickly be expanded to euthanasia as has
occurred in the Netherlands (Van der Maas et al., 1996). Despite
legislative safeguards restricting PAS to those who are able to make
decisions for themselves, it seems unlikely that those who are demented or delirious could be deprived of the right to have their
lives ended if that right is afforded to those who are decision-capable.
Finally, many ethicists have expressed concern that those who are
poor or dependent might seek PAS simply so as not to be a burden
to their families. PAS could become a means for a country with a
rapidly growing number of frail elderly persons to decrease the cost
of caring for its most vulnerable citizens.

The issue of the constitutionality of laws banning PAS has gone
before the United States Supreme Court. In a decision handed down
in June 1997, the justices held that there is no constitutional right
to physician-assisted suicide. The justices also found that there is no
constitutional requirement that PAS be prohibited. Individual states,
in their view, have the right to pass legislation either authorizing or
banning PAS (Burt, 1997). To date, only Oregon has passed a law
legalizing PAS (Alpers & Lo, 1995). After testing in the courts and
subjection to two public referenda, the law went into effect in 1998.
It provides for a decision-capable individual to request a prescription
from a physician for purposes of committing suicide. Safeguards
against abuse include a requirement for psychiatric assessment of
the patient and a 2-week waiting period before the prescription is
granted. Other states are actively considering PAS legislation.

Whether PAS becomes legal in other parts of the United States,
the major focus of physicians caring for patients near the end of
life should be their comfort (Field & Cassel, 1997). Aggressive control
of symptoms often associated with dying, such as pain, dyspnea, and
nausea, is critical. Anxiety and depression are other major issues
near the end of life and should be dealt with both medically and
nonpharmacologically with the help of social workers, psychiatrists,
or pastoral counselors.

RATIONING HEALTH CARE

Decisions about how much and what kind of care are appropriate for elderly individuals influence public policy as well as bed-side care. Given that 30% of all Medicare payments go to care during the last year of life, 50% of which is spent on the last 60 days of life (Lubitz & Riley, 1993), many have argued that care of elderly persons should be rationed. A lively debate has centered on the question of whether rationing should be on the basis of age alone (Callahan, 1987), whether rationing should be on the basis of functional status (Thomasma, 1993), or whether rationing should be avoided. Cost-savings through elimination of administrative waste and through rationalization of medical therapy have been advocated as an alternative to rationing (Eddy, 1994).

Ethical and economic incentives may coincide if physicians and patients actively participate in advance medical planning before illness strikes and consider limiting care when acute illness occurs. While studies to date have been unable to demonstrate that offering patients advance directives saves money (Schneiderman, Kronick, Kaplan, Anderson, & Langer, 1992), patients in these studies typically contemplated limitations of care only in the final days of an intensive care unit stay, shortly before death. Earlier and more comprehensive planning holds the promise of reducing costs while at the same time sparing frail elderly patients invasive treatments that are unlikely to prolong their lives and almost certain to impair their functioning (Gillick, 1994b).

OTHER ETHICAL ISSUES IN THE GERIATRIC PATIENT

Another ethical challenge in the geriatric population relates not to medical decision making but to the difficulties of enhancing autonomy in older individuals. Everyday ethics deals with a variety of types of decisions in people whose autonomy is limited by dementia or whose ability to exercise their autonomy is limited by physical impairments (Kane & Caplan, 1990). Individuals living in nursing homes are at high risk of being denied the opportunity to make choices about such issues as when they get up, what they eat, and where they sit in the dining room. These concerns turn out to be more important to quality of life than the medical decisions that are at the forefront of ethical discussions (Kane et al., 1997). Moreover, the liberal view of autonomy as grounded exclusively in the individual breaks down in the institutional setting (Agich, 1993). Ethical approaches that look at the individual as a member of a community (whether the nursing home, assisted living facility, or elderly housing complex) and as a member of a family are necessary to enhance freedom in the dependent elderly individual (McCullough & Wilson, 1995).

In conclusion, the same issues of informed consent, participation in medical decisions, and maximization of autonomy arise in caring for older patients as in a younger population. Ethical dilemmas arise with greater frequency because older people often differ in their goals of care, are at greater risk of complications, and frequently suffer from cognitive impairment. Cognitive deficits often impede the older person's ability to be involved in medical decision making, leading to increased reliance on advance directives and health care proxies. Cognitive deficits also challenge the ability of caregivers to promote autonomy in daily life. Physicians caring for geriatric patients must therefore be sensitive to and knowledgeable about ethical issues.

REFERENCES

Agich, G. J. (1993). *Autonomy and long-term care.* New York: Oxford University Press.

Alpers, A., & Lo, B. (1995). Physician-assisted suicide in Oregon: A bold experiment. *Journal of the American Medical Association, 274,* 483–487.

Annas, G. J. (1991). The health care proxy and the living will. *New England Journal of Medicine, 324,* 1210–1213.

Appelbaum, P. S., & Grisso, T. (1988). Assessing patients' capacities to consent to treatment. *New England Journal of Medicine, 319,* 1635–1638.

Blackhall, L., Murphy, S., Frank, G., Michel, V., & Azen, S. (1995). Ethnicity and attitudes toward patient autonomy. *Journal of the American Medical Association, 27,* 820–825.

Blendon, R. J., Szalay, U. S., & Knox, R. A. (1992). Should physicians aid their patients in dying?: The public's perspective. *Journal of the American Medical Association, 267,* 2658–2662.

Bok, S. (1976). Personal directions for care at the end of life. *New England Journal of Medicine, 295,* 367–369.

Brett, A. S. (1991). Limitation of listing specific medical intervention in advance directives. *Journal of the American Medical Association, 266,* 825–828.

Brock, D. (1989). Death and dying. In R. Veatch (Ed.), *Medical ethics* (pp. 329–336). Boston: Jones and Barlett.

Burt, R. A. (1997). The supreme court speaks: Not assisted Suicide but a constitutional right to palliative care. *New England Journal of Medicine, 337,* 1234–1236.

Callahan, D. (1987). *Setting limits: Medical goals in an aging society.* New York: Simon and Schuster.

Cassel, C. K., & Meier, D. E. (1990). Morals and moralism in the debate over assisted suicide. *New England Journal of Medicine, 323,* 750–752.

Eddy, D. M. (1994). Rationing resources while improving quality: How to get more for less. *Journal of the American Medical Association, 272,* 817–824.

Emanuel, L. L., & Emanuel, E. J. (1989). The medical directive: A New comprehensive advance care document. *Journal of the American Medical Association, 261,* 3288–3293.

Emanuel, E. J., & Emanuel, L. L. (1992a). Proxy decision making For incompetent patients: An ethical and empirical analysis. *Journal of the American Medical Association, 267,* 2067–2071.

Emanuel, E. J., & Emanuel, L. L. (1992b). Four models of the physician-patient relationship. *Journal of the American Medical Association, 267,* 2221–2226.

Field, M. J., & Cassel, C. K. (1997). *Approaching death: Improving care at the end of life.* Washington, DC: National Academy Press.

Foley, K. M. (1997). Competent care for the dying instead of physician-assisted suicide. *New England Journal of Medicine, 336,* 54–58.

Fried, T., Gillick, M., & Lipsitz, L. (1997). Short-term functional outcomes of long-term care residents with pneumonia treated with and without hospital transfer. *Journal of the American Geriatrics Society, 45,* 302–306.

Gillick, M. (1994a). *Choosing medical care in old age: What kind, how much, when to stop.* Cambridge, MA: Harvard University Press.

Gillick, M. (1994b). The high costs of dying: A way out. *Archives of Internal Medicine, 154,* 2134–2137.

Gillick, M. (1995). A broader role for advance medical planning. *Annals Internal Medicine, 123,* 621–624.

Gillick, M., Serrell, N., & Gillick, L. (1982). Adverse consequences of hospitalization in the elderly. *Social Science and Medicine, 16,* 1033–1038.

Kane, R. A., & Caplan, A. L. (1990). *Ethical issues in the everyday life of nursing home residents.* New York: Springer.

Kane, R. A., Caplan, A. L., Urv-Wong, E. K., Freeman, I. C., Aroskar, M. A., & Finch, M. (1997). Everyday matters in the lives of nursing home residents: Wish for and perception of choice and control. *Journal of the American Geriatrics Society, 45,* 1086–1093.

Lambert, P., Gibson, J., & Nathanson, P. (1990). The values history: An innovation in surrogate medical decision-making. *Law, Medicine, and Health Care, 18,* 202–212.

Lubitz, J. D., & Riley, G. F. (1993). Trends in medicare payments In the last Year of life. *New England Journal of Medicine, 328,* 1092–1096.

Lynn, J. (1988). Conflicts of interest in medical decision-making. *Journal of the American Geriatrics Society, 36,* 945–950.

Marson, D. C., Hawkins, L., McInturff, B., & Harrell, L. E. (1997). Cognitive models that predict physician judgments of capacity to consent in mild Alzheimer's Disease. *Journal of the American Geriatrics Society, 45,* 458–464.

McCullough, L. B., & Wilson, N. L. (1995). *Long-term care decisions: Ethical and conceptual dimensions.* Baltimore: Johns Hopkins University Press.

Menikoff, J. A., Sachs, G. A., & Siegler, M. (1992). Beyond advance directives: Health care surrogate laws. *New England Journal of Medicine, 322,* 1165–1169.

National Conference of Catholic Bishops (1995). *Ethical and religious directives for Catholic health care services.* Washington, DC: U.S. Catholic Conference.

President's Commission for the Study of Ethical Problems in Medicine and Biomedical and Behavioral Research (1982). *Making health care decisions: The legal and ethical implications of informed consent in the patient-practitioner relationship.* Washington, DC: U.S. Government Printing Office.

President's Commission for the Study of Ethical Problems in Medicine and Biomedical and Behavioral Research (1983). *Deciding to forego life-sustaining treatment.* Washington, DC: U.S. Government Printing Office.

Schneiderman, L. J., Jecker, N. S., & Jonsen, A. R. (1990). Medical futility: Its meaning and ethical implications. *Annals of Internal Medicine, 112,* 949–954.

Schneiderman, L. J., Kronick, R., Kaplan, R. M., Anderson, J. P., & Langer, R. D. (1992). Effects of offering advance directives on medical treatments and costs. *Annals of Internal Medicine, 117,* 599–606.

Thomasma, D. (1993). Functional status care categories and national health policy. *Journal of the American Geriatrics Society, 41,* 437–443.

Truog, R. D., Brett, A. S., & Frader, J. (1992). The problem with futility. *New England Journal of Medicine, 326,* 1560–1564.

van der Maas, P., van der Wal, G., Haverkate, I., de Graaff, C. L., Kester, J. G., Onwuteaka-Philipsen, B. D., van der Heide, A., Bosma, J. M., & Willems, D. L. (1996). Euthanasia, physician-assisted suicide, and other medical practices involving the end of life in the Netherlands, 1990–1995. *New England Journal of Medicine, 335,* 1699–1705.

Weir, R. F., & Gostin, L. (1990). Decisions to abate life-sustaining treatment for non-autonomous patients. *Journal of the American Medical Association, 264,* 1846–1853.

CHAPTER 19

Community-based and Educational Services

Carolyn L. Bottum and Alan L. Balsam

For older persons and their families, the most important providers of elder services are likely to be community-based. Community-based agencies provide a vast array of direct services to individuals, usually with the goal of enabling elders to remain independently in their homes for as long as possible. These agencies may include councils on aging, area agencies on aging, informal social clubs, senior centers, multiservice centers, home care corporations, home health agencies, and social day care centers, among many others. Though in many ways the operation of community-based agencies reflect the fragmentation and lack of resources of the elder services system as a whole, agencies with adequate staff, understanding of the needs of their clients and available local resources, and an innovative approach to service design and delivery can bring together services into integrated care plans and effectively meet a continuum of needs.

The term senior center, with its image of card tables of suburban retirees playing bridge and bingo, belies the breadth and sophistication of services provided by community-based agencies. In fact, in

1990, older adults received over a billion dollars worth of services from such agencies funded by the Administration on Aging alone (O'Shaugnessy, 1990). This network of aging services has almost 30 years of experience serving older adults and is acutely aware of their special emotional and physical needs as well as of the most effective means to reach and care for them.

MISSION AND FUNDING

In 1965, as part of the program for Lyndon Johnson's "Great Society," Congress passed The Older Americans Act, creating the Administration on Aging and funding demonstration senior center programs. Among the goals of the Older Americans Act, as amended in 1988, is assisting older people to "secure equal opportunity to the full and free enjoyment of . . . the best possible physical and mental health which science can make available and without regard to economic status . . . " (The Older Americans Act, 1988). This and other goals have been pursued by funding an array of services that are the backbone of the aging services network. Not only do these services reduce institutionalization costs, but they also enhance the physical and mental well being of the older adults.

Funding is provided through the Administration on Aging to the 57 state and territorial units on aging (National Association of Area Agencies on Aging, undated) on a formula basis that targets services to those in "greatest economic" and "greatest social" need, especially low-income, minority older adults. These agencies of state government are mandated by the Older Americans Act to oversee all aging services in their state or territory. The state agencies coordinate services, create plans, provide technical assistance to agencies providing services, and serve as an advocate for older adults in the state (The Older Americans Act, 1988).

Funding is provided to the state agencies on aging by the Administration on Aging through various titles of the Older Americans Act. These titles fund different services, including nutrition, supportive services like transportation, in-home services, preventive health services, employment programs, research, and ombudsman programs. Of particular interest is Title III-B, which provides money for the establishment and maintenance of senior centers, through which elders may receive transportation, health education, health screenings, fitness programs, recreation, counseling, information and referral services, housing assistance and home repair, chore services, shopping services, legal assistance, elder abuse prevention programs, and other services (The Older Americans Act, 1988).

As part of their function, the state units on aging designate area agencies on aging. For very small states, the state unit on aging may be the area agency on aging. In general, however, the state unit on aging divides the state into regions and names a nonprofit organization, a municipal or county government agency, a regional planning and development commission, or other organization, to be the area agency on aging for that region.

The nation's 670 area agencies on aging develop plans for and administer funding for nutritional, home care, and other supportive services and the establishment of senior centers, among other activities (National Association of Area Agencies on Aging, undated).

Some area agencies on aging provide services directly at the community level, while others, especially those in large urban areas, further subcontract with councils on aging or senior centers to provide nutritional, health, and other services. In other cases area agencies on aging may administer these programs but hold them in community-based sites.

For virtually all services, federal funds are joined with state and local funding and private contributions. At a minimum, state units on aging must provide 15% of the funds for their programs (The Older Americans Act, 1988). However, in reality, particularly as the amount of federal funds available has dropped, state and local governments provide substantially more funds for services. Private nonprofit organizations also support senior services, either by contributing to agencies that serve elders, or by establishing their own services. Finally, while no senior is required to contribute to the services they receive, all elders are encouraged to make a small donation.

A more important source of support for community-based agencies is volunteers. Volunteers deliver meals to homebound clients, prepare and serve congregate meals, conduct friendly visits, drive seniors to medical appointments, make telephone reassurance calls, work in the office of the agencies, organize activities and events, lead social trips, assist in bill paying and health benefits counseling, and many, many other functions. A very small agency may have 50 volunteers while larger agencies must recruit, supervise, and maintain literally hundreds.

This reliance on volunteer support is the cause of some concern among managers of community-based agencies because many volunteers are in their seventies or eighties and will soon be in need of volunteered services themselves. Younger seniors in their sixties are more likely to be employed full or part-time and take part in more self-fulfilling activities that leave little time for volunteer commitments. Many of the homemakers who were also a large part of the volunteer corps in the past are now working and unavailable. A significant challenge to today's community-based agency is redesigning volunteer jobs and recruitment methods to ensure that enough volunteers serve to enable community-based agencies to operate.

THE SERVICES OF COMMUNITY-BASED AGENCIES

For an adult turning 60 today, "retirement" frequently lasts 20 or more years (Rogers, Rogers, & Belanger, 1990). Community-based agencies are charged with providing services needed for the widely divergent populations ranging from active, healthy adults who are, in reality, in late middle age, to the oldest-old, who require extensive services to remain precariously in their homes. Those who assess needs, plan programs, and deliver services in community-based agencies usually have years of experience and a strong commitment to their population rather than formal advanced degrees in gerontology (Prohaska & Wallace, 1996).

Perhaps the most important commonality of all community-based agencies is their diversity. A senior center in one town can be radically different in resources, target population, and services from a center in a virtually identical town a few miles away. Local history, attitudes of the municipality's officials and population towards the aging, other demands on resources, personalities and experience of individual agency directors, and many other factors all contribute to the wide-ranging nature of community-based agencies. Some of the elements that result in similarities include federal and state-funded programs and services, national or regional demographic trends, and strong leadership by state agencies on aging or elder services professional organizations, among others.

As diverse as the structure and services of community-based agencies are the professionals who administer them. Some agencies are operated by those with advanced degrees in gerontology (Prohaska & Wallace, 1996). More often, directors have social work or, sometimes, nursing degrees. For a significant portion, however, experience has provided the foundation of their qualifications. Those who began many community-based agencies were truly pioneers, forging a service system for a population that few had tried to serve. As this original generation of directors and founders retires, a new wave of administrators who have benefitted from the emerging educational opportunities in and professionalization of gerontology is changing the face of the community-based elder service agency, increasing the range and number of services and reaching out to new elder populations. While few agencies will be able to provide all of the services below, and some provide other services, what follows is a summary of common services available for community-living elders and their families.

Services for Family Caregivers

For many consumers of elder services, their first contact with a community-based elder services agency comes when they seek services for aging parents. Currently, it is estimated that 80% of long-term care outside of nursing homes is provided by family members (Binstock, 1996). In some cases, these people, usually in their forties or fifties, are seeking services for both parents and grandparents simultaneously. Even when an elder calls for assistance, the community-based agency must usually consult with and counsel the elder's spouse, children, and grandchildren as formal and informal services are coordinated into comprehensive care plans, and children or grandchildren express concerns about finances, the ability of the elder to remain independent, and how the elder's needs affect the family as a whole. Family dynamics can be the most difficult part of coordinating and monitoring services, especially when the elder's situation is used as a means to play out long-standing dysfunctional relationships and resentments. Most family caregivers provide care without compensation, but in some states these caregivers, or others in the community who take elders into their homes and offer the same support as family caregivers, can receive a stipend through foster care programs.

As the importance of family caregivers as a resource has become better understood, services have been put into place to enable caregivers to continue in their physically, mentally, and emotionally demanding roles. The most directly beneficial to caregivers is respite care. Respite care is care provided in the home or in a facility that allows the caregiver a few hours or days away from their caregiving responsibilities so that they may take care of their own medical or emotional needs, shop, care for other members of the family, or go on a vacation. Respite care can be provided by volunteers, paid but untrained companions, or professionals and be administered by virtually any of the types of community-based agencies mentioned above. Respite care services are usually paid for by the caregiver but are sometimes subsidized by public funding.

Services for "Young" Elders

Upon reaching age 60, older adults are suddenly eligible for a wide range of services provided by community-based agencies. The minimum age for eligibility for most federally funded programs, including nutrition and home care, is 60, and many community-based agencies have adopted the same minimum age requirement. For a large portion of this population services are not needed or wanted. Many will continue to work, remain healthy, and have strong social networks for many years to come. In general this group does not seek community-based services (Sabin, 1993).

While some agencies target the most needy among the elderly population, who tend to be older and frailer than the "young-old," others actively seek this young-old population because of their political influence and affluence and because of declining attendance at activities designed for older seniors. Community-based agencies that focus on self-development and social activities attract the younger seniors (Sabin, 1993). Activities initiated to meet the needs of this population may include vigorous fitness classes, massage therapy and other complementary therapies, personal training on fitness equipment, and investment clubs and seminars. These are provided free or for a small program fee.

Many senior centers, especially in suburban and rural areas, offer trips as a way for younger elders to be introduced to elder services and to provide opportunities for elders to increase their socialization and meet new people. These trips, which are sometimes subsidized by municipal or other funding, go to restaurants, theaters, concerts, museums, historic sites, casinos, and shopping malls. While these trips may seem unrelated to the more basic mission of community-based agencies of serving the most needy elders, they can be almost literally life saving when they serve to build social networks of elders who may have recently lost a spouse or are severely socially isolated.

Services for Independent Community-Living Elders

Most services for independent community-living elders in their "middle elderly years"—70 and above—assume deficits in physical, mental, and social abilities and financial status and attempt to assist the elder in managing or overcoming the deficit. Among the most universal of these programs is the nutrition program. Each weekday, elders in almost every community gather at senior centers or other sites for hot lunches, and, less frequently, breakfast and dinner. In 1993 about 127 million meals were served at congregate meal sites (Administration on Aging, 1994). Not only nutritionally beneficial, these meals also give older adults a chance to socialize and attend educational and recreational programs.

Included as an integral part of the congregate meals program is nutrition education, mandated by The Older Americans Act (The Older Americans Act, 1988). Education may include printed materials distributed at meal sites or handed to home-delivered meals clients by meal deliverers or presentations by nutritionists.

Increasingly, community-based agencies are taking on the role of a health center complementary to the senior's regular medical care. Many agencies offer clinic services, usually including blood pressure screening, influenza immunization, podiatric, and other services. Health education programs on a variety of topics, including chronic disease management, prevention of illness, treatment alternatives, stress reduction, and mental wellness enhance elders' ability to manage their well being. In many communities these services are offered by the local health department in conjunction with the elder service agency or are administered by the health department at the elder service agency site. These are usually offered free or for a small program fee. Most social service agencies such as senior centers are not Medicare-certified and so cannot be reimbursed by Medicare for health services. The Older Americans Act funds a portion of these that are in priority areas that include health screening, education, counseling, information and referral, and nutritional and health risk assessment, among others (The Older Americans Act, 1988).

Increasingly state health agencies are beginning to focus on health services for older adults (Balsam & Bottum, 1996). In general, state health departments orchestrate health education campaigns or clinic-style health services and screenings through community-based agencies. Frequently the impetus for these programs comes from the federal Centers for Disease Control, which have initiated grant programs to address such conditions as breast and prostate cancer, diabetes, and incontinence, which are overwhelmingly more prevalent among elderly persons. These programs may include both public and professional education and screenings.

Muddying the health programming waters in those areas of the country experiencing the most penetration of managed care is the entrance of Medicare-based HMO plans for elders. Through these plans Medicare pays private HMOs or other insurers to provide coverage to Medicare beneficiaries. Frequently these plans market themselves by providing health-related programs, including health promotion classes or seminars and fitness programs. In some cases these are presented at community-based agencies and in others they duplicate programs already provided by community-based agencies. Hospitals, also seeking to increase their older patient population or because of a commitment to community-based health, also offer health seminars and screenings focused on the needs of older adults.

Fitness has long been understood to be essential to maintaining health and independence. Thus, exercise programs are among the oldest services offered to seniors at community-based agencies, free or for a small fee. These classes range from less strenuous aerobics classes to strengthening classes using weights, based on recent research showing that weight exercises can significantly increase mobility, to Tai Chi, an Asian form of martial arts adapted to be a gentle form of exercise popular in senior centers nationwide. Many states and communities participate in Senior Olympics, with events especially for older adults. One concern about many of the fitness programs offered in community-based agencies is that they are taught by those who are trained to teach younger people and who may not understand the special needs of the aging body, thus exposing the elder participants to injury.

Mental wellness is an essential component of maintaining physical and mental well being (Bruce, Seeman, Merrill, & Blazer, 1994). Social isolation can be especially severe for the very old, who may have lost their family and friends to death and may be immobile and older retired widowers who may never have developed a social network outside of their work and immediate family. Mental wellness programs aim to provide opportunities for socialization as well as offer more direct mental wellness services.

A significant portion of the services of many community-based agencies is termed "recreational." These may include free bingo, bridge, pool, other games, movies, and crafts. While the much-maligned stereotype of senior centers is that of a bingo parlor, these services are one of the few socialization services that elders will accept and participate in. Some community-based agencies design special programs for special populations, including men. Recreational programs for older men may include "fix it shops," golf classes, and woodworking shops.

Older adults are less likely to take part in more traditional mental health services such as group or individual counseling. Many community-based elder service agencies do offer some support groups, usually focusing on bereavement, care giving, or coping with chronic illnesses. These groups are also offered to older adults by community mental health agencies and hospitals.

Recently, community-based agencies have begun to add the spiritual dimension to their services due to the realization that an elder who is spiritually distressed cannot benefit from physical and mental wellness services no matter how well provided. For the most part, this means attempts at coordination with local religious organizations and the introduction of educational and discussion programs at the agencies.

Legal services for low-income elders are funded by The Older Americans Act and are provided to elders free by legal services corporations or other legal services organizations on a community level. Services are provided free to elders who qualify. Housing, guardianship, elder abuse, and other matters that threaten the independence of elders are the highest priority of these programs.

Some community-based services offer their clients money management programs for those who have lost their ability to handle their personal finances. These free or low-cost programs provide bonded professionals or volunteers who work on a one-time or continuing basis to ensure that an elder is not forced from his or her home due solely to a lack of capacity to pay bills or manage income. These services are also provided for higher fees by individual professionals who may have an expertise in accounting or law.

For some elders, their financial problem is not an inability to pay bills, but a lack of retirement income. For those who are physically and mentally capable, full- or part-time work can be essential. Employment services, offering both job training and job matching, are offered through community-based agencies. Federally funded programs that are contracted to community agencies include one that pays an elder to work 20 hours per week in a public or nonprofit agency with the expectation that the elder will either be hired by the agency or receive enough job experience to find work elsewhere and another that offers 2 weeks' salary for an elder to work at a private company as a incentive for the employer to hire the elder. These programs are only for those with very low incomes. Community-based agencies also offer job matching without federal support to those who do not meet income requirements.

More recently services have begun to be initiated to assist elders without deficits in taking the most advantage of the special freedoms that older age can offer. These might include arts and culture classes offered in community-based agencies. Perhaps the most important, however, is the opportunity for elders to partake of the riches of educational institutions. These services may vary from free tuition on a space-available basis to entire programs especially for elders. One example is the Gerontology Institute of the University of Massachusetts. This certificate program enrolls older adults who learn about gerontology and elder services, conduct research on service needs and prepare publications about elder issues and resources, among other activities.

Elderhostel is an important resource that exists on the national level but is organized on a local level for education for elders. This organization sponsors trips that include educational presentations and courses of study at universities during times regular classes are not in session. Besides its educational function, Elderhostel offers tremendous socialization opportunities to those who participate.

Services for Frail Elders

Services for frail elders mirror services for independent elders in that they provide for the physical, mental, and social well being of elders with the aim of maximizing independence for as long as possible. When a frail person is referred to an elder service agency, ideally a package of services or care plan is developed by a case manager or outreach worker, usually a social worker. The elder and the family may choose to arrange and monitor services, or this may be done on a continuing basis by the agency. A new profession of independent consultants, called "geriatric case managers," offers this service privately to those who can pay the $40 to $100 per hour fees.

As for independent elders, nutritional services are key to maintaining independence. Homebound older adults receive hot or cold meals delivered 5 days a week, with weekend meals funded sometimes by private sources also available in some areas. More than 103 million meals were delivered in 1993 (Administration on Aging, 1994). The home deliverer can use the meal delivery as an opportunity to check on the health of the older person, as well as provide some conversation and human contact.

Certified home health agencies, including both those that are private or nonprofit such as visiting nurse associations, home health agencies, and hospitals all provide nursing and other health and medical services such as physical and occupational therapy in the home. These are sometimes covered under Medicare and insurance plans. Local county or municipal health departments may also offer nursing services, especially blood pressure screenings and other monitoring in the agency's offices or in the client's homes.

Nonmedical services are frequently offered by these same agencies. These are rarely covered by Medicare or other insurance providers. The range of these services is staggering, including chore services such as shopping, escorts for those who are able to shop for themselves with assistance, homemakers who clean and cook, personal care assistants who provide bathing and toileting aid, home health aides who offer basic health services, and companions who simply stay with an elder for socialization.

Though homebound, frail elders sometimes have frequent medical appointments. Thus, transportation to medical appointments can be a significant service in areas that do not have public transportation that is accessible to frail elders. Churches and other religious institutions, organizations such as the American Cancer Society, and community-based elder service agencies all provide transportation to medical appointments free or for a small charge through vans or volunteer or stipend drivers.

Mental wellness programs of community-based agencies concentrate less on counseling than on providing social networking in the elder's home. Friendly Visitor programs recruit and train volunteers to visit elders weekly in their homes while telephone reassurance programs offer daily or weekly phone calls from staff or volunteers. These programs, offered by the range of community-based agencies as well as churches and other religious organizations, and services through which a computer calls an elder daily, also ensure that the elder is safe at home. If the elder fails to answer, emergency services are alerted.

Those elders who can no longer remain at home may benefit from social or medical day care programs offered by nonprofit organizations, nursing homes and assisted living facilities, and community-based agencies. Social day care programs offer recreational activities and social services in a supervised setting while medical day care provides both recreational and social and medical services.

Finally, to prevent the physical, emotional, and financial abuse of older adults by professional or family caregivers and others, The Older Americans Act authorized special funds for states to use to educate the public and professionals about elder abuse and how to detect it and to operate programs to receive and refer complaints of elder abuse to law enforcement agencies and other agencies responsible for protecting older adults (The Older Americans Act, 1988). In addition, most states have now enacted laws initiating programs to assist victims and requiring reporting of suspected abuse cases by such professionals as doctors, nurses and social workers.

These programs can be administered by state, county, or local agencies (American Association of Retired Persons, 1987).

Services for Special Populations

The services outlined above are those that are basic and offered in most locations and settings. Different communities have special needs, however, and community-based agencies will inevitably differ based on the needs of the elders served. Elders in urban areas, for example, frequently cite fear of crime as a major concern. Urban agencies, therefore, may, in addition to the programs above, offer victim assistance and crime and violence prevention programs. Services include advocating for aged crime victims, including replacing stolen funds or property; accompanying crime victims through court proceedings; organizing crime watch groups; and offering intensive education about crime and violence prevention.

Urban agencies will also most likely serve a more heterogeneous population and so must be sure that their programs are conducted in the languages of their population and are culturally appropriate. One successful program to make elders from a particular culture feel welcome offered one meal per week from that culture's cuisine at the agency and also organized lunch clubs in which elders brought food from their culture for potlucks in private homes (Balsam & Rogers, 1987).

For rural agencies, transportation may be a significant barrier to providing services (Miner, Logan, & Spitze, 1993). It may not be possible for elders to travel 20 or 30 miles to receive services and so other ways (such as broadcasting educational programs using the mass media) to bring the service to the senior must be found. An additional difficulty for some rural agencies is that the towns they serve are too small to support a full range of services. One solution has been to join several towns into region-based agencies that offer services at branch locations that are coordinated centrally.

Some immigrant and Native American populations find that mainstream community-based agencies cannot meet their elders' needs and offer elder services as part of larger social service, community, or tribal organizations. In many cases these services mirror those offered through elder service agencies and include social and recreational activities, health promotion, counseling and case management, and nutrition. In some cases, these services are offered through the elder service agencies at culturally appropriate sites such as community centers and temples. Mental wellness is a special concern for immigrant elders who, at a time in their lives when they expected to be settled and revered in their own culture, are instead frequently isolated because they do not speak English, depend on younger family members, and suffer the effects of extremely traumatic past experiences.

Finally, gay and lesbian elders may also find that services offered by elder service agencies do not meet the range of their needs. They may find or fear rejection from other seniors attending programs should their sexual preference become known and feel that their life experiences are too different from heterosexual elders to share the social life of the senior center or other agency. Organizations specifically for older gay and lesbian people provide volunteer friendly visiting, counseling and support groups, education, and other services for older gay men and lesbians.

CASE STUDY: BEDFORD, MASSACHUSETTS

No community can be considered typical of those in which community-based elder services are offered. However, some of the dynamics and realities involved in offering elder services on a daily basis in communities can be examined by reviewing the history and current elder services system in one town.

Bedford, Massachusetts is a suburb of Boston with a population of about 12,000. About 3000 residents, or 25% of the population, are aged 60 or over. The per capita income is $24,590, with 3% of the under 65 population having an income of $20,000 or below. The elder population is significantly less wealthy, with 28% of those 65 or over having an income of less than $20,000. Most elders live in their own modest homes, with about 100 residing in elder housing, while about 300 others live in a continuing care community in town.

The focal points of elder services in town are the municipal Council on Aging (COA) and the local area agency on aging, Minuteman Home Care. Many other agencies and organizations, including the Bedford Board of Health and the local churches and synagogues, also provide significant services. This network of services has grown according to need and the capacity of each provider to serve its clientele, with many formal and informal interconnections forged by individuals as well as by various systemic efforts.

Minuteman Home Care was begun in 1975 and has grown to an organization with an annual budget of over 5 million dollars. Their total number of clients in fiscal year 1995 was 16,819. Minuteman Home Care has a home office staff of over 100 who divide their time among 15 towns besides Bedford with additional site coordinators for meals and other services. Among the diversity of services offered by Minuteman Home Care are congregate meals, home-delivered meals, case management and in-home services for income-eligible frail elders, information and referral, money management, nursing home assessment and ombudsmanship, protective services for abused and neglected elders or those who live alone and are at risk for self-neglect, and health benefits counseling, among others.

The Council on Aging was begun in the 1960s with a board that conducted sporadic activities such as an information campaign about the new Medicare program. In 1979, a part-time director began operating from half a desk in town hall. By 1986, the Council on Aging had acquired a senior center, which was two classrooms in an elementary school that had been renovated into a community center. The director was hired full-time, and an assistant was hired part-time. Social and recreational activities, trips, information and referral, medical transportation, individual client counseling, and health programs were soon offered. In 1986 about 3500 visits were made to the senior center.

Currently, the Council on Aging staff consists of a director, an outreach worker to provide services for frail elders, an assistant, and a part-time volunteer coordinator. The first three staff are paid through town funds while the last is supported through a grant from the state's Executive Office of Elder Affairs. Augmenting this staff are about 200 volunteers who provide rides, friendly visiting, presentation of informational programs and classes, service on boards, and office assistance.

Even as the demand on Bedford's community-based services for elders is increasing, the amount of support from the Administration on Aging and state-based elder services system is stagnant or increasing only slowly. Minuteman Home Care clients are currently limited to about 3 hours of services per week, though they are among the most frail and vulnerable. As the needs have increased the sources of support for community-based elder services has diversified. Only services provided through Minuteman Home Care are funded by any part of the Older Americans Act funding, and 75% of Minuteman Home Care's services are state-funded. An increasing source of funds for Minuteman Home Care are grant funds raised from the community through corporate grants and fund-raising activities and private foundations. The Council on Aging's $100,000 budget comes mainly from the town, but it also receives automatic grant funds of about $12,000 annually from the Executive Office of Elder Affairs, as well as grants totally about $15,000 per year and donations of equipment, furniture, computers, and other items from local businesses and corporations. The Friends of the Bedford Council on Aging, a non-profit organization, raises about $3000 each year to purchase objects for the senior center and pay for programming.

Services for Well Elders

The senior center now consists of four classrooms, two of these added in 1996 and 1997. In fiscal year 1999, 14,500 visits were made to the center. Bedford seniors come to the center for socializing, game playing, three kinds of fitness classes, weekly health promotion talks, a weekly informational series about benefits and other topics related to aging, a sing-along group that performs at community functions, art and humanities classes, book discussion groups, employment counseling, health services including massage and podiatric care, health screenings, office hours by state legislators, and trips, among others. Among these, social events and trips garner the greatest attendance per session, with up to 100 participating. Informational programs attract about 25 people per session, while other activities serve smaller groups.

Altogether about 900 individuals come to the senior center each year for activities. A small group of about 100 come several times a week, sometimes for a day or half-day's worth of activities. Another growing group may come once a week or once every 2 weeks for particular programs, while others may come two or three times a year. An increasing number of those who come for particular events, especially Tai Chi, arts and humanities, and discussion groups, are part of the younger elder population, aged 60 to 75, who have other social support networks and more family responsibilities than the very old seniors. This younger group, which may have become involved in the Council on Aging because of parents in the older group, are becoming a major source of volunteers. The major service provided to well elders by Minuteman Home Care are congregate meals, which 264 elders received in 1995.

These services for well elders are provided through the collaborative efforts of the public and private sectors in Bedford and the region. Besides services provided by Minuteman Home Care and the Council on Aging, informational programs at the Council on Aging are provided by local hospitals and nursing homes, the Bedford Library, the Bedford Adult Education Department, the Bedford Fire Department, the Bedford Police Department, and many, many volunteers. The Bedford Board of Health offers general health education, health screenings, and immunization clinics. Mental health services are beginning to be offered by the town's Department of Youth and Family Services.

A variety of other organizations also serve well elders. The Friends of the Bedford Council on Aging, a nonprofit organization that raises funds for the Council on Aging and the Golden Age Club, a social organization, both offer social events and trips. Churches provide informational programs at their sites as well as significant counseling to members. Local corporations provide information about resources and public benefits to their retirees. The region's Air Force base, Hanscom, offers benefits assistance, health and fitness facilities, and informational programs to the more than 400 military retirees in Bedford. Finally, the local Veterans Administration hospital provides mental and physical health services to eligible Bedford veterans.

Services for Frail Elderly Persons

By far the fastest-growing segment of the Council on Aging's services has been outreach to frail elders. In 1999, about 8,500 contacts with about 300 elders, including in-person, phone, and home consultations, were provided. These contacts include information about avail-

able services, counseling on aging-related services, coordination of
in-home services, monitoring of the well being of frail elders, and
crisis management. The ability to meet the growing need for outreach services has been achieved gradually. In fiscal year 1996, the
outreach worker was hired part-time for 6 months through a grant
paid for by the state Executive Office of Elder Affairs. The following
year the town, at its annual meeting during which any legal resident
may cast a ballot, voted to pay for an additional 20 hours per week.
The next year the town voted to fully fund the outreach worker's
salary.

For those who are income eligible, case management services are
provided through Minuteman Home Care. In 1995, 47 elders took
advantage of this opportunity. Two elders who may have been abused
or were at risk for self-neglect also received protective services in
that year.

The town has also provided significant services to frail elders
through other means. The five Public Health Nurses in the Bedford
Board of Health provide monthly home visits to over 100 seniors.
They offer in-home health assessments, evaluation, information and
referral, emotional support and reassurance, and other non-hands-
on services. The Board of Health also provides essential assistance
in cases of self-neglecting elders who are not able to maintain their
homes or themselves safely.

The police and fire departments also know many of the frail
elders in town well through responding to crises. These departments
regularly report cases of suspected self-neglect for follow-up by Minuteman Home Care, the Board of Health, and the Council on Aging.
Other departments, including the Town Clerk, Tax Collectors, and
others who have regular contact with elders also notify the Council
on Aging or the Board of Health about seniors in whom they have
noticed significant changes in capacity.

Most of the actual in-home services coordinated by the Council
on Aging and Minuteman Home Care, including nursing, personal
care, chore, and home health aide assistance, are provided by three
nursing agencies, two independent and one attached to a local hospital. For those who are income eligible through Minuteman Home
Care, the agencies contract directly with Minuteman. A smaller number of care providers are independent, though these are most likely
to be companions and homemakers rather than health professionals.

This increase in outreach services signals a significant change in the operation of community-based agencies, especially those that include senior centers. Increasingly those who provide services in Bedford are becoming multigenerational service centers as families become increasingly involved in the care of elders. Enhancing the quality and quantity of services has become increasingly important to all generations in communities. In the years since outreach services were begun at the Council on Aging, the involvement of families has evolved from one family member being the contact with the council to having several members involved with a resulting increase in complicated family dynamics. In addition, families that once sought to move elders nearer to them are more often asking for assistance in placing their relative in nursing facilities in Bedford, perhaps reflecting the reality that families have greater stress than before and cannot shoulder the burden of caring for family members in their homes.

The same organizations outside the elder services network that provide services to well elders also offers assistance to frail elders. In addition to the services mentioned above, churches and synagogues also provide transportation to medical appointments, friendly visiting, and a tremendous amount of pastoral care for frail elders. The local housing authority, which oversees Bedford's elder housing complex of 80 units, also provides social events and informational programming to its mainly frail residents.

Frail elders have a variety of community resources available to them, and it is in coordination of their care that the fragmented services systems are brought together by skillful Council on Aging outreach workers or Area Agency on Aging case managers. Regular communication among the many care providers of a frail elder is essential, yet daunting. For example, a Bedford elder with moderate in-home care needs may receive services from the following:

- The Council on Aging
- Minuteman Home Care
- The local police and fire departments, who may have provided emergency services
- The Bedford Housing Authority, in whose building the elder may live

- The Bedford Board of Health, whose nurses may visit the elder regularly
- The clergy of the church or temple to which the elder may belong and that may provide medical transportation, friendly visiting, pastoral care, and other services
- The home care agency offering in-home care
- Independent in-home workers
- Family, friends, and neighbors who may provide significant informal services

In addition, services are coordinated through a bimonthly meeting of the Council on Aging, Board of Health, visiting nurse, and other staff convened by the council, a monthly meeting of town departments providing human services, and daily telephone contact between service providers on individual cases.

Some of the trends evident in this case study of Bedford signal current and emerging realities for those providing community-based care. Among these are:

- Community-based care is provided by a daunting variety of providers, many of whom are rarely mentioned in discussions of the formal aging services network
- Most care is informal, provided by families with the assistance of the aging services network
- Most support for aging services comes from state or local sources with only a small portion of budgets supported through the Older Americans Act
- Localities support their elders and the concept of the importance of multigenerational communities through the combined efforts of many individuals and sectors, including government, businesses, nonprofit organizations, and religious and social organizations

Few service systems have grown and changed as quickly as that providing community-based elder services. The lives and successful aging of elders depends on the effectiveness of these services and the ability and willingness of local communities to support them. While policymakers and others make decisions based on aggregates of millions of elders, it is in the local sector that the battles for independence and dignity are fought and won, one elder at a time.

ACKNOWLEDGMENTS

The authors would like to acknowledge the contribution of Joan Butler-West of Minuteman Home Care, Wendy Aronson, Lenore Dichard, Donna Argon, and Joanne Balkovish of the Bedford Town Council on Aging, David Black of the Bedford Board of Health, and Rick Reed, Bedford Town Administrator, for their contributions to the case study section.

REFERENCES

Administration on Aging (1994). *Title III elderly nutrition program data.* Washington, DC: U.S. Administration on Aging (OPCA). 94–63.

The American Association of Retired Persons (1987). *Domestic mistreatment of the elderly: Towards prevention.* Washington, DC: The American Association of Retired Persons.

Balsam, A. L., & Bottum, C. L. (1996). Understanding the aging and public health networks. In T. Hickey, M. S. Speers, & T. R. Prohaska (Eds.), *Public health and aging* (pp. 17–36). Baltimore, MD: The Johns Hopkins University Press.

Balsam, A., & Rogers, B. (1987). *Service innovations in the elderly nutrition program: Strategies for meeting unmet needs.* Medford, MA: Tufts University School of Nutrition.

Binstock, R. H. (1996). Issues of resource allocation in an aging society. In T. Hickey, M. S. Speers, & T. R. Prohaska (Eds.), *Public health and aging* (pp. 53–72). Baltimore, MD: The Johns Hopkins University Press.

Bruce, M. L., Seeman, T. E., Merrill, S. S., & Blazer, D. G. (1994). The impact of depressive symptomology on physical disability: The MacArthur studies of successful aging. *American Journal of Public Health, 84,* 1794–1796.

Miner, S., Logan, J. R., & Spitze, G. (1993). Predicting the frequency of senior center attendance. *The Gerontologist, 33,* 650–657.

National Association of Area Agencies on Aging (undated). *Area Agencies on Aging.* Washington, DC: Author.

The Older Americans Act (1988). Washington, DC, U.S. Government Printing Office.

O'Shaugnessey, C. (1990). *The Older Americans Act Nutrition Program.* Washington, DC: Congressional Research Service, Library of Congress.

Prohaska, T. R., & Wallace, S. P. (1996). Implications of an aging society for the preparation of public health professionals. In T. Hickey, M. S. Speers, & T. R. Prohaska (Eds.), *Public health and aging* (pp. 275–292). Baltimore, MD: The Johns Hopkins University Press.

Rogers, R. G., Rogers, A., & Belanger, A. (1990). Active life among the elderly in the U.S.: Multistate life-table estimates and population projections. *Milbank Quarterly, 67,* 370–411.

Sabin, E. P. (1993). Frequency of senior center use: A preliminary test of two models of senior center participation. *Journal of Gerontological Social Work, 20,* 97–114.

CHAPTER 20

Maximizing the Contributions of Older People as Volunteers

Francis G. Caro and Robert Morris

The United States finds itself with two parallel phenomena that invite convergence. On one hand the country has vast unmet community service needs; on the other hand, the United States draws only partially on the large and growing productive potential of older people. This chapter will explore the possibilities that the United States might achieve substantial gains in its community services by enlisting larger numbers of older people in major roles as volunteers. Two sets of issues are involved. One set concerns the manner in which responses to community service needs are defined and organized. Of concern are such matters as the priorities that are attached to addressing human needs, the role of nonprofit organizations in addressing those needs, and the division of labor within those organizations between paid workers and volunteers. The second set of issues concerns the ability and willingness of older people to volunteer. Of concern is the extent to which the productive efforts of older people take the form of volunteering for organizations.

The focus of this discussion throughout will be on the role that formally organized services play in addressing community service needs. In the background will be recognition of the vast importance of nuclear and extended families and the informal assistance that often takes place among neighbors in meeting human needs. Some older people will continue to be highly productive but in sectors other than volunteering for organizations. They may be engaged in paid work or may provide unpaid assistance to others informally within their families or neighborhoods.

The argument that will be developed here is that substantial expansion of community service by older people in the community service will depend first on the manner in which the nation defines its community needs and the manner in which community problem-solving efforts are organized. If the nation makes improved services a priority, if nonprofits play a central role in these efforts, and if volunteers play a major role in these efforts, the potential for older volunteers to play a major role will be very great. A large number of older people will be available who have the potential to make substantially greater contributions as volunteers. The question, then, will be the extent to which they can be mobilized to serve.

THE POLITICAL CONTEXT FOR VOLUNTEERING IN THE UNITED STATES

The United States has become a highly complex society that relies heavily on specialized institutions. While families remain important in addressing many needs, contemporary life depends on a vast array of commercial and noncommercial services. The thickness of the yellow pages in major metropolitan areas is an indicator of the extent to which contemporary life is dominated by commercial services. The fact that information and referral services are now ubiquitous is a parallel indicator of the size and complexity of health and social services. Within two centuries the United States has become transformed from an agricultural society dominated by somewhat self-sufficient family farms to a thoroughly urbanized society heavily dependent on specialized formal services.

The political culture of the United States is at a crossroads with respect to the manner in which community services are provided and financed. Most community services in the United States originated as strictly volunteer efforts (Ellis & Noyes, 1990). The pattern was particularly prominent in areas of new settlement, where civic institutions were usually organized by volunteers. On the frontier, such services as education, law enforcement, fire fighting, and civil defense initially relied heavily on volunteers. In urban areas, hospitals and social service agencies began as volunteer efforts.

Religious organizations have been important as a source of volunteers and in the organization of community services. Religious congregations often responded to need for services by founding hospitals, schools, orphanages, and so on. Often at the outset they relied heavily on volunteers to provide staffing. In an earlier period the Catholic Church was particularly successful in attracting men and women to religious orders in which they were committed to lives of volunteer services in such fields as health and education. Churches themselves have also tended to rely heavily on volunteers to sustain their own activities.

Over time, community services have come to be dominated by paid personnel. In various community service organizations, only when demand for services increased and the supply of volunteers was insufficient were paid personnel introduced. The early paid staff were often coordinators of volunteers. With the hiring of full-time personnel came emphasis on the expertise that paid professional could bring; because they were regarded as amateurs, the efforts of volunteers then were often devalued. In this way, paid personnel have come to dominate most community service organizations, and volunteers have been relegated to marginal duties.

With the Great Depression, the federal government became increasingly active in providing financing to address human needs. Programs like Social Security were important in their own right, but they also spawned other programs at all levels of government to address various community needs. The expansion of federal programs reached its peak in the 1960s with Lyndon Johnson's Great Society programs. A pattern was established in which Americans looked increasingly to formal community services to address human needs, expected that services be provided by paid professionals, and expected that much of the financing would come from public sources. Various levels of government came to be involved in financing community services. Local governments with some assistance from state governments carry most of the financial responsibility for public elementary and secondary education; states and the federal government share major responsibility for financing income supports and health care for poor families; and the federal government finances the major income security and health programs that serve older people.

Perhaps it was inevitable that a taxpayer revolt would slow down the expansion of public expenditures for community services. Demand for services continued to expand; service workers wanted to be paid more adequately; yet, the economy was stagnant. Publicly funded services could continue to expand only if taxpayers were willing to pay a greater proportion of their income to finance them. Signs of increasing concern about the financing of public services were evident in the 1970s. By the 1980s pressures to contain public spending became greater than pressures to expand services. Public discourse in the 1990s was so dominated by concerns about fiscal constraint that advocates for services have been forced to make major downward adjustments in their aspirations.

Adding to the pressure on publicly funded services has been a combination of an increase in income inequality and increased preference on the part of the more affluent for private solutions to their own service needs. The United States is moving more and more toward a two-tiered system in which the more affluent obtain services privately and the less affluent rely on inferior publicly funded services.

Evidence of the weaknesses of services that rely on public funding is everywhere. They include schools and hospitals that are understaffed; working families that cannot find affordable child care; and public places that are run-down and littered. The consequences of weak service systems are serious. The unprecedented involvement of children in violent crime illustrates the inadequacies of our social services in the face of persistent poverty, racial discrimination, and serious weaknesses in nuclear families. At the other end of the age spectrum, frail, confused older people who live alone are often left to manage with only sketchy service supports.

The situation invites consideration of the extent to which a revival of voluntarism might stem the deterioration of community services. It can be argued that the country would prefer to have strong community services; the nation is only reluctant to pay for community services through taxes. If more volunteers can be enlisted, can we have stronger services without increasing taxes?

Any increase in volunteering will depend on the social climate, the availability of volunteers, and the nature of the assignments for volunteers. The opportunity to contribute to an important cause is an important motivation to volunteer. Commitment to either a very specific cause or a general concern about community can be a major element in volunteer motivation. The United States does not currently have any overriding popular causes that are likely to attract volunteers in large numbers. In earlier periods, world wars, the Civil Rights movement, and the antipoverty effort in the Great Society era did have that effect. In fact, in the current era, increasing economic and ethnic diversity in the United States coupled with privatization diminish any national sense of purpose that might inspire volunteering. In this period, only specific causes such as reproduction issues, environmental matters, youth recreation, or hunger are likely to attract substantial numbers of volunteers.

For people in midlife, contemporary economic pressures discourage volunteering. In an earlier period, one working professional could sustain a middle-class life style for a family. In the current era, two professional wage earners are required to meet the income needs of typical middle class families. As a result, the well-educated, middle class women who used to provide the backbone of community service volunteering are much less available as volunteers. If there is to be a resurgence of volunteering, other groups will have to step forward.

The commercialization of services also discourages volunteering. Volunteers are much more likely to be attracted to nonprofit than for-profit enterprises. The increasing commercialization of health care, for example, discourages volunteering in the health sector. Volunteers are more likely to be attracted to hospitals sponsored by churches or other nonprofit organizations than they are when they are owned privately—and particularly by large chains. Contributing time to a nonprofit organization is akin to contributing money to a charity. When services are provided by for-profit organizations, potential volunteers may well aspire to be paid workers instead of volunteers. Would-be volunteers might ask, "If the owner is making a profit, why shouldn't I get paid, too?"

A resurgence of volunteering will also require a redefinition of the symbolism that is associated with money. In work settings, money is important not only as an economic incentive but as a status symbol. Compensation tends to be the single most important measure of worth in organizations. When volunteers and paid personnel are part of the same organization, the financial compensation for paid staff tends to set them above volunteers. If volunteers are not to be recognized with money, some other substantial forms of recognition are needed to symbolize the importance that organizations attach to their efforts.

A good case can be made that in some sectors service organizations may have moved too far in replacing volunteers with paid personnel. Volunteers can be seen as a labor resource that competes with paid personnel. To the extent that volunteers compete with paid personnel, it is in the interest of paid personnel to discredit the capabilities of volunteers to justify greater rewards for themselves. In school settings, for example, volunteers are not likely to be available to assume the responsibilities of teachers. However, volunteers may take on responsibilities similar to those of teachers' aides. In some school systems the use of volunteers in schools is likely to be underdeveloped because of pressures from organized representatives of teachers' aides. At the same time these schools may be experiencing difficulties in hiring of both teachers and teachers' aides in adequate numbers and at adequate rates of compensation. The challenge in instances like this is the capacity of sponsoring organizations to create useful positions for volunteers that complement the contributions of paid school personnel.

THE YOUNG-OLD AS A VOLUNTEER RESOURCE

The young-old offer the potential for substantial expansion of the supply of volunteers. The pool of older people who could make significant contributions as volunteers is large and growing. People are living longer; between 1900 and 1986 life expectancy at birth in the United States increased for White women from 49 to 79 years and for White men from 47 to 72 years (Taeuber, 1989). More important than longevity is the fact that most older people are in good health. Only about 10% of those 65 to 74 years of age report that chronic illness prevents them from carrying out their usual responsibilities (Taeuber, 1989). Further, among noninstitutionalized people 65 years of age and older, the National Health Interview Survey found that 71% reported themselves to be in excellent, very good, or good health (National Center for Health Statistics, 1989).

For most older people, employment is not an obstacle to making major time commitments as volunteers since most are out of the workforce. Among men 65 years of age and older, only 16.6% are employed. Among women age 65 and older, 8.4% are employed (U.S. Senate, Special Committee on Aging, 1991). Productive activity is not foreign to older people. Substantial proportions of older people are already engaged in unpaid productive activities. A number of surveys have documented the extent of volunteering among older people; for recent reviews of the surveys, see Fischer and Schaffer (1993) and Chambre (1993). In fact, there is evidence that rates of volunteering have increased in the past few decades (Chambre, 1993).

The Commonwealth Fund's Productive Aging study (a survey of a 2999 people, representative of the noninstitutionalized population 55 years of age and older in the United States) is particularly useful in documenting the extent of unpaid productive activity in a number of separate sectors (Caro & Bass, 1995a). The study showed that 26% of older people were volunteering for organizations, 29% were helping the sick and disabled informally, and of those having grandchildren, 38% were spending some time helping them. In fact, the data indicated that 72% of older people were active in at least one of these forms of productive activity.

However, caution is needed in interpreting these percentages. Most of those reporting unpaid productive activity indicated that they did so at low intensity levels; for example, among those who volunteered for organizations, 60% reported contributing fewer than 5 hours a week. Volunteers who assist an organization occasionally for a few hours are often greatly appreciated for the help that they provide, but their contribution is usually of a lesser magnitude than that of those who devote substantial numbers of hours on a regular basis. The small minority of older people who contribute extensive time in unpaid productive activity, those volunteering 20 hours a week or more—the equivalent of at least half-time employment— deserve special attention. Considering the three sectors just described together, the data indicate that 13.5% of people 55 years of age and older engage in some combination of these unpaid productive activities a minimum of 20 hours a week. A slightly smaller percentage (12.2%) engages in one of the three forms of unpaid productive activity for at least 20 hours a week. More specifically, 1.8% of all people 55 years of age and older volunteer 20 or more hours per week to work in a formal agency without pay; 6.4% devote 20 or more hours informally to helping grandchildren; and 4.6% informally help the sick and disabled with activities of daily living 20 or more hours a week.

The greater prevalence of informal productive activities than volunteering for organizations is noteworthy. The difference may largely be explained by a greater sense of obligation associated with family than civic roles. Expectations of mutual aid are strongly built into family systems (Becker, 1981; Rossi & Rossi, 1990). Participation in informal long-term care, in particular, is often thrust on older people by the long-term care needs of a spouse. The assumption of an unpaid role with a community organization is more clearly discretionary.

THE POTENTIAL FOR INCREASED VOLUNTEERING

The potential for increasing volunteering among elderly persons is substantial. On the basis of the findings of two earlier national surveys, and using 1981 data, Kieffer estimated that 12.6 million people ages 55 and older were volunteering and another 6.4 million were interested in doing so (Kieffer, 1986). The Commonwealth Fund Productive Aging study found that of those respondents not already volunteering, 15% were willing and able to do so (Caro & Bass, 1995b). In other words, for every two older people who were volunteering, another older person indicated a willingness and ability to volunteer. While these reports of receptivity to volunteering may be somewhat optimistic, they do suggest a potential for substantially increasing the number of older people who are active as volunteers.

Working with the same data, Caro and Bass (1997) found particular potential for increasing volunteering in the period immediately after retirement. Findings of the Commonwealth Productive Aging Study were similar to other studies in showing that employment status among older people had no effect on the likelihood of volunteering. Those who were retired were not more likely to be volunteering than those who were employed. However, among those who were volunteering, those who were not working tended to contribute slightly more hours per week as volunteers than those who were working. The intriguing finding of their analysis is that nonvolunteers who had recently left the workforce more often reported that they were willing and able to volunteer than their counterparts who were working or had been out of the work force for a long time. The findings suggest that in the period immediately after retirement there is a heightened receptivity to volunteering that does not translate into higher rates of volunteering. The finding invites attention to strategies to enlist more of these relatively young, healthy, recent retirees into volunteer assignments.

VOLUNTEERS AS A HUMAN RESOURCE

Formal organizations have reason to consider volunteers as complementary to paid staff in pursuing certain aspects of their mission. Service organizations have particular reason to rethink their use of resources because on a long-term basis a wide variety of social problems have been growing more severe during a period in which resources for funding of programs to address those problems have contracted. Resource shortages are particularly great for services that are labor intensive. Many nonprofit organizations in both the public and private sectors have experienced a substantial decline in their purchasing power with respect to paid personnel. If they are to maintain services, an important option for many nonprofit organizations is to draw increasingly on volunteers. Well-designed public policies can influence the ways in which these organizations draw on older volunteers in pursuing their mission.

In many organizations, established views concerning volunteering should be challenged. While many service organizations began as efforts of volunteers, they are now dominated by paid personnel (Ellis & Noyes, 1990). The dominant contemporary perspective of human-service delivery organizations is that more serious responsibilities must be carried out by paid personnel. Volunteers, characteristically, are trusted only to perform limited enhancing roles. Frequently, volunteers are asked to take on peripheral, low-priority responsibilities for which paid staff lack time. We believe that organizations should be encouraged to revise their thinking about volunteers, opening up possibilities for older volunteers to make more significant contributions. We believe that public policies should encourage service organizations to regard volunteers as highly valuable resources to help meet their overall staffing needs; under some circumstances volunteers will be highly cost-effective alternatives to staffing that otherwise relies entirely on paid personnel.

For many organizations, the barriers to more extensive use of volunteers are substantial. The reasons for the marginal roles of volunteers are varied. One is that many organizations prefer to give major responsibilities to those who are continually available during normal business hours and who make long-term commitments. Because volunteers tend to help on a low-intensity and often temporary basis, these organizations tend to assign less substantial duties to volunteers.

A second reason for the marginal status of volunteers may be a subtle consequence of the fact that the volunteer contribution is regarded as a gift. Many organizations are reluctant to ask a great deal of volunteers because their effort is freely given. In contrast, the perception of these organizations is that paid personnel can be asked to do more because they are paid.

An important third reason is that paid personnel may regard volunteers with parallel responsibilities as an economic threat to them. Paid staff may ask themselves whether their employer will retain them if their job can be done adequately by volunteers. Further, even if they are not worried about losing their jobs, paid personnel may find it difficult to negotiate effectively for improved compensation when duties similar to theirs are being performed by volunteers.

The typical volunteer experience may also discourage many potential volunteers. People who are accustomed to carrying substantial responsibilities in their work roles are often reluctant to make major commitments to volunteer assignments that involve only light responsibilities. The combination of light duties and modest time commitments widely associated with volunteering by older people may therefore represent a self-fulfilling prophecy. If greater responsibilities were built into volunteer assignments, better-educated and more capable older people might be attracted to them and might be willing to make greater time commitments.

INVESTMENTS IN VOLUNTEERING

More adequate capitalization is needed for the volunteer sector. Discussions of measures to increase volunteering have tended to focus on strategies to recruit, place, and recognize volunteers (Fischer & Schaffer, 1993; Glickman & Caro, 1992). Less attention has been given to the investment of resources that organizations need to make to develop and support significant volunteer work. Organizations are accustomed to making significant investments in recruitment, training, and supervision of paid personnel, to say nothing of expenditures for fringe benefits. Expenditures that will enhance volunteer productivity are also needed. Of particular interest here is the organizational investment in the structuring of more significant roles that would attract more capable volunteers willing to make major time commitments.

What combinations of paid personnel and volunteers are likely to be most cost effective? Under some conditions, well-trained, supervised, and highly motivated volunteers may be good alternatives to organizations for paid personnel. This is particularly the case when resource limitations make it impossible to rely entirely on paid personnel. In a pioneering formal cost-effectiveness analysis of paid personnel and volunteers, Brudney and Duncombe (1992) compared paid, volunteers, and mixed-staff fire departments in New York state. They found that departments with all-paid staff were most effective. In other situations, volunteers may be an attractive option from a cost-benefit perspective even though they are less effective than paid personnel. Yet, for many communities, volunteer departments remain a preferred option because of the combination of low cost and acceptable quality. (Fire department staffing is of interest only as an example of a serious comparison of paid and volunteer units; we are not suggesting this as a field for significant volunteering for older people.)

Formal cost-effectiveness studies are sometimes useful in demonstrating the value of volunteer programs. An example of a volunteer program that can be examined in cost-effectiveness terms is Tax-Aide, an established community-service program administered by the American Association of Retired Persons [AARP] (Morris & Caro, 1996). The nationwide program offers free personal income tax assistance to older people. According to its own data, Tax-Aide in 1992 helped to prepare more than 1.6 million tax returns with the efforts of 30,000 volunteers. The program is funded by the Internal Revenue Service through a $2.7 million grant. The Internal Revenue Service also provides training to volunteers. Data provided by AARP suggest that Tax-Aide volunteers prepared tax returns at an average cost of $1.70. An informal survey of commercial tax preparation services in the Boston area suggested that a typical person filing a basic tax return might have to expect to pay approximately $40 for tax preparation. By that standard, if it is assumed that users of the Tax-Aide service would otherwise have been forced to use a commercial service, the volunteer program appears to be a dramatically less expensive alternative from a consumer perspective. While this brief example illustrates the importance of cost-effectiveness analysis, it does not address some of the critical questions concerning the quality of the service and the complexity of the returns, for example, that might be raised in a serious comparison with commercial services.

SIGNIFICANT VOLUNTEERING

A direction deserving more attention is *significant volunteering*, that is, volunteer assignments that require both high levels of responsibility and extensive time commitments (Morris & Caro, 1996). In the absence of explicit demonstration programs to encourage the development and testing of models of significant volunteering, the Gerontology Institute at the University of Massachusetts at Boston has been exploring one version of significant volunteering. The Institute has created an Elder Leadership program (O'Brien & Norton, 1997) that enlists mature people who commit themselves to at least 40 weeks of high responsibility service with an extensive weekly time commitment.

In its first formulation, the Elder Leadership program focused on the challenges faced by councils on aging in suburban communities in addressing the needs of the frail, noninstitutionalized elderly persons. Councils on aging are local public entities with a mandate to serve older people. Councils on aging are eligible to receive certain funds made available by the Older Americans Act. Local governments enjoy a great deal of discretion in the scope of activities of their councils on aging. Elder leaders were trained to serve as volunteer coordinators and were assigned to councils on aging and other aging service organizations. Councils on aging Massachusetts have a mandate to provide services to frail elders but usually have to rely extensively on volunteers if they are to offer more than nominal services. All too often, councils on aging have a minimal capacity to organize projects for volunteers, recruit volunteers, and to provide them with the training, supervision, and recognition that they need if they are to be effective. Elder leaders worked with council on aging directors to develop projects, recruit volunteers of all ages, place volunteers in assignments, and train and supervise volunteers. Projects developed by elder leaders included shopping assistance, friendly visiting, telephone reassurance, and outreach to frail isolated elders. Because the Elder Leadership program was launched with funds from the federal AmeriCorps program, it was able to provide Elder Leaders with living allowances equivalent to the minimum wage. However, Elder Leaders had to work a minimum of 20 hours a week and commitment themselves for at least 40 weeks.

A second phase of the program is being introduced entirely with local support. In this formulation, elder leaders will continue to serve as volunteer coordinators. Some will address the needs of the frail elderly population through councils on aging. Others will seek to strengthen child care and after-school programs offered by branches of the YMCA. Instead of living allowances, members will receive much more modest expense payments. Work obligations will be reduced to 2 days per week.

The Elder Leadership program is illustrative of the initiatives that are needed to create significant volunteer assignments for skilled older people who are willing to make a substantial commitment to volunteering if the assignments are meaningful. Other initiatives to stimulate significant volunteering are needed that address other causes and with other roles for volunteers. This form of volunteering will be particularly attractive to older people with secure incomes for whom challenging responsibilities are the most important aspect of a volunteer assignment.

STRATEGIES TO PROMOTE
SIGNIFICANT VOLUNTEERING

The literature on volunteering provides some insights about the circumstances in which significant volunteering initiatives are likely to be viable. In general, the principles that underlie effective volunteer administration generally also will apply to significant volunteering among older people (see, for example, Brudney, 1990 and Fischer & Schaffer, 1993). The need to provide volunteers with sufficient incentive, for example, can be addressed in three ways: (1) the assignments must carry enough responsibility so that volunteers can gain the intrinsic satisfaction to justify their extensive, persistent effort; (2) the volunteers should receive immediate and continuing recognition of the value of their exceptional efforts; (3) the volunteer experience should have other attractive qualities such as opportunities for congenial social interaction; and (4) the volunteers might be offered tangible rewards such as stipends (which may reduce the difference between those positions and conventional paid work). Working relationships between these volunteers and paid staff may be enhanced if these volunteers are part of a peer group of volunteers in which all are making extensive commitments. If peers are also working without pay, volunteers will be less likely to complain that they are working without pay while others are being paid for similar responsibilities. In fact, significant volunteering may prove to be particularly viable in young, growing organizations that rely entirely or almost entirely on volunteers.

The threat to paid staff of job displacement associated with significant volunteering may be minimized if paid personnel are convinced that without volunteers task could not be carried out at all. Potential resentment of paid staff may also be avoided if the work done by volunteers is distinctly different from that done by paid staff. In some instances potential conflict can be managed effectively by placing significant volunteers in cadres that are spatially separated from certain groups of paid staff in their work assignments. Because of rigidities in the patterns of work in some public sector organizations, Brudney (1990) goes so far as to suggest that public agencies obtain the services of volunteers by contracting out certain tasks to private organizations that are dominated by volunteers.

CONCLUSION

The key to increasing levels of volunteering among older people rests in the manner in which the nation addresses its human and environmental needs. If the nation escalates it efforts to improve the lives of disadvantaged citizens, improve the environment, and make its communities more livable; and if the nation invigorates its efforts to address its needs through nonprofit organizations; and if more significant roles for volunteers can be created in nonprofit organizations, older people will respond. Because they are very much a part of the political culture, older people will contribute to any collective decision that the nation makes to do more to address community needs; older people are also part of the public discourse about the role of nonprofit organizations in community problem-solving. Older people can also be part of the debate within nonprofit organizations about the division of labor between paid personnel and volunteers.

Older people have the potential to make a much greater impact as volunteers. The numbers of older people who are healthy and permanently out of the work force at relative early ages will continue to increase. The rise in educational levels among new cohorts of older people also suggests increasing potential for older people to be attracted to opportunities for significant volunteering.

No doubt there are limits to the extent to which older people can be enlisted as volunteers. Health problems, preferences for paid work or leisure, and family obligations all draw older people away from volunteering. These limits will be much better understood when it is possible to examine the response of older people in a nation that places greater emphasis on community needs, that underscores the role of the nonprofit sector, that reemphasizes the role of volunteers in the nonprofit sector, and that provides challenging opportunities to those who make substantial commitments as volunteers.

REFERENCES

Becker, G. (1981). *A treatise on the family.* Cambridge, MA: Harvard University Press.

Brudney, J. (1990). *Fostering volunteer programs in the public sector.* San Francisco: Jossey-Bass.

Brudney, J., & Duncombe, W. (1992). An economic evaluation of paid, volunteer, and mixed staffing options for public services. *Public Administration Review, 52,* 474–481.

Caro, F., & Bass, S. (1995a). Dimensions of productive engagement. In S. Bass (Ed.), *Older and active: How Americans over 55 are contributing to society.* New Haven, CT: Yale University Press.

Caro, F., & Bass, S. (1995b). Increasing volunteering among older people. In S. Bass (Ed.), *Older and active: How Americans over 55 are contributing to society.* New Haven, CT: Yale University Press.

Caro, F., & Bass, S. (1997). Receptivity to volunteering in the immediate post-retirement period. *Journal of Applied Gerontology, 16,* 427–441.

Caro, F. G., & Morris, R. (1992). Retraining older workers: An >emerging economic need. *Community College Journal, 63,* 22.

Chambre, S. (1993). Volunteerism by Elders: Past trends and future prospects. *The Gerontologist, 33,* 221–229.

Ellis, S., & Noyes, K. (1990). *By the people: A history of Americans as volunteers.* San Francisco: Jossey-Bass.

Fischer, L., & Schaffer, K. (1993). *Older volunteers: Enlisting the talent.* Newbury Park, CA: Sage.

Glickman, L., & Caro, F. (1992). *Improving the recruitment and retention of older volunteers.* National Eldercare Institute on Employment and Volunteerism. College Park, MD: Center on Aging, University of Maryland.

Kieffer, J. (1986). The older volunteer resource. In Committee on an Aging Society (Eds.), *America's aging: Productive roles in an aging society* (pp. 51–72). Washington, DC: National Academy Press.

Morris, R., & Caro, F. (1996). Productive retirement: Stimulating greater volunteer efforts to meet national needs. *Journal of Volunteer Administration, XIV,* 5–13.

National Center for Health Statistics (1989). *The National Health Interview Survey.* Washington, DC: Author.

O'Brien, J., & Norton, J. (1997). *Serving communities through elder leadership.* Boston: Gerontology Institute, University of Massachusetts.

Rossi, A., & Rossi, P. (1990). *Of human bonding: Parent-child relations across the life course.* New York: A. de Gruyter.

Taeuber, C. (1989). Diversity: The dramatic reality. In S. Bass, S. Kutza, & F. Torres-Gil (Eds.), *Diversity in aging: Challenges facing planners and policymakers in the 1990s* (pp. 47–72). Glenview, IL: Scott, Foresman, & Co.

U.S. Senate. (1991). *Aging America: Trends and projections.* Special Committee on Aging, U.S. Department of Health and Human Services. Washington, DC: U.S. Government Printing Office. Publication No. 91-28001.

Index

Sue E. Levkoff, Sc.D., M.S.W., S.M., is Associate Professor of Psychiatry at Brigham and Women's Hospital and Associate Professor of Social Medicine at Harvard Medical School, and Associate Professor of Health and Social Behavior at Harvard School of Public Health. She is the former recipient of a National Institute on Aging Special Emphasis Research Career Award and currently, the recipient of a National Institute on Aging Senior Academic Leadership Award. She has conducted research on excess disabilities in cognitively impaired aged persons, delirium, substance abuse, and mental health, in efforts to develop an integrated clinical and behavioral approach to geriatric care. Dr. Levkoff directs the Harvard Upper New England Geriatric Education Center, funded by the Bureau of Health Professions of the Health Resources and Services Administration, which provides specialized training for academically based faculty and primary care practitioners from the medical, dental, nursing, and allied health professions to expand and improve geriatric health care with particular emphasis on minority elders. Dr. Levkoff is also the Director of the Inter-Faculty Working Group on Aging, a Harvard University-wide interdisciplinary working group examining a broad array of issues related to aging in the 21st century. She also is the Principal Investigator of a Coordinating Center funded by the Substance Abuse and Mental Health Services Administration, the VA Administration, and HRSA that is examining the delivery of substance abuse and mental health services to older persons in primary care in a 11-site multi-center randomized trial.

Yeon Kyung Chee, Ph.D., is Instructor in the Department of Social Medicine and Division on Aging, Harvard Medical School. She received her Ph.D. in Family and Child Development with a Graduate Certificate in Gerontology from Virginia Polytechnic Institute and State University. She was a Post-Doctoral Research Fellow in the Department of Social Medicine at Harvard Medical School, conducting research on ethnicity, family relations, and dementia, behavioral health in later life, and the continuum of long-term care from life course and cross-cultural perspectives. Since 1996, she has co-directed teaching programs on Successful Aging and Dementia Specialist Training in academic settings. She has participated in the Colalborative of Ethnogeriatric Education with support from the Bureau of Health Professions of the Health Resources and Services Administration, develolping a multidisciplinary curriculum in ethnogeriatrics for health professionals. She is also a co-investigator of a multi-site study on aging, substance abuse, and mental health in primary care funded by the Substance Abuse and Mental Health Services Administration, the VA Administration, and the HRSA. Dr. Chee is the recipient of the Training Award from the National Institute on Aging and Brookdale Foundation's Summer Institute on Aging Research.

Shohei Noguchi, B.A., is founder of three colleges: Mejiro Human Science College, Mejiro Life Science College, and Chuo College of Law. He is Visiting Professor at Shanghai University of Traditional Chinese Medicine and Visiting Scholar at Shanghai Jiaotong University in China. Professor Noguchi is the Vice Chairman of the Board of the Trustees of Toshima Social Support Center and also serves as Vice Chair of the Board of the Trustees of the Nice Heart Foundation, which is dedicated to the commemoration of the International Year of Disabled Persons in Tokyo, Japan. He has worked closely with the Japanese Government to establish social and public policy for the elderly. He is interested in developing and implementing training programs for health care workers to better enable the Japanese health care industry to provide appropriate services to the elderly and their family caregivers.